Patient Safety

Principles and Practice

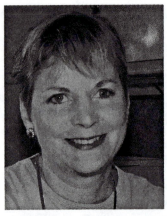

Jacqueline Fowler Byers, PhD, RN, CNAA, CPHQ, is an Associate Professor, School of Nursing, College of Health and Public Affairs, at the University of Central Florida. She has over 25 years experience in health care in varied clinical, educational, and administrative roles. In all of these roles, Dr. Byers has pursued evidence-based practice and improved patient experience and outcomes. She has been actively involved in quality management, outcomes research, and patient safety for 10 years. Dr. Byers received her doctorate from the University of Florida in 1996. Her master's degree is from Vanderbilt University, and her bachelor's degree is from Duke University. She was in the inaugural class of the Robert Wood Johnson Executive Nurse Fellowship Program. Dr. Byers is the Research Editor of the *Journal for Health Care Quality* and serves as a peer reviewer for several journals. She is active in the National Association for Healthcare Quality and the American Association of Critical Care Nurses. Dr. Byers has received a number of awards and has over 60 publications and 100 presentations to her credit in the areas of health care administration, quality management, critical care, and outcomes and efficacy research.

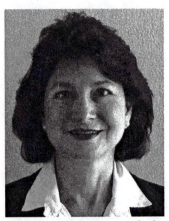

Susan V. White, PhD, RN, CPHQ, FNAHQ, is the Associate Chief of Nursing/Quality Improvement at the James A. Haley Veterans Hospital. Prior to this position she was the past Vice President/Quality Management of the Florida Hospital Association. She has over 20 years of experience in the health care field in administration, management, and clinical roles. She was the Associate Executive Director and Director of Nursing in a community hospital and developed the quality management program for a hospital in a network. Dr. White has health care experience in acute care including clinical, administrative, and informatics. She has a master's degree in nursing as well as her doctor in philosophy from the University of Florida. Her recent work has included Joint Commission activities, quality initiatives, clinical performance improvement and patient perception, educational programs, newsletters, and patient safety. Dr. White is a sixth year Sterling Examiner for the Florida Sterling Council and teaches part-time at the University of Phoenix. She is a member of multiple professional organizations and is a Fellow in NAHQ. She is a member of the editorial board for the *Journal for Healthcare Quality*.

Patient Safety

Principles and Practice

Jacqueline Fowler Byers,
PhD, RN, CNAA, CPHQ

Susan V. White,
PhD, RN, CPHQ, FNAHQ

Editors

 Springer Publishing Company

Springer Publishing Company, Inc.
536 Broadway
New York, NY 10012-3955

Acquisitions Editor: Ruth Chasek
Production Editor: Sara Yoo
Cover design by Joanne Honigman

04 05 06 07 08 / 5 4 3 2 1

Library of Congress Cataloging-in-Publication Data

Patient safety : principles and practice / Jacqueline Fowler Byers, Susan V. White, editors.
        p. ; cm.
    Includes bibliographical references and index.
    ISBN 0-8261-3346-0
    1. Medical errors—United States—Prevention. 2. Medical care—United States—Quality control. 3. Health services administration—United States.
    [DNLM: 1. Patient Care Management. 2. Safety Management. 3. Evidence-Based Medicine. W 84.7 P2978 2004] I. Byers, Jacqueline Fowler. II. White, Susan V.
R729.8.P385 2004
610 68'5—dc22   2004007715

Printed in the United States of America by Integrated Book Technology.

Contents

PART III: PATIENT SAFETY IN SPECIFIC
SETTINGS AND POPULATIONS

Contributors

Christy L. Beaudin, PhD, MSW, CPHQ, is Director, Quality Improvement for PacifiCare Behavioral Health in Van Nuys, California. She has extensive experience in managed behavioral health care and has worked with health plans and hospitals in NCQA and JCAHO survey preparation and accreditation surveys.

Monica C. Berry, BSN, JD, LLM, DFASHRM, CPHRM, is Vice President of Risk Management and Loss Control for Rockford Health System in Rockford, Illinois. She is a well-recognized national speaker on various risk management topics and is Past President of the American Society for Healthcare Risk Management (ASHRM).

Mary Lou Brunell, MSN, RN, is Executive Director of the Florida Center for Nursing (FCN) in Orlando, Florida. The FCN was established by the Florida legislature during the 2001 session to address issues of supply of and demand for nurses in the state. Prior to her work with the FCN, Ms. Brunell served in faculty and administrative roles.

Tania Daniels, MBA, PT, is Director, Health Policy for Minnesota Hospital and Healthcare Partnership in St. Paul, Minnesota. She is a patient safety specialist and is responsible for convening and providing a forum for patient safety stakeholders statewide.

Jo Ann Miller, MSN, RN, is employed by the Florida Center for Nursing, which addresses issues of recruitment, retention, and the utilization of nurse workforce resources. She is also a staff nurse on a busy medical surgical unit in Daytona Beach, Florida.

Janice Z. Peterson, PhD, RN, is an Assistant Professor at the University of Central Florida in Orlando, Florida, where she is actively involved in work with the elderly, recently completing a funded project to increase awareness about depression in the elderly.

Debra Roach, RN, BA, is a consultant for Jupiter Medical Center in Palm Beach Gardens, Florida, with over 20 years experience in healthcare informatics. She has experience with Point of Care Bar Code Medication Administration applications, Nursing Documentation Systems, Enterprise Wide Scheduling Systems, Nurse Triage Call Center Systems, Surgery Systems, Acuity methodologies and Nurse Staff Scheduling Systems.

Beatrice A. Schafhauser, BSN, RN, CPN, is a Nurse Clinician for the Acute Pediatrics and Pediatric Hematology/Oncology Units at the Arnold Palmer Hospital for Children and Women in Orlando, FL. Her 25 years of experience encompasses both neonatal and pediatric nursing in the inpatient setting.

Lynn Unruh, PhD, RN, is an Assistant Professor in Health Services Administration at the University of Central Florida. Her publications and research interests are in the areas of hospital organization, responses of hospitals to market forces, the job of nursing, nurse staffing in hospitals and nursing homes, and the relationship between nurse staffing and the quality of patient care.

List of Acronyms

AARP	American Association of Retired Persons
ADE	Adverse Drug Event
AE	Adverse Event
ADM	Automated Dispensing Machine
AHA	American Hospital Association
AHRQ	Agency for Healthcare Research and Quality
AONE	American Organization of Nurse Executives
APIC	Association of Practitioners in Infection Control
APSF	Anesthesia Patient Safety Foundation
ASHP	American Society of Health System Pharmacists
ASRS	Aviation Safety Reporting System
BPOC	Bar Coding at Point of Care
CDC	Centers for Disease Control and Prevention
CMS	Center for Medicare and Medicaid Services
CPOE	Computerized Provider/Physician Order Entry
FDA	Food and Drug Administration
FMEA	Failure Mode and Effects Analysis
HFMEA™	Healthcare Failure Mode and Effects Analysis
HHC	Handheld Computers
IHI	Institute for Healthcare Improvement
IOM	Institute of Medicine
ISMP	Institute for Safe Medication Practices
JCAHO	Joint Commission on Accreditation of Healthcare Organizations
NCCMERP	National Coordinating Council for Medication Error Reporting and Prevention
NCHC	National Coalition for Health Care
NCQA	National Committee on Quality Assurance
NHSN	National Healthcare Safety Network
NNISS	National Nosocomial Infection Surveillance System

NPSF	National Patient Safety Foundation
NPSG	National Patient Safety Goal
NQF	National Quality Forum
P4PS	Partners for Patient Safety
PDA	Personal Digital Assistant
POCS	Point-of-Care Systems
PSRS	Patient Safety Reporting System
QuIC	Quality Interagency Coordinating Council
RCA	Root Cause Analysis
SE	Sentinel Event
SEA	Sentinel Event Alert
USP	United States Pharmacopoeia
VHA	Veterans Health Administration

Acknowledgments

We thank all of the contributors to this book, and appreciate the contributors' expertise, effort, and commitment to patient safety. We also thank Mary Fobell for her assistance with the finalization and compilation of this manuscript. Your calm and persistence were appreciated.

J.F.B. and S.V.W.

Thanks to my friends and family for your support in the pursuit of writing this book and my professional dreams.

J.F.B.

I want to thank my husband, Hugh Richard, for his love, support, and assistance during the countless hours of writing this book. He is the wings beneath my feet.

S.V.W.

Introduction

The patient safety movement was significantly spurred by the Institute of Medicine's report, *To Err is Human: Building a Safer Health System*, and has received global attention across the United States, England, Australia, Japan, and other countries. Many national and federal initiatives have been created to advance patient safety bringing together a critical mass to make changes in improving patient care and reducing both risk and harm to patients. While major advances have been made in patient safety, there remain many questions about safety practices and the best way to implement them. On the other hand, there is sound evidence for a number of activities that can be implemented today to improve patient care and safety.

The goal of this book is to provide the reader with both theoretical knowledge regarding patient safety as well as to provide tools and exemplars for application in various clinical settings. This book brings together a thorough view of patient safety for health care providers and quality professionals. Foundational patient safety principles and evidence-based patient safety practices are presented to assist health care providers and organizations in developing a cutting edge patient safety program. This approach assists practitioners in understanding medical errors, using a framework for a multifactorial approach to patient safety, and accessing key resources for using best practices. Health care providers in clinical and leadership positions will find value in the knowledge of and tools for use in patient safety issues and interventions in a format that is comprehensive and addresses the continuum of care. An emphasis throughout this book is to provide readers with key knowledge to develop a principle- and evidence-based comprehensive patient safety program in their organizations.

The first section of the book provides an overview of concepts and principles related to why errors occur, considers human factors and process characteristics, and provides strategies to address various error-prone situations and processes. This linkage between principles and strategies allows the practitioner to put these principles into practice.

The next section focuses on putting patient safety principles into practice. These chapters consider the impact on patient safety of other nursing issues such as staffing and work culture. The current work environment and workforce shortages made it critical to include discussion of these topics and their influence on patient outcomes. Critical to this section is the chapter on using evidence-based practice for improving patient safety. This section also highlights the patient's active involvement in care and a variety of resources to inform patients about how to ask the right questions about their care and how to use resources wisely. This book provides examples and practices throughout each chapter to give the reader many opportunities for practical interventions. The framework also describes how to leverage technology to improve patient safety, including the most current applications such as CPOE, bar coding, and smart infusion pumps. The authors then present key risk management concerns woven around the aspects of reporting and disclosure.

Specific clinical examples for different patient populations are discussed in section three, building on real-world examples that can be used as models. This section examines special patient populations including issues and potential intervention strategies. The chapters include acute care, ambulatory care, behavioral health, pediatric, geriatric, and research populations. Case studies and exemplars within these special populations help practitioners focus attention on their unique practice setting while using a principle-centered approach. The book concentrates the research and strategies for various patient populations into different chapters so that practitioners can utilize general concepts and see applications that are similar as well as those that are unique for different patient groups. This section also summarizes the myriad initiatives underway across the country and their impact on patient safety across the care continuum.

Our goal was to provide a comprehensive patient safety resource for health care professionals. We hope that this book provides guidance for health care professionals to implement and prioritize patient safety programs in their work setting in order to improve patient outcomes.

Jacqueline Fowler Byers, PhD, RN, CNAA, CPHQ
Susan V. White, PhD, RN, CPHQ

Part I

Overview of Concepts and Principles

Chapter 1

Patient Safety Issues

Susan V. White

NATIONAL ATTENTION ON PATIENT SAFETY

Ask "What happened?" not "Who did it?"

Patient safety is not a new concept for health care practitioners, but the attention focused on it by the Institute of Medicine (IOM) report, *To Err is Human: Building a Safer Health System* galvanized public and media attention as well as policymakers (Kohn, Corrigan, & Donaldson, 2000). While safety issues are not new for most caregivers, knowledge of how mistakes and errors occur has been advanced by studying other high-risk industries, such as aviation, space, and nuclear power, and learning from a special discipline called human factors engineering (Kohn, Corrigan, & Donaldson, 2000). This chapter provides an overview of how national attention recently became focused on a topic that springs from ancient Greek times in which the phrase associated with caring for the ill is "First, do no harm." Recent attention on safety is inextricably linked with quality of care initiatives, so the chapters in this book will also address patient safety concepts within a larger quality framework.

A number of different events have sharpened the focus on patient safety beginning with Ernest Codman who is considered the father of outcomes management (Joint Commission on Accreditation of Healthcare Organizations [JCAHO], 2002c). While Codman did not specifically describe patient safety initiatives, he was concerned with patient outcomes, complications, and measurements to monitor outcomes. Codman's contribution to patient safety is the advancement of the concepts of measuring patient outcomes and reporting those outcomes to improve care. What becomes clear as each major event is described is how it contributes to our current understanding of patient safety, including the dimensions of quality of health care, the importance of measurement and reports, and the use of research or evidence to reduce variation in practice and improve patient outcomes.

An overview of the events and initiatives in patient safety during the last 15 to 20 years is provided (Table 1.1) to explain how different initiatives have coalesced and new alliances and collaborations have been formed to focus on this topic. Specific information about many of these initiatives will be presented in chapter 2. In the years 1995–1996 interest in medical errors and patient safety across multiple specialties peaked. The first Annenberg Conference on patient safety was convened during this time period, the National Patient Safety Foundation (NPSF) was formed (NPSF, 2002), and President Clinton established the Advisory Commission on Consumer Protection and Quality in the Health Care Industry to address issues of quality of health care (Advisory Commission on Consumer Protection and Quality in the Health Care Industry, 1998).

Even earlier than the 1995 peak in patient safety interest, the Anesthesia Patient Safety Foundation (APSF) had been formed in 1984 as a result of the increasing mortality rate in surgical patients. At the 1984 meeting of the American Society of Anesthesiologists, Dr. Ellison C. Pierce, the society's president, inaugurated the Anesthesia Patient Safety Foundation (APSF) (Siker, 2001). At that time there were many issues associated with mortality related to surgery or the anesthesia administered. However, discussion of these issues started as early as 1954 with the publication of a paper by Beecher and Todd, *A Study of the Deaths Associated With Anesthesia and Surgery*. As a result of the concern about mortality rates, a concerted focus on research was made, and standardization and safety controls were applied in anesthesia machines, monitoring, and tubing circuits. This was an early example in health care in which the concept of patient safety, specifically related to the preventable problem of mortality, was addressed. A key learning from the anesthesia investigation and analyses of mortality was that a scientific base was essential for demonstrating which changes were effective in improving patient care. As a result, individual practitioners were not singled out as bad performers to be eliminated, and systems of care and their potential failures were redesigned so the entire field of anesthesia care improved. Mortality rates plummeted over the next 10

TABLE 1.1   Landmark Events Related to Patient Safety and Quality

Date	Event
1955	Ernest Codman focused on patient outcomes
1984	Anesthesia Patient Safety Foundation formed
	Harvard Medical Practice Study in New York
1992	Medical Practice Study in Colorado/Utah
1995	First Annenberg Conference on Patient Safety
1996	National Patient Safety Foundation formed
	Joint Commission issues Sentinel Event Policy
	President Clinton establishes Advisory Commission on Consumer Protection and Quality in the Health Care Industry
	National Coalition on Health Care in conjunction with the IOM commissions RAND to review academic literature for articles to provide evidence of quality of care in US
	First Executive Session on Medical Error and Patient Safety at Harvard University
1997–1998	Institute of Medicine Technical Advisory Panel on the State of Quality commissions an update to include studies published between 1997–1998
	President Clinton establishes Quality Interagency Coordination Task Force
	Quality of Healthcare in America Project initiated by the Institute of Medicine as a result of the Advisory Commission on Consumer Protection and Quality
	Vice President Gore creates the National Forum for Health Care Quality Measurement and Reporting
	Institute of Medicine National Roundtable on Health Care Quality meets and describes three types of quality problems (overuse, underuse, misuse)
	The Committee on Quality of Care in Medicine of the IOM publishes *To Err is Human: Building a Safer Health System.*
2000	Agency for Health Care Policy and Research changes to Agency for Healthcare Research and Quality
	Leapfrog Group is established by the Business Roundtable
	Institute of Medicine publishes *Crossing the Quality Chasm*
	Joint Commission publishes Safety Standards
	Partners for Patient Safety (P4Ps) formed and sponsored Patient Safety Conference
	CQuIPS formed under the Agency for Healthcare Research and Quality
	Patient Safety research agenda established by QuIC and AHRQ

(continued)

TABLE 1.1   *(continued)*

Date	Event
2001	National Patient Safety Task Force formed (FDA, AHRQ, CDC, CMS)
2002	Institute of Medicine publishes *Envisioning the National Health Care Quality Report*
	Joint Commission publishes Six National Patient Safety Goals
	Centers for Medicare and Medicaid Services publishes conditions of participation requiring quality assessment and performance improvement including reduction of medical errors
2003	Joint Commission announces new survey process of Shared Vision—New Pathways and publishes *Weaving the Fabric: Strategies for Improving Our Nation's Health Care*
	Institute of Medicine publishes *Priority Areas for National Action*
	Centers for Medicare and Medicaid Services publishes conditions of participation requiring programs for quality and performance improvement including reduction of medical errors
	The Patient Safety and Quality Improvement Act of 2003 (HR 877) is approved by House Committee
	FDA issues rules to require bar coding on medications
	Agency for Healthcare Research and Quality publishes book of patient safety indicators and launches web-based quality measures resource
	Institute for Healthcare Improvement develops online interactive quality resource

years providing clear evidence that a systems approach was essential. Anesthesiology has addressed a high-risk system with redesign efforts to reduce its error rate from 25–50 per million to 5.4 per million and is now approaching six sigma (see chapter 3 for a discussion of six sigma) in anesthesia-related mortality (Agency for Healthcare Research and Quality [AHRQ], 2000; Merry & Brown, 2002).

Several major studies of anesthesia mortality have been conducted in the United Kingdom and Australia, which have anonymous reporting systems. In the 1980s, there were two deaths per 10,000 for anesthesia; and studies now demonstrate only one death in every 200,000 to 300,000 cases (Pierce, 1995). Studies in this country have been far fewer due to legal and risk issues. Eichhorn studied over one million anesthetics in ASA class

I and II in Harvard hospitals from 1976–1985 (Pierce, 1995). He found 11 intraoperative anesthesia accidents. After monitoring standards were implemented, there were no major preventable intraoperative anesthesia injuries in the next 300,000 cases. The processes of delivering anesthesia care were analyzed, root causes contributing to mortality were identified, and actual and potential failures were eliminated. Examples from this systemic analysis seem common today such as the use of anesthesia checklists, improved patient monitoring, and pin indexing on gasses.

The initiatives described to this point were promoted primarily by private professional organizations. Another body that was busy during the same time in the mid nineties was the Joint Commission on Accreditation of Healthcare Organizations [JCAHO]. In 1996 the JCAHO issued its Sentinel Event Policy that provides four options for voluntary reporting of sentinel events. "A sentinel event is an unexpected occurrence involving death or serious physical or psychological injury, or the risk thereof. Such events are called 'sentinel' because they signal the need for immediate investigation and response" (JCAHO, 1996, Revised 2000; JCAHO, 2002a, paragraph VIII). The JCAHO also developed safety standards in 2001 (JCAHO, 2001), followed by publication of six national patient safety goals in 2002 (JCAHO, 2002d). More about the goals are presented in the chapter 11 discussion on acute care. In its most recent work, the JCAHO (2003) has integrated all of its safety initiatives and strategies into a single summary that demonstrates the linkage of the various activities and the accreditation survey process.

FEDERAL INITIATIVES TARGETING PATIENT SAFETY

While numerous activities were taking place at the national level, the federal government was leading a similar movement on medical errors, patient safety, and consideration of national reports. The Advisory Commission on Consumer Protection and Quality in the Health Care Industry was established by President Clinton in 1997. This commission worked through the Institute of Medicine [IOM] to initiate the Quality of Healthcare in America Project, which was to improve the quality and accountability of care as well as produce reports. Through the IOM's Committee on Quality of Care in Medicine, the first report issued was *To Err is Human: Building a Safer Health System* (Kohn, Corrigan, & Donaldson, 2000). This report is widely known and has become a landmark work, since it presented the problem of medical errors, and therefore patient safety issues, in terms that the lay public could easily understand. With a focus on medical errors, patient safety was defined as the absence of error, or freedom from accidental injury (Kohn, Corrigan, & Donaldson, 2000).

Every person has a health story to tell—a national poll indicates that 42% of those responding had been affected by a medical error, with 32% indicating the error had a permanent negative effect on their or a family member's health (Gordon, 2002). Surprisingly, while 42% of the public report errors in care, they do not see medical errors as one of the most important problems in health care. The public tends to believe that the number of hospital deaths due to preventable errors is actually lower than that reported by the IOM (Blendon, et al., 2002). While many people have been affected by medical errors, there are several well-known celebrity cases that bring a personal face to the problem and have contributed to an appreciation of errors in specific categories.

Examples of Medical Errors

The Florida case of Willie King brought to light the issue of wrong site/limb surgery, while the Lehman and Gargano cases identified fatal chemotherapy medication overdoses at Dana Farber. The issue of pediatric medication overdose was noted in the 1997 Houston case of a newborn that received a tenfold overdose of digoxin, and the case of Miguel Sanchez, who received a tenfold overdose of penicillin G benzathine by intravenous administration. The practice in surgery of marking and administering of solutions that have been removed from their original containers was identified in the 1995 Ben Kolb case in Florida, and the issues of drug-drug interactions and resident supervision were noted in the Libby Zion case in New York (Cook, Woods, & Miller, 1998). In 2003, as a result of an error, Jesica Santillan, a 17-year-old girl, received a heart and lung transplant at Duke University Hospital that was incompatible with her type O-positive blood, reminding us of the importance of system issues identifying all patient information accurately (Holmes, 2003). In the same month an infant at Children's Medical Center in Dallas received an organ transplant from the wrong donor.

Often the types of experiences shared are based on problems encountered in the health care system and involve all types of settings and practitioners. The experiences are significant to the individual patient and color future interactions with health care organizations. In a national survey (Gordon, 2002) Americans indicated they are very concerned about medical errors including the fear of receiving the wrong medication and having complications from procedures. The patient's role in health care decisions will be discussed further in chapter 5, and disclosure related to medical errors and unanticipated outcomes will be discussed in chapter 9.

The IOM report estimated that 44,000 to 98,000 people die each year as a result of a preventable adverse event—but each error happened to a real person and we can never lose sight of the personal impact of errors. Studies conducted after the release of the IOM report (Hayward & Hofer, 2001) provide a different analysis of errors, and the issues identified in these studies should be further explored to provide the research base for practice. This book focuses on the fact that medical errors are problematic regardless of the exact number. Therefore efforts to improve patient safety must become everyone's responsibility and part of everyday life for caregivers.

The IOM issued several additional reports that continued the focus on quality health care, but not specifically on patient safety. The second report was *Crossing the Quality Chasm* (Committee on Quality of Health Care in America, 2001a), followed by *Envisioning the National Health Care Quality Report* (Committee on Quality of Health Care in America, 2001b). While these reports focus less on patient safety, they are important for the broader quality framework that supports all dimensions of care. In fact, one of the six dimensions of care proposed in *Crossing the Quality Chasm* is patient safety. The other characteristics that are proposed for patient care include: patient-centeredness, timeliness, efficiency, effectiveness, and equity (Committee on Quality of Health Care in America, 2001b). The 2003 report, *Priority Areas for National Action* (Adams, & Corrigan, 2003) includes 20 areas for action, of which several target patient safety including care coordination, medication management, and nosocomial infections.

While the president established a national initiative on health care quality in 1998, he also established the Quality Interagency Coordination Task Force (QuIC) to address the multiple federal agencies that provide health care (Clinton, 1998). This was one way in which specific actions could be mandated for federal agencies, since the IOM has no regulatory authority and any recommendations would need to be transformed by policymakers to become mandatory (IOM, n.d.). A few policy changes have begun to occur. Responding to the IOM report and media attention, the Centers for Medicare and Medicaid Services (CMS) (2003) updated the conditions of participation to require providers to implement quality assessment and performance improvement programs to identify patient safety issues and reduce medical errors. In early 2003 the Patient Safety and Quality Improvement Act was introduced by a congressional committee demonstrating action at the federal level to advance legislation.

Several other changes occurred during this time period spurred by the IOM report. The Agency for Health Care Policy and Research (AHCPR) changed both its name and role in 2000. This entity became the Agency for Healthcare Research and Quality (AHRQ) with the Healthcare Research and Quality Act of 1999. This change was significant for patient safety as AHRQ became a key funding source for research aimed at patient safety, reducing medical errors, setting a research agenda for patient safety, and using technologies to improve care (AHRQ, 1999).

Another addition to the scene in 2000 was the creation of The Leapfrog Group (Leapfrog) by the Business Roundtable, a coalition of major employers of Fortune 500 companies. Leapfrog proposed three major goals for hospitals to achieve based on expected reductions in morbidity and mortality associated with risk for errors. The reduction in morbidity and mortality translates into significant savings for employers and improved health for employees. These three goals include: (1) Computer Physician Order Entry (CPOE) in which physicians enter orders into a computer rather than writing them down so that orders can be automatically checked against the patient's information profile for potential mistakes, (2) Evidence-based Hospital Referral (EHR) in which patients select hospitals based on outcomes or the hospital's experience with specific conditions or procedures associated with a high risk of death or complications, and (3) ICU Physician Staffing (IPS) with physicians specially trained to care for critically ill patients (Leapfrog, 2000). Since its inception in 2000 Leapfrog has increased the volume of participating hospitals working on these goals (Leapfrog, 2000). These three goals have been controversial among certain groups because of the cost of implementation of CPOE, the shortage of specialists, and limited access to care in areas that do not have the required volumes of procedures specified by Leapfrog (Pollack, 2002). These three goals are among the many that have been suggested in relation to patient safety. A variety of other tools and activities will be discussed in more detail later.

Patient safety is not a new concept, but there is increased interest and the realization that it is a problem. The efforts in the past were not coordinated or focused, and there is no single agency in this country that has oversight for patient safety. Multiple coalitions and alliances have recently been created at both the national and federal level since patient safety initiatives require resources to achieve a critical mass for change. Traditionally, health care groups have led the charge on clinical issues, but now other stakeholders such as employers are forcing change efforts.

TYPES OF ERRORS

In order to provide a context for discussion, it is important to provide definitions of medical errors. According to James Reason (1990), an expert in accident causation, errors are of two kinds. These kinds of errors have also been described by the IOM (Kohn, Corrigan, & Donaldson, 2000) in their report to define errors. Either the correct action does not proceed as intended (an error of execution), or the original intended action is not correct (an error of planning). So there are two major distinctions in types of errors—(a) planning and (b) performing (Table 1.2). Errors of planning take place in cognitive problem-solving activities. The practitioner intentionally develops a plan and orders treatment for the patient. At this point the error is not observable until it becomes apparent that the desired outcome has not been achieved for the patient. It is important to understand this first distinction about errors since the focus in the planning phase is the practitioner's knowledge about the individual patient and the patient's condition, as well as treatment modalities, therapies, and medications. The strategy to minimize errors of planning is based on using research and evidence-based practice as discussed in chapter 4 to build the foundation for developing the best care plans on the front end to minimize risk and improve patient outcomes. Errors in planning may or may not harm the patient but these errors will lead to suboptimal outcomes. For example, the early administration of aspirin to acute myocardial infarction (AMI) patients on admission and discharge from the hospital has been documented to reduce mortality (Ryan, et al., 1999; Marciniak, et al., 1998). Not prescribing aspirin for an AMI patient who meets criteria for this treatment would be an error in planning. In the same way, prescribing an antibiotic to which a patient has demonstrated an allergy is an error in planning, and prescribing an antibiotic to which the organism is not sensitive is an error in planning. Other examples in which planning the patient's care promotes safe practices include appropriate antibiotic prophylaxis, appropriate use of prophylaxis to prevent thromboembolism, and continuous aspiration of subglottic secretions to prevent ventilator associated pneumonia (AHRQ, 1999). Practice based on research and evidence will reduce this type of error and improve patient safety.

The second type of error, performing or execution, occurs quite unintentionally during automatic performance of activities. When this type of error occurs it is almost always visible at the patient-caregiver interface. This patient-caregiver interface is called the *sharp end*; whereas, the *blunt end* of an error is the compilation of system issues that contribute to the error

TABLE 1.2   Types of Errors

Phase	Definition	Issue	Visibility	Focus	Example
1. Error of planning	Use of a wrong plan to achieve an aim	Intentional aspect of problem solving or planning patient care	Not readily observable	Knowledge about the patient, condition, treatment modalities. Use of evidence-based research	Physician prescribes an antibiotic to which the organism is not sensitive. This is the wrong treatment plan.
2. Error of performing or execution	Failure of a planned action to be completed as intended	Unintentional or automatic performance of patient care. Slips and lapses *Rules based errors (policies and procedures) *Knowledge-based errors (unfamiliar situations) *Skill-based errors (lack of education, experience)	Observable at the sharp end or patient and caregiver interface	Reliance on automatic functioning. Distractions, stress, forgetting.	The nurse administers the wrong antibiotic. The treatment plan was correct but performed incorrectly. The reasons for the error could be many such as inadequate labeling.

by shaping the environment and influencing caregiver behavior (Reason, 1990; Kohn, Corrigan, & Donaldson, 2000).

The errors of performing or execution occur due to "slips and lapses" (Reason, 2001). These slips and lapses occur everyday and usually don't cause many problems. Slips account for approximately 90% of errors in health care with certain conditions predisposing a person to make a slip (Turnbull, 2002). In health care these slips and lapses can cause minor or major consequences for the patient. For example, administering Humalog® mix instead of Humulin® insulin, putting a decimal point in the wrong place thus creating a tenfold overdose, or not recognizing that a liquid medication in a syringe was for oral use and not for intravenous administration.

Errors of performance or execution are the result of many factors such as distractions, interruptions of routines, breakdowns in communication, stress, or forgetfulness (Merry & Brown, 2002). They occur due to several major reasons. The first is that the rules, policies, or procedures do not provide sufficient support to minimize the error. For example, if a policy does not address checks on calculations for high-risk medications, then it is possible during medication administration to miscalculate a dose. Second, there may be lack of knowledge about a particular aspect of care or an unfamiliar situation in which the caregiver finds him or herself. Without enough information an error may then be made. For example, a nurse may be assigned to a unit where he/she does not routinely work and encounters a different infusion pump than one that he/she has been trained to use. Although the model looks similar, the device is an older model without free-flow protection. One can now anticipate the scenario. The nurse turns off the infusion pump when the patient's condition improves, but the remaining intravenous solution infuses due to an error of execution based on lack of knowledge and equipment design features. Finally, the caregiver may not have the necessary skills needed for a particular intervention due to lack of education or experience, and an error may result from incorrect performance (Reason, 1990).

These examples prompt us to describe several other ways to think about errors. Errors may also be classified as active or latent (Table 1.3). Active errors are most familiar to people because they are visible at the sharp end with immediate consequence to the patient. Latent errors are error-provoking situations that occur at the blunt end, meaning they are part of organization factors such as structure, environment, equipment, processes, culture, regulations, and administration (Reason, 2001). Latent errors may lie dormant for years, often deeply rooted in organizational culture, until

TABLE 1.3   Active and Latent Error

Type	Location	Visibility	Consequence	Example
Active error	Error occurs at the sharp end (patient and caregiver interface)	Visible	Usually immediate consequences to the patient. Severity depends on the error.	Pharmacist dispenses wrong medication. Nurse gives medication via wrong route. Physician operates on wrong limb.
Latent error	Error occurs at the blunt end (management or system)	Rarely visible	Usually dormant for a long time until local forces act.	Informal practice does not require separation of look-alike medications. No special designation of oral and parenteral syringes. No policy on marking surgical site.

the right mix of circumstances allows the error to pass through safety defenses. Examples of latent errors in medication delivery might include: (1) purchasing practices from a single vendor with look-alike packaging of medications; (2) inconsistent pharmacy practices on storage of look-alike and sound-alike medications; (3) lack of policies for labeling of medications with generic and brand names; (3) no policies on dosage calculations for high-risk medications or vulnerable patients; (4) staffing patterns; and (5) frequent use of per diem staff without training. This list can be quite extensive if we continue to address each aspect of patient safety, but one can quickly see how each latent error is waiting to become active under the right set of circumstances. Latent errors are often what we think of as "accidents waiting to happen". While active errors are often the focus of a root cause analysis, they rarely present a complete picture of contributory causes. Rarely is a single root cause found; more often, several contributory causes are found. This concept will be important in the next section that discusses how errors are traditionally viewed. Analysis strategies will be presented in chapter 3.

The last distinction in error types (Table 1.4) includes separating errors of planning and performing in which the error is unintended, from those that are intentional violations of rules (Reason, 2001). Intentional violations often arise from issues of morale and motivation and are linked to leadership/management systems or the organizational culture. The violations may be routine practices to cut corners and save time during high workloads and time pressures or they may be willful disregard for rules, regulations, or laws. Violation of rules has been described by the Veteran's Administration (VA) National Patient Safety Center (Department of Veterans Affairs, 2002) which distinguishes errors based on whether they are violations due to a criminal act, a purposefully unsafe act, an act related to alcohol or substance abuse, impaired provider/staff, or events involving alleged or

TABLE 1.4 Unintentional Error Versus Violation of Rules

Type	Intention	Common Problem	Example
Error (Planning and Performing)	Unintentional	Information • Incomplete information • Distraction • Forgetting	Pharmacist dispenses wrong medication with only generic name on the label. Nurse does not know generic name and administers wrong medication.
Violation of rules	Intentional • Routine (cutting corners) • Personal gain (for kicks) • Situational (not covered in current policy)	Motivation • Low morale • Poor supervision • Nonsupportive culture	Nurse is in a hurry to end her shift and does not follow policy for double checking dose calculation on insulin.

suspected patient abuse of any kind. These special cases are handled by management and the appropriate legal authorities rather than by traditional root cause analysis of systems and process issues.

Not all errors result in harm. "Errors that do result in injury are sometimes called preventable adverse events. An adverse event is an injury resulting from a medical intervention, or in other words, it is not due to the underlying condition of the patient. While all adverse events result from medical management, not all are preventable" (Kohn, Corrigan, & Donaldson, 2000, p. 4) (see Glossary of Terms). Sometimes adverse events are considered synonymous with errors so definition is important in interpreting research findings and using error rates or adverse event rates for any comparisons. In health care, preventable injuries from care have been estimated to affect between 3% to 4% of hospital patients (Brennan, et al., 1991). A preventable injury might include administering medications to a patient who has demonstrated an allergy to the ordered medication. It would also include not administering preoperative prophylactic antibiotics when empirically indicated. A nonpreventable injury might include administering a new medication to a patient, who has not received the medication previously, but subsequently demonstrates a reaction.

WHY ERRORS HAPPEN

Multiple Defenses

Traditionally, errors have been viewed as a single event (active error) occurring at the patient/caregiver interface (sharp end) and analyzed after the event has occurred (hindsight). The current approach to viewing errors is based on different concepts. The newer approach is based on models from aviation, the nuclear power industry, long-distance trucking, and human factors engineering (Kohn, Corrigan, & Donaldson, 2000). The first concept in our approach is the existence of multiple system defenses designed to prevent or minimize errors, not a single-factor failure. This concept has been likened to Swiss cheese (Reason, 1990) (Figure 1.1). Each slice of cheese can be thought of as a safety defense or system. Each cheese slice can be a strong defense with a few tiny holes that allow errors to penetrate. Or the safety defenses can be weak with many large holes that allow errors to occur often. When the holes in the cheese align, then a number of slips occur so that an error finally reaches the patient. This concept supports the need for a systems perspective with many interlinking

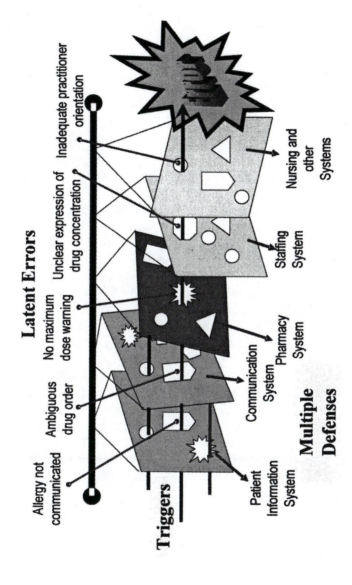

FIGURE 1.1   Swiss Cheese Model illustrating multiple defense systems.
Reason, 1990. Reprinted with permission of the Cambridge University Press.

systems and recognizing multiple contributory causes related to patient safety. The JCAHO has provided analysis of several major errors and identified a number of system issues. In wrong-site surgery (JCAHO, 1998) contributory system issues were unusual time pressures, multiple surgeons, multiple procedures on a single case, unusual equipment, and unusual physical traits of the patient. Similarly, when events of retained foreign objects were studied there were a variety of contributory system issues such as emergency cases, complications while on the operating table, and obesity (Gawande, Studdert, Oray, Brennan, & Zinner, 2003).

Visibility

The second concept relates to the visibility of the error. The sharp end, or caregiver, is seen by others as the single person who made the error and is typically blamed without consideration of the blunt end or the myriad system issues and defense systems that play a role in contributing to the error. The blunt end is not observable and tends to shape the environment and influence behavior by the way resources, constraints, incentives, and demands are handled (Reason, 1990; Kohn, Corrigan, & Donaldson, 2000). There are multiple factors involved in a single error rather than the isolated error of a single practitioner, but only the action of the practitioner is really visible. It is important to recognize that there are many unseen or invisible systems and processes that contribute to an error, and blaming a person does little to resolve the latent errors, which will persist until the next person makes the same error. The nurse who administers the wrong blood product to a patient is quickly identified and blamed for the error, while what is not visible is the process of delivering and storing multiple blood products on the nursing unit, the method of identification of patient and blood product, or multiple patients receiving blood at the same time.

Simplified Analysis

The third concept in our approach to understanding errors is to avoid a limited, oversimplified analysis due to hindsight bias. After the error occurs it seems easy to determine that a different course of action should have been taken; it isn't so simple when one is in the midst of a complex patient care situation with conflicts, work pressures, changes, and unexpected events. Risk in health care systems is inherent and always emerging so that each analysis of error cannot be oversimplified.

SCOPE OF THE PROBLEM

Frequency, Type, and Cost of Errors in Healthcare

The magnitude of the problem of medical errors can be described in several ways. The IOM report provides a generalization from two large-scale studies using hospital records to describe the number of deaths from medical errors in this country. The first study was conducted in New York in 1984 using records from 30,000 discharges from five hospitals with an adverse event occurrence rate of 3.7%. In the Colorado/Utah study in 1992 using 15,000 discharges, the adverse event occurrence rate was 2.9%. The researchers concluded that over half of the adverse events were preventable, 58% in New York and 53% in Colorado/Utah (Kohn, Corrigan, & Donaldson, 2000; Brennan, et al., 1991; Leape, et al., 1991; Thomas, et al., 2000).

In the Colorado/Utah study 6.6% of these adverse events led to death while in New York, 13.6% of adverse events led to death. The study authors then multiplied the percentage of deaths by the number of hospital discharges in 1997 of 33.6 million, as reported by the American Hospital Association. This calculation led to the figure that 44,000 Americans die each year as a result of medical error, and the data from the New York study imply that number may be as high as 98,000 (Table 1.5) (Brennan, et al., 1991; Leape, et al., 1991).

The cost of medical errors, based on these two studies translates into $17 to $29 billion in lost income, disability, and health care costs. Using the 98,000 figure places preventable deaths from adverse events as the fifth leading cause of death in this country (Kohn, Corrigan, & Donaldson, 2000). These reports illustrate that there are sizeable numbers of patients who are harmed from medical errors. Furthermore, preventable adverse events are a leading cause of death in the United States. In a study of patients admitted to two intensive care units and one surgical unit at a large teaching hospital, 45.8% were identified as having had an adverse event, where adverse event was defined as "situations in which an inappropriate decision was made when, at the time, an appropriate alternative could have been chosen" (Andrews, et al., 1997). For 17.7% of patients the adverse event was serious, resulting in disability or death. The likelihood of

TABLE 1.5   Calculation of Deaths From Preventable Adverse Events

New York	
Hospital Admissions 1997	33,600,000
Adverse Occurrence Rate	× .037
National Extrapolation	1,243,200
Preventable Rate	× .58
National Extrapolation	721,056
Death Rate	× .136
National Extrapolation	98,064
Colorado/Utah	
Hospital Admissions 1997	33,600,000
Adverse Occurrence Rate	× .029
National Extrapolation	974,400
Preventable Rate	× .53
National Extrapolation	516,432
Death Rate	× .088
National Extrapolation	45,446

Brennan, et al., 1991

experiencing an adverse event increased about 6% for each day of hospital stay (Kohn, Corrigan, & Donaldson, 2000).

This description of the scope of the problem provides a high level aggregate picture of the patient safety problem related to the frequency, type and cost of medical errors primarily in hospitals. There are several ways to provide additional details about medical errors and their impact on safety, but it is important to note that the research is limited both in the types of problems addressed as well as the health care setting. The IOM report and many other studies describe research conducted in hospitals (see chapter 11 on acute care). While hospitals provide the most acute level of services, health care is primarily provided in other settings (Kohn, Corrigan, & Donaldson, 2000). Most health care is provided in ambulatory settings such as physicians' offices, clinics, and ambulatory surgery centers in which thousands of patients are seen daily.

In other settings, home care involves patients and families in many complex interventions and technologies with self-care as an integral component. Retail pharmacies play a major role in filling prescriptions for patients. Settings such as long-term care provide care to vulnerable populations for which little data are collected about medical errors and patient safety.

Although many of the available studies have focused on the hospital setting, medical errors present a potential problem in any setting, and the gap in knowledge about patient safety problems and the incidence of errors in these other settings is evident.

The AHRQ has begun to fund research in settings other than hospitals (AHRQ, 2001), but there are many interventions and strategies that can be applied now to reduce risk of problems and improve practice. Therefore, the dollar value associated with medical errors is probably underestimated since hospital patients represent only a small proportion of the population and hospital costs are a fraction of the total costs.

SCOPE OF THE PROBLEM

Frequency, Type, and Cost of Medication Errors

The picture of medical errors presented so far is a high-level view of the errors in health care including the costs associated with the errors. Research has been conducted to further delineate types of medical errors. Based on the Harvard Medical Practice Study (Brennan, et al., 1991; Leape, et al., 1991) the authors found that approximately 19.4% of medical errors are medication errors. Since medication delivery crosses multiple settings and comprises a large percentage of the total number of medical errors, there have been a number of studies specifically about medication errors, and many improvement initiatives have targeted medication safety such as the Massachusetts Coalition for the Prevention of Medical Errors, the Institute for Safe Medication Practices (ISMP), the Health Research and Education Trust (HRET), and the American Hospital Association's (AHA) Pathways for Medication Safety (2002). Studies about medication errors and patient safety provide another perspective of the scope of the larger problem of medical errors.

Medication errors are the most frequently cited cause of errors and a report by MedMARx[SM] of 2000 data indicates that relatively few medication errors in hospitals result in harm, according to the United States Pharmacopeia Center for the Advancement of Patient Safety (2002), which showed that 2.4% of errors resulted in harm. Of those resulting in harm, 353 required initial or prolonged hospitalization, 70 required interventions to sustain life, and 14 resulted in death. The United States Pharmacopeia (USP) is a private not-for-profit organization that has developed the Med-MARx[SM] program for a national medication errors database. Errors are categorized as harm, no harm, and potential harm. In 2000, as with the 1999 data, the majority (97%) of actual errors did not result in patient harm. This is similar to work in which it was found that most medication errors are harmless, but 1%–2% cause injury. In the 1991 Harvard Medical Practice Study, 1% was fatal, 12% were life-threatening, 30% were serious, and 57% were significant (Bates, Cullen, & Laird, 1995).

In hospital emergency departments (ED), the failure to prescribe or authorize the correct medication, failure to administer a prescribed medication, and administering the incorrect dose of a medication are the three most common medication errors (see www.usp.org). The USP has also provided recommendations for preventing errors in emergency situations after analyzing medication error data. In 2001, hospitals reported more than 2,000 ED-related medication errors. According to the USP, the combination of interruptions, intense pressure, and a fast-paced environment lead to medication errors and fewer error interceptions. In fact, the USP found that 23% of errors in the ED were detected before reaching patients, as opposed to 39% detected in other areas of the hospital.

Even though medication errors that result in death or serious injury occur infrequently, increasing numbers of people are affected because of the extensive use of medications in all health care settings. Nearly 2.5 billion prescriptions were dispensed in U.S. pharmacies in 1998 at an estimated cost of about $92 billion (National Wholesale Druggists' Association, 1998). In a study by AHRQ (2000) 2.4 million prescriptions are filled improperly each year in Massachusetts alone. Of the total medications administered, errors are estimated to account for 7,000 deaths a year, in and out of hospitals (American Society of Hospital Pharmacists, 1993; Classen, Pestotnik, Evans, Lloyd, & Burke, 1997). Adverse events occur frequently in hospital settings, and problems related to medications continue into the home setting such that 1%–4% of all visits to emergency rooms are related to inappropriate use of medications (Schneider, Gift, Lee, Rothermich, & Sill, 1995).

Activities that can improve medication delivery will be discussed in chapter 3, but the risks and strategies for medication safety in different settings and for different patient types are addressed in chapters 10–14 in the discussion of the vulnerabilities of different populations. Not all patients have the same level of risk for errors. For example, a study of an intensive care unit revealed an average of 1.7 errors per day per patient, of which 29% had the potential for serious or fatal injury (Leape, 1994). A 1990 study of prescribing errors in teaching hospitals found 3.13 errors per 1,000 orders written, and a rate of 1.81 significant errors per 1,000 orders

(Lesar, et al., 1990). A 1996 study at an urban community hospital found that medication delivery was a problem 79% of the time (Hackel, Butt, & Banister, 1996).

Further delineation of medication errors into four major phases of (1) ordering, (2) dispensing, (3) administering, and (4) monitoring allows one to identify error-prone phases and suggestions to reduce errors for each phase (Figure 1.2). Errors in the ordering and administering of medications

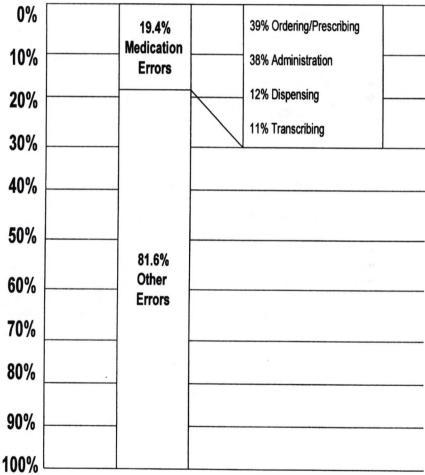

FIGURE 1.2   Medical errors by type.

Leape, et al., 1991.

are common in hospitals. According to the American Society of Healthsystem Pharmacists (ASHP) on average, one patient per hospital per day will experience a medication error (Brown, 1992). Some estimates of the total cost of medication errors to hospitals are as high as $15 billion per year (Brown, 1992). A 1997 study of 4,108 admissions to two hospitals over 6 months found that the annual costs attributable to all adverse drug events (ADE) were $5.6 million and preventable ADEs were $2.8 million. These results were obtained by determining average increased hospital costs associated with ADE of $4,700 per admission. If these findings are generalized, the increased hospital costs of preventable adverse drug events for inpatients could amount to $2 billion for the country (Bates, et al., 1997). Medication-related errors occur frequently in hospitals and although not all result in actual harm, those that do are costly.

Another study (Classen, Pestotnik, Evans, Lloyd, & Burke, 1997) found that an ADE is typically associated with a prolonged hospital stay, excess costs of around $2,000 per case, and an almost twofold increased risk of death. In a review of adult admissions to 11 medical and surgical units at two tertiary care hospitals, Bates, Cullen, and Laird (1995) identified 247 ADEs for an event rate of 6.5 ADEs per 100 nonobstetrical admissions, and a mean number per hospital per year of approximately 1,900 ADEs.

Children are at particular risk of medication errors primarily due to the multiple weight-based calculations that must be done for each child. Many medications do not come prepared in the doses required for infants and neonates thereby adding an additional step of preparation. A case in Denver in which an error with a decimal point created a tenfold overdose of intramuscular penicillin G benzathine by intravenous route, proved to be fatal for the child (Dana & McKendrick, n.d.). Pediatric populations create vulnerabilities that are in many ways different from adults. This issue will be further discussed in chapter 10.

Other Errors

Patient safety problems of many kinds occur during the course of providing health care. Figure 1.2 illustrates the frequency of medication errors in hospitals in relation to the total number of medical errors as well as the breakdown by the four phases of medication delivery. Figure 1.3 further illustrates the types of other medical errors that were found in the Harvard Medical Practice Study (Brennan, et al., 1991; Leape, et al., 1991). Medical errors were separated into two major categories—operative and nonopera-

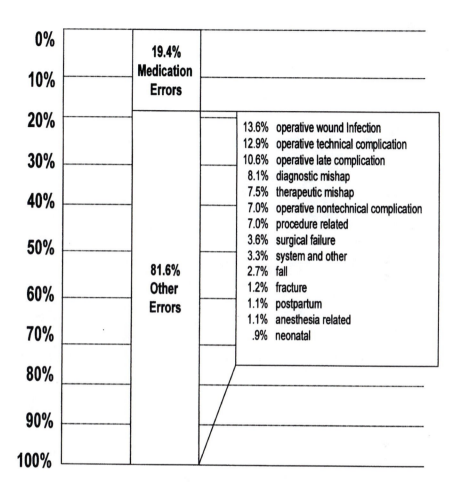

FIGURE 1.3 Medical errors by type.
Leape, et al., 1991.

tive. Operative errors constituted 47.7% of the total errors and nonoperative errors were 52.3% (Table 1.6). The value of identifying the frequency of error types is to combine this information with the severity of the errors, the level of risk, and the organization-specific services to help prioritize resource allocation as safety initiatives are implemented.

There are few methods in the literature used to categorize errors that may be useful to organizations in trying to capture and sort information

TABLE 1.6   Categories and Percentages of Error-related Injuries Identified in the 1991 Harvard Medical Practice Study Based on Operative and Nonoperative Categories

Operative	
Wound infection	13.6%
Technical complication	12.9%
Late complication	10.6%
Nontechnical complication	7.0%
Surgical failure	3.6%
Subtotal	47.7%
Nonoperative	
Drug related	19.4%
Diagnostic mishap	8.1%
Therapeutic mishap	7.5%
Procedure related	7.0%
Fall	2.7%
Fracture	1.2%
Postpartum	1.1%
Anesthesia related	1.1%
Neonatal	0.9%
System and other	3.3%
Subtotal	52.3%
Total	100%

Leape, et al., 1991

about errors, but these methods are probably more useful to the researcher (NCCMERP, 2001; U.S.P. Center for the Advancement of Patient Safety, 2002; American Hospital Association (AHA), 2002). The most defined method of error classification is found for medications (National Coordinating Council for Medication Error Reporting and Prevention (NCCMERP), 2001). Other categories are more likely used by risk and quality managers in organizing error reports but there is no national mandatory system for reporting of errors with standardized categories. Currently, most reporting systems are voluntary except those mandated by certain state agencies. Use of NCCMERP, Medwatch, or MedMARx[SM] are voluntary systems. Discussion has been generated regarding potential federal reporting of errors for a national database but no proposed legislation has been enacted to date.

The JCAHO has categorized errors via the sentinel event reporting database (JCAHO, 2002b). The number and type of sentinel events are found in Table 1.7. The findings from these sentinel events have been used to develop recommendations for safety improvement published in the *Sentinel Event Alerts* (JCAHO, 2000a) and to generate the focus for six national patient safety goals (JCAHO, 2000d). The JCAHO has had a policy for reporting of sentinel events since 1995 and often similar events must be reported to state agencies as well.

Major Settings for Errors

Different patient populations have different risk factors. Based on the patient's underlying condition and the intensity of the treatment provided, certain units in hospitals are more likely to be error-prone settings. For example, intensive care units have processes with many tight time con-

TABLE 1.7   Joint Commission Summary of Sentinel Events 1995–2003 as of May 7, 2003

Type of Sentinel Event	Number	Percent
Patient suicide	328	16.1%
Operative/postoperative complication	252	12.4%
Wrong-site surgery	240	11.8%
Medication error	234	11.5%
Delay in treatment	122	6.0%
Patient fall	97	4.8%
Patient death/injury in restraints	99	4.9%
Assault/rape/homicide	79	3. 9%
Transfusion error	55	2.7%
Perinatal death/loss of function	49	2.4%
Patient elopement	43	2.1%
Fire	37	1.8%
Anesthesia-related event	31	1.5%
Medical equipment-related	29	1.4%
Ventilator death/injury	29	1.4%
Maternal death	28	1.4%
Infant abduction/wrong family	24	1.2%
Death associated with transfer	15	0.7%
Other less frequent types of sentinel events	243	11.9%

© Joint Commission on Accreditation of Healthcare Organizations (JCAHO), 2002. Reprinted with permission.

straints and processes in which steps must take place in a defined manner (see chapter 11 on acute care). Patients receiving more medications, tests, and treatments have more complexity and variable input. Patients receiving multiple high-alert medications may be at greater risk, and patients who require special calculations and dosing for medications are also at greater risk for error. When errors were separated by hospital unit the frequency was the following: medical intensive care units (ICU) 19.4%, surgical ICU's 10.5%, medical units 10.6%, surgical units 8.9%, pediatrics 9.1%, obstetrics and gynecology units 6.2%, and emergency departments 5.0% (Leape, et al., 1991).

COMPREHENSIVE APPROACH TO PATIENT SAFETY

Approaching patient safety within health care organizations requires a multifaceted approach since patient safety includes numerous aspects. Table 1.8 presents a comprehensive approach to consider patient safety in combination with selected factors for safety to the caregiver as well. There are a number of factors to be analyzed and a variety of tools to assist. More about tools and strategies will be described in chapter 3. The approach provided is a guide for organizations as they develop a safety plan and prioritize actions and allocation of resources. This comprehensive approach presents six major areas: (1) structure, (2) environment, (3) equipment/technology, (4) processes, (5) people, and (6) leadership systems/culture (Spath, 2000b; Turnbull, 2002; Merry & Brown, 2002). Within these six areas there are overlapping items since safety issues are pervasive in all aspects of care, but this approach will provide an organized way to analyze different areas using current knowledge, evidence-based research, and consensus and best practices, where research does not exist. By using this approach, and understanding those characteristics that contribute to greater risk for errors, one can apply concepts and principles to reduce risk and promote safety. These six areas will vary by patient type. For example, the equipment used in neonatal units is quite different from that used in a geriatric unit or primary care clinic. As one works with different patient populations it is possible to use the approach for general concepts and then apply knowledge about specific patient types to develop and implement safe practices. Special patient populations will be addressed in chapters 10–14.

Structure

The first area of the approach is structure. Structure includes the basic components of an organization. The structure of work can be described

TABLE 1.8 A Comprehensive Approach to Assess Safety

Structure	Environment	Equipment/ Technologies	Processes	People	Leadership/ Culture
Policies and procedures for organization	Lighting	Design features (including flaws or failures)	Work design	Attitude, motivation	Philosophy of safety
Facilities	Surfaces	Functionality and intuitiveness	High risk characteristics	Physical health	Communication channels
Supplies	Temperature	Safety features including controls	Cycle time	Emotional and mental health	Reporting culture
	Noise	Override features	Efficiency	Human factors—interaction with technology and environment	Staffing—workload, hours and personnel policies
	Space, access	Default modes	Effectiveness	Cognitive and psychological factors	Teamwork
	Design	Labels/ instructions		Training/ education	Hierarchy
	Functionality (rails/ bars)	Alarms		Communication methods, perceptions, interpretations	
	Ergonomics				

in terms of physical facilities, supplies, and the policies and procedures that govern operations and work. Structure is the foundation of the organization and its operations. Already one can see that policies and procedures have an element of philosophy or culture of the organization and therefore overlap with other areas, so the approach we have suggested should not be thought of as exhaustive or exclusive.

In assessing how structure contributes to errors, it is necessary to think about each area either proactively in terms of problems that could occur, or retrospectively after an error happens to determine those problem areas needing correction. For example, how are the general facilities built and designed to promote safety? Then one must determine if the right supplies are available when needed or if substitutions are made, assess the visibility of patients on nursing units, and consider the proximity of specialty units such as emergency department and radiology or critical care and surgery for rapid access to these services. Finally, one must check to be sure policies and procedures address operations and general safety considerations. These issues will assist in analyzing how basic elements support safety, and they will also prompt further analysis of patient flow or processes. Again, the overlapping and linking of patient safety areas is evident.

Environment

Perhaps the easiest aspect of the approach to understand is the environment. Factors in the environment that must be considered relative to patient safety from both the patient's perspective, as well as the practitioner include: Lighting, surface types, temperature, noise levels, design, functionality, and ergonomics. It is easy to see how lighting and surface type may contribute to patient falls and injuries, or how noise levels can distract the nurse during medication administration. Noise levels can also detract attention from alarms signaling a change in the patient's condition. Temperature is an important consideration during surgery procedures so that optimal cooling is done yet timely rewarming occurs. Certain orthopedic procedures require specific temperatures so the cement used in joint replacements does not harden too quickly. This must be balanced with cooling levels of the patient. Another key aspect of the environment, especially in surgical areas, is the oxygen-rich environment, which may increase the risk of fires or burns.

Only a few possible scenarios or examples are provided to assist in thinking about different facets and their importance to patient safety.

Functionality and ergonomics are other areas that can have an impact on performance. How could these factors play a role in safety? Since these factors are often linked, let's think of them together in several common examples. Observe the arrangement of the bed, bedside table, and other furniture to determine if the nurse can easily and safely access and move the patient. If a patient transfer from one bed to another is needed and the beds don't align well (either by bed type, height, or other factor), the staff may have difficulty safely transferring the patient, increasing the risk for a patient fall or a staff injury. Are patient lifts available to assist caregivers and reduce the risk of dropping or injuring a patient? Some hospitals are implementing no-lift policies to protect the staff—which requires implementation of special lifting devices for patients. Positioning the bed properly using lift devices allows caregivers to perform activities without straining and putting both the caregiver and patient at risk. Check the location of grab bars, breakaway bars, and corridor rails for access. Think of other examples you have encountered in your work setting in which the environment plays a crucial role.

Equipment/Technology

Equipment and technology cover a wide array of items; technology will specifically be discussed in chapter 8. The focus here is not to identify every possible type of equipment or technology that is used in health care, but to think about these tools from a larger perspective. For example, caregivers must identify the type of equipment that is used and how the equipment is designed. A critical review of equipment should reveal if there are visible flaws or potential failures such as those noted in free flow infusion devices (JCAHO, 2000b; ISMP, 1998). Are there default modes on the equipment/technology that are considered to be the safe mode or must the caregiver have specialized training to understand how to operate the equipment? Labels and instructions should be clearly marked with hints for troubleshooting readily available. For equipment that may need to be shut off quickly is the on/off switch clearly designated? Safety features should be designed into the equipment to automatically protect the patient or user, or warn the user that a potentially dangerous condition exists. While new equipment or computers are often seen as the solution to many problems, each new piece of equipment or technology brings its own set of issues and potential opportunities for error (Turnbull, 2002).

Systems and Processes

Systems and processes are the core of how work is actually designed and accomplished. Systems comprise multiple processes in which many steps are taken for a specific task and how each step is designed and connected shapes the level of risk for error and the final outcome. There are certain characteristics associated with error-prone processes. By understanding these characteristics, processes can be redesigned to be safer or strategies added if the process cannot be redesigned. The six process characteristics are (1) complexity, (2) variable input, (3) inconsistency, (4) human intervention, (5) tight time constraint, and (6) tight coupling (Croteau & Schyve, 2000; Spath, 2000a).

Complexity refers both to the number of steps involved in a particular process as well as the rules or algorithm choices that apply for each step. If there are multiple choices and decision arms for an action then it becomes complex for the individual user to remember the correct step. Complex processes increase the risk of an error as the caregiver may forget a step, perform the step incorrectly, or not select the correct decision arm.

Variation has long been known to exist in every process, but the greater the variation the greater the risk for error and undesired outcomes. In manufacturing there may be multiple inputs into a process. In health care, people are the input and they come in all shapes, sizes, ages, and conditions. People can be considered as variable input. While all diabetic patients have common characteristics with similar treatment methods, each diabetic patient is different with a specific type of diabetes, onset, medication, diet, and activity. The challenge is to recognize that patients will be similar and different at the same time and determine how the caregiver can accommodate the differences into a plan that will be safe.

Processes that are designed without adequate research basis or sufficient description will be inconsistent as each person determines his/her own way to perform. This inconsistency prevents the best practice or research-based practice to be implemented in patient care. As each caregiver performs differently there is a greater chance for an error to be made.

Processes that rely heavily on human intervention rather than automation are subject to the weaknesses of humans such as fatigue, ability to be distracted, and short-term memory lapses (Merry & Brown, 2002; Cook & Woods, 1994). Little leverage in making improvement can be achieved by reminding individuals to be careful and follow a particular procedure. Instead, methods to minimize reliance on human frailties such as automatic reminders for tasks or automated completion of tasks will reduce the risk of error.

Tight time constraint and tight coupling are actually two separate characteristics but are often found together so they will be presented in one discussion. Tight time constraint refers to the time intervals between two consecutive steps in a process. When this time interval is short it is called "tight". A good example to illustrate tight time constraints is a cardiac arrest emergency. There is very little time between steps in resuscitation. Medications and fluids are administered. The patient is defibrillated and intubated almost simultaneously. Multiple caregivers are notified at the same time as the family. With everything happening quickly a mistake could occur more easily than if time were not a critical factor. An emergency is a good way to describe coupling as well. Coupling refers to the way that steps in a process are linked. If a step follows the preceding step in a specific way but also in a defined time interval then the coupling is "tight". If the order the steps follow is not dependent on certain actions being accomplished, then the steps are "loose". Processes with tight coupling are more prone to error. In our resuscitation example, defibrillation is tightly coupled with rhythm identification, equipment preparation, paddle placement, pressure application, clearance, and defibrillation. Success is dependent on each step being followed in a specific sequence, in a short time. Any deviation can result in an inadequate patient outcome or potential injury to a bystander.

Time constraints can impact patient care in another way. Shift change is a vulnerable time for patients because nurses are frequently unavailable due to reporting and completion of other activities. This transition time between caregivers exposes the patient to additional risk for safety problems such as falls.

An additional feature of processes is cycle time. Usually, cycle time refers to the time required to complete a particular step in a process or the process. It refers to all aspects of time performance (Baldrige National Quality Program, 2003). This time plays an important role in turnaround time for diagnostic reports, administration time of medications such as thrombolytics and prophylactic antibiotics, or treatment times. If the cycle time is overly long it can contribute to delays in diagnosis or treatment. The nature of the diagnostic report, severity of the patient's condition, and window for treatment must all be considered as to appropriate cycle time. Rarely is cycle time too short. Often, cycle time is prolonged with costly delays, or if not actually prolonged, then it is prolonged in being communicated to the right caregiver or in being acted upon. There are many cases in which a test result was completed timely but placed on the wrong medical record or the physician not notified so that the delay still occurs for the patient.

The last two factors of processes that should be considered for patient safety are effectiveness and efficiency. A process may be well designed but if it requires significant resources to be achieved it may not be efficient for organizations that are facing shortages in manpower and financial resources. Similarly, a process may be well designed but does not achieve the desired outcome for the patient and is, therefore, not effective. So while it is important to focus on the process don't forget the importance of the "end process" result or outcome.

Considerable attention will be focused on systems and processes. Deming (1986) noted that most organizational problems were due to these factors rather than individual performance, so improvement efforts should be primarily targeted at process and performance improvement. This approach is also evident in accreditation standards of the JCAHO, in International Organization for Standardization (ISO) standards (Gardner, 2001; Godwin, 2002), and in Six Sigma techniques (Merry & Brown, 2002) to reduce variation and errors.

People

While attention will be focused on systems and processes, the characteristics of people working within systems are also key to understanding how errors occur. We have addressed human intervention as a contribution to error prone processes and will further discuss some of the characteristics that support this. First, one's attitude or motivation will affect performance level, attention span, and distraction. These factors are linked to the management systems and often influenced by organizational policies, supervision, and personal life. When attitude or motivation influences negative performance then errors are more likely to occur. Performance is also affected by both physical and mental health. Illness, fatigue, and sleep deprivation will have an impact on performance by reducing alertness and reaction time (Rosekind, et al., 1996). One's mental and emotional health can also impact performance when attention is focused on other personal needs or problems. Without full attention to the patient, there is a greater chance that symptoms will be missed and an error will occur. People are subject to limited memory capacity, limited mental processing capacity, and limited ability to multitask (Spath, 2000a). Chapters 6 and 7 will provide further discussion about these issues as they affect staffing, the nurse's work environment, and strategies to improve patient safety.

Training and education are critical for practitioners to stay abreast of new medications, treatments, tests, equipment, and policies. Without education, or with inadequate education, practitioners may not have all of the information needed when confronted with a new situation or problem. This information need can range from recognition of conditions not often seen, such as smallpox, anthrax, or West Nile virus, to operating a new infusion device, or entering orders online. Each situation has a different level of risk and opportunity for error. Additional knowledge about people and how they think, perceive, and act comes from human factors engineering. Human factors engineering is a science devoted to the interaction of people and equipment and their environment (Merry & Brown, 2002; Food and Drug Administration (FDA), n.d.). Human factors research studies human performance and ways to reduce the likelihood of error and patient injury. This is achieved by understanding the needs of users, including their abilities, limitations, and work environments, and recognizing the limitation of all of these factors. The application of human factors knowledge helps with designing and using equipment or devices in a way that is intuitive with low reliance on human intervention, coupled with easy-to-read displays, easy-to-use controls, safe connections, effective alarms, and easy repair (FDA, n.d.). Many of the concepts on the human interface with equipment and technology have already been applied in the aviation model and are only now being used in health care.

Cognitive functioning also plays a significant role in understanding how errors occur (Merry & Brown, 2002). Attention allocation, pattern recognition, and decision making are some of the concepts to be considered. These key concepts include our ability to attend to a limited number of items, distraction due to other stimuli, seeing what we expect to see, using past solutions to solve new problems, confusion encountering unfamiliar situations, perception of oral and written communication within our frame of reference, and use of automatic functioning (Cook & Woods, 1994). Here are some common examples:

Ability to Attend to a Limited Number of Items

During a busy day a nurse usually has a team of patients to care for which includes medications, treatments, monitoring, lab tests, orders, and new admissions or discharges. If a new admission arrives in serious condition with multiple orders and treatments to be administered immediately, the nurse can only complete one item at a time and during this time the nurse is not able to provide focused attention to other patients.

Distraction Due to Other Stimuli

A busy day at the hospital often finds the nurse dealing with phone calls, lab reports, patient requests, and physician orders. If the nurse is distracted by these other events during medication administration it is easy to see how the wrong medication can be administered or given to the wrong patient.

Seeing What We Expect to See

Our brains help us cope with a complex world in many different ways. One way is that our brains adjust what we actually see to match our expectations. This is not uncommon when we are accustomed to having a syringe of lidocaine at the bedside of a cardiac patient. We expect lidocaine, so we see lidocaine because it is located where we expected. If for any reason a syringe of another medication such as epinephrine had been placed in the location the results could be deadly. This same phenomenon occurs in cases in which staff who are familiar with an antibiotic that is packaged in a foil wrapper "see" what they expect when a new paralyzing agent is also packaged in a foil wrapper.

Using Past Solutions to Solve New Problems

Our brains help in another way. We draw upon past learnings and experiences to solve a problem even if the problem is not the same. For example, patients undergoing a MidCAB procedure for occluded coronary arteries may need to have different monitoring from patients undergoing the traditional coronary artery bypass graft surgery (CABG). Without understanding the new procedure (MidCAB) used to treat the same cardiac condition and its unique potential complications, we might tend to treat these patients exactly alike assuming that heart surgery is the same regardless of approach. However postoperative assessment and management vary due to the CABG patient undergoing heart lung bypass, whereas the MidCAB patient does not.

Encountering Unfamiliar Situations

When we encounter an unfamiliar situation, our brain starts to look for a recognizable pattern that will help us deal successfully with the situation. We may try a solution for a similar experience based on our past experience, but find we need new information. This has occurred many times in health care as new strains of diseases develop and global transference of people with conditions once limited to certain regions or races takes place.

Perception of Oral and Written Communication

Errors arise from both oral and written communication. While communication entails many aspects, two common misperceptions often occur. With oral communication we often hear something different from what was said or the sender says something different than what was intended. Either way this oral method is prone to many misinterpretations. Errors with verbal orders are common and a key reason for the JCAHO's goal on elimination of verbal orders (JCAHO, 2002d). Likewise, written communication is often illegible with many abbreviations and shorthand used in health care. Unfortunately, many abbreviations have led to unfortunate medication errors (Cohen, 1999) and frequently the person who wrote the information is not available when the caregiver must interpret illegible handwriting. This has given rise to multiple interpretations from others. The patient may indeed be lucky if the written material is interpreted correctly or could be seriously harmed if it is not. Numerous examples of errors have been reported to the ISMP due to illegible notations of look-alike medications such as Celebrex and Celexa, Axert and Antivert, Valtrex and Valcyte.

Automatic Functioning

If you have ever taken vital signs, administered medications, and performed multiple patient care tasks without stopping to think about each step, it is because of the ability to function in an automatic mode. There are many things a person can do this way so as not to consciously think about every detail of every action. This mode helps us manage day-to-day activities, but this mode can interfere with safety when vigilance is needed, such as an unexpected change in a patient's condition, a complex procedure, or administration of high-risk medications or blood.

Leadership Systems and Culture

The area of leadership systems and culture plays an important role in our approach to understanding errors and patient safety. The first aspect of leadership is the philosophy and values that leaders create. Leadership support for patient safety is critical for a successful program and is evident in the type of resources allocated, the analysis of processes, the implementation of changes, the response to error reporting, and the use of evidence-based practice (see chapters 4 and 7 for further discussion on work culture and evidence-based practice).

Communication channels are important in how leaders communicate these values and philosophy about patient care and safety, as well as how staff communicate problems and report errors. Communication channels are not the same as communication methods among individuals described earlier. Certainly communication channels include communication methods but the major difference is that communication channels include lines of communication—who talks to whom, is the message supported by action, what is the consistency of message, and how communication occurs across different units or divisions? Communication from leaders and managers determines the philosophy and actions of reporting errors. If errors are recognized as system and process issues to be addressed, then leaders will want errors to be reported and will reward this behavior. If errors are seen as individual failures and a poor reflection on the organization then reporting will be punished, either directly or indirectly. Punitive responses may include: private or public reprimand, remedial education, a point system for errors in the personnel file, error data in personnel files, or blaming the individual. Blaming is a universal phenomenon. It is natural in our culture, emotionally satisfying, and often legally convenient. However, blaming is a knee-jerk response due to pressure and usually occurs as a result of hindsight bias when only the single error is visible (Turnbull, 2002).

Another important area of leadership systems and culture is human resource policies on staffing and personnel management including hours worked, workloads, and management of fatigue, stress, and illness. All health care organizations are facing workforce shortages and are challenged to create a work environment that provides adequate qualified staff to provide safe patient care. More on the relationship of staffing, work culture, and patient safety issues will be discussed in chapters 4 and 6 with identification of frameworks found to demonstrate improved performance, safety, and satisfaction.

Teams and teamwork are important components of health care. All patient care involves members from different professions who must coordinate care across multiple settings during various stages of health and illness. The ability to communicate and work together is essential for continuity of care. The most effective teams have a common goal for their work (Merry & Brown, 2002). Team members must be able to function efficiently and effectively to reap desired patient outcomes. Current research based on the aviation model demonstrates the importance and responsibility of each team member in participating in the team activities. Some of the best examples of high performing teams are illustrated in situations of crisis or where rapid action is needed. For example, in the emergency department when a trauma patient arrives, team action is needed to diagnose injuries, implement emergency life saving treatment, and prepare for additional procedures. Accurate and timely documentation of events requires all team members to communicate actions, administer medications and fluids, and describe findings so that everyone understands the patient's condition at all times. Lack of effective teamwork creates many opportunities for errors to occur.

The last factor of hierarchy is often seen in health care. Hierarchy may be evident in management positions with the chief executive officer, vice president, director, manager, supervisor, and staff level. It is also seen in medical staff positions with the attending physician, resident, intern, and medical student or the health care team including physician, nurse, and nursing assistant hierarchies. These hierarchies usually impede communication flow from a person of lower position to one of higher position. Again, other models have taught us that these levels often create unnecessary barriers in which serious mistakes can be made. In health care one example is that of surgery site verification. Several reports of sentinel events to the Joint Commission indicated that surgery technicians had knowledge that a problem existed but did not notify the surgeon. The results were wrong-site procedures for patients (JCAHO, 1998). More about wrong-site surgery will be presented in chapter 11 on acute care.

It is easy in a hierarchy for those in lower positions to assume that those in higher positions could not be wrong in the decision regarding a patient. Rarely is a person thinking about any of the possible factors that might be involved in the case such as "this physician worked all night and is tired" or "the nurse got distracted while taking care of several patients" or "the pharmacist did not hear the order correctly" or "that policy changed last month". The newer way of thinking about hierarchies is that everyone must be accountable to speak up if an unsafe or potentially unsafe practice is evident, regardless of position (Turnbull, 2002). The long-standing traditions within health care make this extremely challenging but important.

CONCLUSION

This first chapter has focused on helping the practitioner understand types of errors and how errors occur, and outlines an approach that will be used to identify strategies to reduce risk for errors. Chapter 2 will begin on a different note. Health care is probably one of the few industries that gauges its performance on negative outcomes (errors) rather than its successful outcomes. Every day practitioners are successful in navigating complex organizations, hazards, miscommunications, and other challenges to produce safe patient care. Certainly latent errors exist in every system but the vulnerabilities change and practitioners exhibit remarkable skill, knowledge and flexibility to prevent problems from reaching patients. In the next chapter strategies and tools will be described that can be used to build reliable organizations with a positive foundation for patient safety.

WEB RESOURCES

Name of Resource/URL	Description
ABC's of Patient Safety *www.npsf.org*	Basic concepts of safety using alphabet
AHRQ web journal *www.webmm.ahrq.gov/*	Online journal with case examples and analysis
American Hospital Association *www.aha.org*	Tools and resources for hospitals on patient safety
AHA/VHA Strategies for Leadership: An Organizational Approach to Patient Safety *www.aha.org*	Tools for organizations to assess safety
Anatomy of an Error *www.mederrors.com*	Continuing education program on errors with references to celebrity cases
Aviation Safety System *www.faa.gov/publicinfo.htm*	Review of aviation system
Beyond Blame Video *www.mederrors.com*	Video that can be purchased outlining several celebrity cases.
GHA—Elements of a Culture of Safety *www.gha.org*	Factors to support positive culture of safety
Identifying and Understanding Medical Device Use Errors *www.fda.gov/cdrh/useerror/ UseErrorChecklist.pdf*	Checklist for assessing medical devices to reduce risk for error
Institute of Medicine Report— Crossing the Quality Chasm *www.national-academies.org*	IOM report on health care quality with six quality aims
Institute of Medicine Report— Priority Areas for National Action: Transforming Health Care Quality *www.national-academies.org*	IOM report outlining 20 national priorities

Institute of Medicine Report—To Err Is Human *www.national-academies.org*	IOM landmark report on medical errors
Institute for Safe Medication Practices *www.ismp.org*	Multiple resources on medication errors and corrective actions
Joint Commission on Accreditation of Healthcare Organizations (JCAHO) *www.jcaho.org*	Sentinel event policy; Sentinel event alerts; Sentinel event statistics
The Leapfrog Group *www.leapfroggroup.org*	Leapfrog three major goals for hospitals
Make Sure the Medical Device You Choose Is Designed for You *www.fda.gov/cdrh/useerror/you_choose_checklist.html*	Checklist for assessing medical devices
Medication Safety Issues Briefs *www.hhnmag.com/asp/downloads.asp*	Medication safety reports
Medication Use System Safety Strategy *www.ashp.org/patient_safety/ms3-1.pdf*	Medication safety use
National Patient Safety Foundation *www.npsf.org*	Compendium of "Best Solutions"
Patient Safety Handbook *www.patientsafety.gov*	Veterans Administration handbook on patient safety
Patient Safety and the Just Culture *www.mers-tm.net*	Culture issues in safety
Patient Safety Reporting System *www.psrs.arc.nasa.gov*	Model of health care error reporting based on aviation model
P4PS—First Do No Harm *www.p4ps.org*	Video that can be purchased with scenarios for analysis and discussion
Redefining the Culture for Patient Safety *www.mhhp.com/ptsafety/psbrochure.html*	Brochure developed by the MHHP using three aspects of culture change
VHA National Patient Safety Center *www.patientsafetycenter.gov*	Multiple resources on safety, FMEA, RCA

REFERENCES

Adams, K., & Corrigan, J. M. (Eds.). (2003). *Priority areas for national action: Transforming health care quality*. Washington, DC: The National Academies Press.

Advisory Commission on Consumer Protection and Quality in the Health Care Industry. (1998). *Quality first: Better health care for all Americans*. U.S. Department of Health and Human Services. Retrieved January 12, 2003, from www.hcqualitycommission. gov/final/

Agency for Healthcare Research and Quality. (AHRQ). (1998). Reducing errors in health care. *Research in Action*. Retrieved January 13, 2003, from www.ahrq.gov/ research/errors.htm

Agency for Healthcare Research and Quality. (AHRQ). (1999). *Reauthorization fact sheet*. Retrieved January 13, 2003, from www.ahrq.gov/about/ahrqfact.htm

Agency for Healthcare Research and Quality. (AHRQ). (2000). *Medical errors: The scope of the problem. Fact sheet* (Publication No. AHRQ 00-P037). Retrieved May 8, 2003, from www.ahrq.gov/qual/errback.htm

Agency for Healthcare Research and Quality. (AHRQ). (2001). *Quality research for quality health care. A report from AHRQ on recent activities and future directions*. Retrieved January 18, 2003, from www.ahrq.gov/about/qr4qhc/qr4qhc-1.htm

American Hospital Association (AHA). (2002). *Pathways for medication safety. Leading a strategic planning effort*. Health Research and Education Trust, Institute for Safe Medication Practices. Retrieved January 20, 2003, from www.hospitalconnect.com/ medpathways/authorize.jsp?page=/medpathways/tools/tools.html

American Society of Hospital Pharmacists. (1993). ASHP guidelines on preventing medication errors in hospitals. *American Journal of Hospital Pharmacy, 50*, 305–314.

Andrews, L. B., Stocking, C., Krizek, T., Gottlieb, L., Kirzek, C., Vargish, T., et al. (1997). Alternate strategy for studying adverse events in medical care. *Lancet, 349*, 309–313.

Baldrige National Quality Program. (2003). *Health care criteria for performance excellence*. Retrieved January 15, 2003, from www.quality.nist.gov/PDF_files/ 2003_HealthCare_Criteria.pdf

Bates, D. W., Cullen, D, J., & Laird, N. (1995). Incidence of adverse drug events and potential adverse drug events: Implications for prevention. *Journal of the American Medical Association, 274*, 29–34.

Bates, D. W., Spell, N., Cullen, D. J., Burdick, E., Laird, N., Petersen, L., et al. (1997). The costs of adverse drug events in hospitalized patients. *Journal of the American Medical Association, 277*(4), 307–311.

Beecher, H. K., & Todd, D. P. (1954). A study of the deaths associated with anesthesia and surgery. *Annals of Surgery, 140*, 2–34.

Blendon, R. J., DesRoches, C. M., Brodie, M., Benson, J. M., Rosen, A. B., Schneider, E., et al. (2002). Views of practicing physicians and the public on medical errors. *New England Journal of Medicine, 347*(24), 1933–1940.

Brennan, T. A., Leape, L. L., Laird, N. M., Hebert, L., Localio, A. R., Lawthers, A. G., et al. (1991). Incidence of adverse events and negligence in hospitalized patients: Results of the Harvard Medical Practice Study I. *New England Journal of Medicine, 324*, 370–376.

Brown, C. (Ed.). (1992). Medication errors: High liability and price for hospitals. *Hospital Risk Management, 14*(10), 129–133.

Centers for Medicare and Medicaid Services. (2003). Hospital conditions of participation: Quality assessment and performance improvement. *Federal Register, 68*(16), 3435–3455.

Classen, D. C., Pestotnik, S. L., Evans, R. S., Lloyd, J. F., & Burke, J. P. (1997). Adverse drug events in hospitalized patients: Excess length of stay, extra costs and attributable mortality. *Journal of the American Medical Association, 277*(4), 301–306.

Clinton, W. J. (1998). *Establishment of the QuIC Task Force.* Retrieved January 13, 2003, from www.quic.gov/about/clintonestablish.htm

Cohen, M. R. (Ed.) (1999). *Medication errors.* Washington, DC: American Pharmaceutical Association.

Committee on Quality of Health Care in America. (2001a). *Crossing the quality chasm: A new health system for the 21st century.* Washington, DC: National Academy Press.

Committee on Quality of Health Care in America. (2001b). *Envisioning the national health care quality report.* Washington, DC: National Academy Press.

Cook, R., & Woods, D. (1994). Operating at the sharp end: The complexity of human error. In M. S. Bogner (Ed.), *Human error in medicine.* Hillsdale, NJ: Lawrence Erlbaum Associates.

Cook, R. I., Woods, D. D., & Miller, C. (1998). *Tale of two stories: Contrasting views of patient safety.* National Patient Safety Foundation, Chicago, IL. Retrieved January 10, 2003, from www.npsf.or/exec/tocr.html

Croteau, R. J., & Schyve, P. M. (2000) Proactively error-proofing health care processes. In P. L. Spath (Ed.), *Error reduction in health care.* San Francisco: Jossey-Bass Publishers.

Deming, W. E. (1986). *Out of the crisis.* Cambridge, MA: Massachusetts Institute of Technology.

Department of Veterans Affairs. (2002). *VHA national patient safety improvement handbook.* Retrieved January 12, 2003, from http://www.patientsafety.gov/NCPShb.pdf

Food and Drug Administration (FDA). (n.d.). *Human factors.* Retrieved February 4, 2003, from www.fda.gov/cdrh/humfac/hfbrochure.html#1

Gardner, R. A. (2001). Resolving the process paradox. *Quality Progress, 34*(3), 51.

Gawande, A. A., Studdert, D. M., Oray, E. J., Brennan, T. A., & Zinner, M. J. (2003). Risk factors for retained instruments and sponges after surgery. *New England Journal of Medicine, 348*(3), 228, 229–235.

Gordon, I. (2002). *Medical errors. The scope of the problem.* Retrieved January 15, 2003, from www.tball.org.

Godwin, P. (2002). Simplifying your quality system. *Quality Progress, 35*(3), 43.

Hackel, R., Butt, L., & Banister, G. (1996). How nurses perceive medication errors. *Nursing Management, 27*(1), 31–34.

Hayward, R. A., & Hofer, T. P. (2001). Estimating hospital deaths due to medical errors. *Journal of the American Medical Association, 286*(4), 415–420.

Holmes, W. L. (2003, February 20). Teen's new heart beating on its own: Second surgery completed for girl who received mismatched organs. *Orlando Sentinel.*

Institute of Medicine. (n.d.). *About the Institute of Medicine.* Retrieved January 15, 2003, from www.iom.edu/iom/iomhome.nsf/Pages/About+the+IOM

Institute for Safe Medication Practices (ISMP). (1998). *IV pump set free flow: When is enough enough?* Retrieved January 24, 2003, from www.ismp.org/msaarticles/free-flow.html

Joint Commission on Accreditation of Healthcare Organizations (JCAHO). (1998). *Lessons learned: Wrong site surgery.* Retrieved January 22, 2003, from www.jcaho.org/about+us/news+letters/sentinel+event+alert/sea_6.htm

Joint Commission on Accreditation of Healthcare Organizations (JCAHO). (2000). *Sentinel event policy and procedures.* Retrieved January 22, 2003, from www.jcaho.org/ptsafety_frm.html

Joint Commission on Accreditation of Healthcare Organizations (JCAHO). (2000a). *A framework for conducting root cause analysis.* Retrieved January 22, 2003, from www.jcaho.org/sentinel/sentevnt_frm.html

Joint Commission on Accreditation of Healthcare Organizations (JCAHO). (2000b). *Infusion pumps: Preventing future adverse events.* Retrieved January 12, 2003, from www.jcaho.org/accredited+organizations/patient+safety/npsg/index.htm

Joint Commission on Accreditation of Healthcare Organizations (JCAHO). (2001). *Revisions to Joint Commission standards in support of patient safety and medical/health care efforts.* Retrieved January 22, 2003, from www.jcaho.org/standard/fr_safety.html

Joint Commission on Accreditation of Healthcare Organizations (JCAHO). (2002a). *Sentinel event policy and procedures revised: July 2002.* Retrieved January 12, 2003, from www.jcaho.org/accredited+organizations/hospitals/sentinel+events/se_pp.htm

Joint Commission on Accreditation of Healthcare Organizations (JCAHO). (2002b). *Sentinel Event Statistics—May 7, 2003.* Retrieved May 28, 2003, from www.jcaho.org/accredited+organizations/hospitals/sentinel+events/sentinel+event+statistics.htm

Joint Commission on Accreditation of Healthcare Organizations (JCAHO). (2002c). *The Codman Award Program Overview.* Retrieved January 12, 2003, from www.jcaho.org/accredited+organizations/codman+award/codman_overview.htm

Joint Commission on Accreditation of Healthcare Organizations (JCAHO). (2002d). *2003 national patient safety goals.* Retrieved January 12, 2003, from www.jcaho.org/accredited+organizations/patient+safety/npsg/index.htm

Joint Commission on Accreditation of Healthcare Organizations (JCAHO). (2003). *Weaving the fabric: Strategies for improving our nation's health care.* Retrieved May 8, 2003, from www.jcaho.org/about+us/weaving+the+fabric.pdf

Kohn, L. T., Corrigan, J. M., & Donaldson, M. S. (Eds.). (2000). *To err is human: Building a safer health system.* Washington, DC: National Academy Press.

Leape, L. L. (1994). Error in medicine. *Journal of the American Medical Association, 272*(23), 1851–1857.

Leape, L. L., Brennan, T. A., Laird, N. M., Lawthers, A. G., Localio, A. R., Barnes, B. A., et al. (1991). The nature of adverse events in hospitalized patients: Results from the Harvard Medical Practice Study II. *New England Journal of Medicine, 324*(6), 377–384.

Leapfrog. (2000). *Leapfrog initiatives to drive great leaps in patient safety.* Retrieved January 12, 2003, from www.leapfroggroup.org/safety1.htm.

Lesar, T. S., Briceland L. L., Delcoure K., Parmalee, J. C., Masta-Gornic, V., & Pohl, H. (1990). Medication prescribing errors in a teaching hospital. *Journal of the American Medical Association, 263*(17), 2329–2334.

Marciniak, T. A., Ellerbeck, E. F., Radford, M. J., Kresowik, T. F., Gold, J. A., Krumholz, H. M., et al. (1998). Improving the quality of care for Medicare patients with acute myocardial infarction: Results from the cooperative cardiovascular project. *Journal of the American Medical Association, 279*, 1351–1357.

Merry, M. D., & Brown, J. P. (2002). From a culture of safety to a culture of excellence: The business of health care. *A Journal of Innovative Management Collection.* Salem, NH: Goal/QPC.

National Coordinating Council for Medication Error Reporting and Prevention. (NCCMERP) (2001). *Types of medication errors.* Retrieved January 14, 2003, from www.nccmerp.org/index.htm?http://www.nccmerp.org/sidebar.htm

National Patient Safety Foundation. (NPSF). (2002). *About NPSF.* Retrieved January 12, 2003, from www.npsf.org/html/pressrel/krawisz.html

National Wholesale Druggists' Association. (NWDA). (1998). *Industry profile and healthcare factbook.* Reston, VA: Author.

Pierce, E. C. (1995). *The 34th Rovenstine Lecture: Forty years behind the mask: Safety revisited.* Retrieved January 13, 2003, from www.apsf.org/foundation/rovenstine/rovenstine.html

Pollack, R. (2002). *AHA comment letter of May 20, 2002.* Chicago: American Hospital Association.

Quality Interagency Coordination Task Force. (2000). *QuIC report to the president: Doing what counts for patient safety: Federal actions to reduce medical errors and their impact.* Retrieved January 12, 2003, from www.quic.gov/report/toc.htm

Reason, J. T. (1990). *Human error.* Cambridge: Cambridge University Press.

Reason, J. T. (2001). Understanding adverse events: The human factor. In C. Vincent (Ed.), *Clinical risk management* (pp. 9–30). London: BMJ Books.

Rosekind, M. R., Gander, P. H., Gregory, K. B., Smith, R. M., Miller, D. L., Oyung, R., et al. (1996). Managing fatigue in operational settings 1: Physiological considerations and countermeasures. *Behavioral Medicine, 21*, 157–170.

Ryan, T. J., Antman, E. M., Brooks, N. H., Califf, R. M., Hillis, L. D., Hiratzka, L. F., et al. (1999). ACC/AHA guidelines for the management of patients with acute myocardial infarction: 1999 update. Retrieved January 13, 2003, from www.acc.org/clinical/guidelines and www.americanheart.org

Schneider, P. J., Gift, M. G., Lee, Y., Rothermich, E. A., & Sill, B. E. (1995). Cost of medication related problems at a university hospital. *American Journal of Health-System Pharmacy, 52*, 2415–2418.

Shojania, K., G., Duncan, B. W., McDonald, K. M., & Wachter, R. M. (2001). *Making health care safer: A critical analysis of patient safety practices* (Publication 01-E058). Rockville, MD: Agency for Healthcare Research and Quality.

Siker, E. S. (2001). *ASPF history.* Retrieved January 13, 2003, from www.apsf.org/foundation/history/history.html

Spath, P. L. (2000a). *Error reduction in health care.* San Francisco: Jossey-Bass.

Spath, P. (2000b). *Patient safety improvement guidebook.* Forest Grove, OR: Brown-Spath and Associates.

Thomas, E. J., Studdert, D. M., Burstin, H. R., Orav, E. J., Zeena, T., Williams, E. J., et al. (2000). Incidence and types of adverse events in negligent care in Utah and Colorado. *Medical Care, 38,* 261–271.

Thomas, E. J., Studdert, D. M., Newhouse, J. P., Zbar, B. I., Howard, K. M., Williams, E. J., et al. (1999). Costs of medical injuries in Utah and Colorado. *Inquiry, 36*(3), 255–264.

Turnbull, J. E. (2002). *Process management and systems thinking for patient safety.* The business of health care: A journal of innovative management collection. Salem, NH: Goal/QPC.

U.S. General Accounting Office. (2000). *Adverse drug events: The magnitude of health risk is uncertain because of limited incidence data.* (#HEHS-00-21; B281822). Retrieved January 12, 2003, from www.gao.gov/new.items/he00021.pdf

U.S. Pharmacopoeia Center for the Advancement of Patient Safety. (2002). *Summary of information submitted to MedMARx in the year 2001: A human factors approach to medication errors.* Retrieved January 22, 2003, from www.usp.gov.

Chapter 2

National Patient Safety Initiatives

Susan V. White

OVERVIEW

The Institute of Medicine's (IOM) report, *To Err is Human: Building a Safer Health System*, (Kohn, Corrigan, & Donaldson, 2000) illustrated gaps in the current system with a high volume of medical errors and adverse events. For example, the system gaps include lack of a single national oversight agency for patient safety, and the oversight that does exist is fragmented by clinical area, such as drugs or infections, and by different agencies. There is no unified mechanism to collect data (either voluntary or mandatory) on adverse events, medical errors or aggregate data across multiple health care settings. There are a few voluntary data collection efforts that will be described.

Attempts have been made to make changes via the legislative process as well as through regulations by specific agencies. Since 2000 a number of federal bills have been proposed to advance patient safety, including the most recent *Patient Safety and Quality Improvement Act* (S. 2590), yet none have passed. This chapter summarizes the major federal and national initiatives related to patient safety. These initiatives provide resources, directions, and best practices for different professions and settings. Table

2.1 summarizes the federal and national agencies involved in these patient safety initiatives.

FEDERAL INITIATIVES

The federal government has undertaken a number of patient safety initiatives through its agencies. A mandate was created for these agencies by the President's Advisory Commission on Consumer Protection and Quality in the Health Care Industry in 1998. Through the Commission, the Quality Interagency Task Force (QuIC) was formed and subsequently drafted a report with recommendations for federal agencies that were adopted by President Clinton. As a result, a number of federal agencies have specific priorities and agendas focused on patient safety. Also, the federal Office of Personnel Management (OPM), which contracts for services and benefits for federal employees, has developed criteria to contract only with groups that meet requirements related to patient safety.

Each agency will be described in relation to its specific focus on patient safety. Many of these agencies have broad areas of responsibility and patient safety may be only one aspect.

TABLE 2.1   Summary List of Federal and National Organizations With Patient Safety Initiatives

Federal	National
AHRQ	AHA
CDC	ASHRM
CMS	AONE
DOD	ASHP
FDA	IHI
IOM	ISMP
OPM	JCAHO
QuIC	Leapfrog
NQF	NCCMERP
VA	NCHC
	NPSF
	P4PS

Agency for Health Care Research and Quality (AHRQ)

The AHRQ is the "lead agency charged with supporting research designed to improve the quality of healthcare, reduce its cost, improve patient safety, decrease medical errors, and broaden access to essential services" (AHRQ, n.d.d). The AHRQ, formerly the Agency for Health Care Policy and Research, was reauthorized by the Healthcare Research and Quality Act of 1999, which changed the name and modified its goals and research priorities (AHRQ, n.d.a). This new name was important because it clarified the role of AHRQ as a research agency rather than a policy setting agency. It also ended the agency's responsibility for developing clinical guidelines. AHRQ no longer develops guidelines, but it supports development of guidelines through evidence-based centers, with dissemination through the National Guideline Clearinghouse™. Finally, the Act established AHRQ "as the lead Federal agency on quality of care research, with new responsibility to coordinate all Federal quality improvement efforts and health services research" (AHRQ, n.d.a). AHRQ's research agenda includes over $50 million in initiatives to increase understanding of when and how errors occur to foster a national strategy to improve patient safety.

Under the leadership of Dr. John Eisenberg, the AHRQ developed many public and private partnerships to conduct safety research. AHRQ leads the federal quality effort through its leadership on QuIC. Specific charges to AHRQ include promotion of patient safety and reduction of medical errors. Methods to achieve these goals include partnerships to promote research to reduce medical errors and the reliance on Centers for Education and Research on Therapeutics (CERTs). These centers are to conduct research "to increase awareness of both the uses and risks of new drugs and drug combinations, biological products, and devices, as well as of mechanisms to improve their safe and effective use" (AHRQ, n.d.d).

The contributions of AHRQ have resulted in a broader understanding of what the patient safety problems are and where they occur in the delivery of health care. AHRQ funded research is leading to a rethinking of what does and does not work at the health care systems level. The research priorities for patient safety include:

- Assess effectiveness of methods of collecting/using information to reduce medical errors and their impact
- Clinical informatics to promote patient safety
- Effects of working conditions on patient safety

- Patient safety research dissemination and education
- Provide reports of research findings

Accomplishments of AHRQ as a result of research and dissemination include:

- Funding of a large number of studies
- Developing numerous fact sheets for practitioners and consumers on health care safety, prevention tips, cost issues, working conditions, and 20 tips on preventing medical errors for adults and one for children
- Creating a national center for patient safety
- Developing an online journal called *Web M&M*, which provides case scenarios and commentaries
- Developing a compendium of patient safety practices produced, by a team of editors at the University of California, San Francisco (Shojania, Duncan, McDonald, & Wachter, 2001).

Centers for Disease Control and Prevention (CDC)

The CDC is the national agency that is responsible for developing and applying disease prevention and control methods, supporting environmental health, and health promotion, and providing education activities to improve the health of the people of the United States. It has been doing this since 1946 (CDC, n.d.a). The CDC's vision for the 21st Century is *Healthy People in a Healthy World—Through Prevention*.

The CDC's primary role in patient safety is in the collection and reporting of data on hospital nosocomial infections through the National Nosocomial Infection Surveillance System (NNISS). The CDC has collected this data since 1970 making a major contribution to reducing infections. The CDC's attention on nosocomial infections is to describe the epidemiology of nosocomial infections, monitor antimicrobial resistance trends, and produce nosocomial infection rates for comparison purposes (CDC, n.d.b). The NNISS has been a uniform data collection process with trained infection control personnel using risk-adjusted data providing a standard methodology. Surveillance protocols, targeting inpatients at high risk of infection, were reported and aggregated into the database. The CDC is now moving into a new electronic era with the National Healthcare Safety Network (NHSN) designed as a web-based knowledge system. The NHSN will integrate three patient and healthcare worker surveillance systems to provide performance measurement data that health care organizations will be able to access in order to compare performance. The NHSN will offer a new portal into a system that offers much information about both patients and caregivers in the realm of safety.

The CDC has issued numerous guidelines and recommendations on infection control practices, which are often adopted by health care organizations, but it has no real authority to mandate these practices. Informational resources developed by CDC address issues of needlesticks, blood-borne pathogens, use of vaccines, reporting and controlling infectious and contagious diseases, emerging infections, and antimicrobial resistance. As new problems arise, the CDC develops recommendations such as the cleaning and disinfecting of bronchoscopes and endoscopes. The most recent priority of the CDC has been on instructional materials on bioterrorism for the safe, prompt identification of the agent, treatment of patients, and treatment/protection of healthcare providers (CDC, n.d.a).

Centers for Medicare and Medicaid Services (CMS)

The CMS is the federal agency responsible for managing health care quality for Medicare and Medicaid beneficiaries. CMS was renamed in 2001 to reflect a more service-centered approach. As part of its responsibility to manage the care of Medicare beneficiaries, the CMS contracts with Quality Improvement Organizations (QIOs), through a Scope of Work (SOW). The SOW is the contract that identifies specific quality goals to be achieved and specific clinical conditions to be addressed over the course of the contract. The specific goals are intended to promote the best medical practices associated with targeted clinical condition, prevent or reduce the incidence of these conditions, and prevent related complications.

The quality improvement projects are currently defined for acute care facilities, home health care, nursing homes, and more recently, doctors' offices. Within the projects, best practices based on research have been developed, such as the early administration of aspirin and use of beta blockers for acute myocardial infarction (CMS, n.d.a; CMS, n.d.b). When these practices are not followed, an error of omission has occurred.

The CMS identifies requirements for health care organizations in Conditions of Participation (COP), which are posted in the *Federal Register*. Recent COPs that relate to patient safety were posted in 1999 and 2003. In 1999 the COP focus was on patients' rights, which also included limitations on restraint and seclusion to keep patients safe (*Federal Register*, 1999). In 2003, the COP updated requirements on quality of care, but added a specific focus on indicators related to improved health outcomes and the prevention and reduction of medical errors (*Federal Register*, 2003). Hospital-wide performance improvement efforts must address priorities for improved quality of care and patient safety. The COPs additionally require health care organizations to monitor the effectiveness and safety of services and quality of care. The performance improvement activities must track medical errors and adverse patient events, analyze their causes, and implement preventive actions and mechanisms that include feedback and learning.

Department of Veterans Affairs (VA)

The VA has led the patient safety movement in the areas of culture change, widespread adoption of bar-coded medication administration (BCMA), and nonpunitive reporting. Dr. Jim Bagian has been instrumental in this movement, capitalizing on his experience in both aerospace and medicine. As a result of concerted efforts, the VA National Center for Patient Safety (NCPS) was established as a unified patient safety program with active participation by all VA hospitals. The center focuses on prevention, human factor analysis and research from highly reliable organizations, which spend attention on identifying and eliminating system vulnerabilities (VA, n.d.). The center's Web site offers any user access to a safety handbook, tools for root cause analysis (RCA), and a model for health care failure mode and effects analysis (HFMEA™). The center has developed numerous resources, online newsletters, and educational programs to share their learnings and programs with other health care organizations. Dissemination of findings about patient safety errors is critical so other organizations or providers will not make the same mistake. Sharing information can be achieved by the VA's system-wide communication, publications, or special reports (VA, n.d.).

The VA operates under regulations that are different from most private health care organizations and has immunity not enjoyed by the private sector. This has contributed to the VA's ability to develop a partnership program with the National Aeronautics and Space Administration (NASA) for error reporting. The Patient Safety Reporting System (PSRS), which was formed in May 2000, is a program to define "procedures and responsibilities for reviewing, reporting, tracking and trending patient incidents as well as other safety related events" (PSRS, 2003). The PSRS allows VA medical facility staff to voluntarily report any events or concerns that involve patient safety. The guiding principles for PSRS are (1) voluntary participation, (2) confidentiality protection, and (3) nonpunitive reporting. It is designed, not as a replacement system, but as a complementary external system to the current internal VA reporting system.

NASA has experience since 1976 with the Aviation Safety Reporting System (ASRS) for the Federal Aviation Administration (FAA). ASRS has been praised for "its strict confidentiality procedures, managed reports, database created for the easy retrieval of information, creation of safety products, and distribution of safety information" (ASRS, n.d.). These characteristics were the reasons the VA selected NASA. NASA is an independent, research organization that does not have a regulatory or enforcement role in medical errors. The knowledge and experience with aviation are now being applied to health care. The PSRS analysts remove from reports all personal identifiers such as names, facilities, locations, and other potentially sensitive information to provide anonymity and confidentiality in reporting.

The PSRS events to be reported include: close calls, unexpected events of death, physical or psychological injury of a patient or an employee, lessons learned or safety ideas, and any safety-related event. There are several types of events not protected under 38 USC 5705, and they are therefore not reported to the PSRS. These include the intentional unsafe acts such as: criminal acts, purposefully unsafe acts, alleged or suspected patient abuse, acts related to alcohol/substance abuse, impaired provider, or alleged/suspected abuse (PSRS, 2003).

Food and Drug Administration (FDA)

The FDA's role in patient safety relates to the approval of new drugs for market, focus on device design, anonymous reporting system for medication error, and labeling of blood products. The FDA has had responsibility for approval of drug use, but also drug names. In years past, the agency had not paid as much attention to names and labeling as it has after the IOM report. The current review process requires an investigation of look-alike and sound-alike names, and packaging similarities, to prevent problems before mistakes are made. This increased vigilance on premarketing will reduce errors postmarketing.

The FDA sponsors a voluntary anonymous reporting system for medication errors called MedWatch. This system is designed to educate health care professionals about the importance of adverse events and to learn about specific medication problems. Information from MedWatch is shared with the Institute for Safe Medication Practices (ISMP), which then shares medication error information through newsletters and online bulletins.

With its attention on improving medication safety, the FDA issued a bar code proposal in 2002 to embrace the use of this technology for medication administration (FDA, n.d.; FDA, 2003). Currently most drugs do not come with unit dose bar codes, nor is there a standardized bar code format. The proposal will likely take several years before finalization. In the meantime, several major pharmaceutical companies have made public commitments to provide bar codes on medications. The FDA proposal would require bar coding not only on drugs, but also on blood products. Under this proposal, bar coding would be required on all prescription drug products, on most over-the-counter drugs, and on vaccines. For drugs, the bar code would contain the drug or National Drug Code (NDC) number. For blood, the bar code would include blood and Rh type, the facility that prepared the unit, and codes that can trace the donor, if necessary. The use of bar coding (see chapter 8) can prevent many medication and transfusion errors, primarily at the administration phase. The FDA's bar coding standards are likely to accelerate the adoption of safety-improving information technologies by hospitals and nursing homes. Benefits will be realized by pharmacies from standard codes that will be used by all prescription manufacturers. Drug manufacturers may benefit from uniform standards, rather than dealing with conflicting requirements from different purchasers that add to the cost of adopting bar coding (FDA, 2003).

The FDA has entered the education arena with *Patient Safety News*, a televised series for health care personnel provided on satellite networks aimed at hospitals and other healthcare facilities. The program features information on new drugs, biologics and medical devices, FDA safety notifications, product recalls, and ways to protect patients when using medical products. This last feature supports the FDA's Medical Products Reporting Program, which addresses device design, and the reporting of injuries related to medical devices. The FDA announced a new framework for innovative programs to identify and manage safety problems associated with FDA-regulated medical products more effectively, using modern information technology, partnerships with health care organizations, and more effective communication tools. The FDA has developed new Web-based communication methods to better inform consumers and health care professionals about the risks associated with medical product use. The FDA is working with the National Library of Medicine to set up *The DailyMed*, a new way to distribute up-to-date and comprehensive medication information electronically for use in information systems that support patient care. By making information about FDA-regulated medical products readily available to patients and health care providers, *The DailyMed* will help to reduce medication errors and improve patient safety (FDA, 2002).

MedSun is the FDA's new Internet-based pilot program to collaborate with health care facilities to ensure the safe use of medical products. MedSun provides the FDA with real-time, electronic information about problems clinicians have identified using medical devices. MedSun also uses the safety data collected to provide health care facilities with information that can be used to improve patient safety (FDA, 2002).

The FDA is proposing to amend certain regulations governing the reporting of safety information by the industry for human drugs and biological products. These proposed standards will improve the quality and usefulness of patient safety data submitted to regulatory authorities and also reduce the reporting burden by allowing organizations to use the same definitions and follow one common set of procedures in reporting safety information. The potential benefits of the proposed rule result from the improved scope, timeliness, and quality of reports of actual and potential adverse drug reactions. Postmarketing safety information is critical to managing risk information, to the safe prescribing and use of new drugs, and to reducing the number and duration of avoidable hospitalizations related to adverse drug reactions (FDA, 2003; FDA, n.d.).

Through this sharing of data the FDA is expecting to receive reports of adverse drug reactions (ADR) that might be caused by the drug of interest in order to be better able to generate warnings of new potential safety problems with drugs and biologic products. When warnings are generated, further investigation can then be undertaken to determine whether an ADR is actually related to a drug. Also this includes medication errors that were averted before administration of the product (near misses) and potential medication errors that do not involve a patient but rather, describe information or a complaint about similar product names, packaging, or labeling. Information will be collected on certain reactions that may put the patient at risk and/or require medical or surgical intervention to treat the patient. All serious adverse reactions for blood and blood products will be collected. Finally, the FDA would require information on resistance to antimicrobial drug products (FDA, 2002). The FDA's new tools for identifying and addressing patient safety will supplement the approach to adverse event monitoring with automatic reporting and electronic communications (FDA, 2003; FDA, n.d.).

Connecting for Health is a public-private partnership led by the FDA aimed at improving quality and patient safety through electronic interchange of patient safety information. Participating health care organizations will use clinical data standards and compatible health information systems to share selected patient safety data confidentially. The FDA is participating in a national pilot project in conjunction with the Markle Foundation for this eHealth Initiative to demonstrate the feasibility and the value of electronic interchange of safety data. The pilot involves hospitals, information technology suppliers, and other organizations interested in promoting patient safety and quality. The FDA has also developed a partnership with a managed care organization and the CMS to access quality data that can be used to analyze safety concerns in large patient populations (FDA, 2002).

Institute of Medicine (IOM)

The IOM is an organization associated with the National Academy of Sciences, which was created by the federal government to be an advisor on scientific and technological matters. The IOM is a private, nongovernmental organization and does not receive direct federal funding. Studies undertaken for the government by the Academy are usually funded out of appropriations to federal agencies. The IOM is an independent body, with volunteer experts who author the reports. Each report goes through institutional review with a formal peer review process, so findings and recommendations are evidence-based. The IOM does not have any regulatory authority to implement the findings or recommendations. Any regulations must be proposed through the legislative process. Since it is not a governmental agency, the committee is not obliged to conduct sessions in a public forum. Committees deliberate, come to consensus, and author the IOM reports, but follow strict institutional processes (IOM, n.d.a).

In the realm of quality and patient safety, the IOM's report *To Err is Human: Building a Safer Health System* (Kohn, Corrigan, & Donaldson, 2000) is widely known and made a huge impact in raising public awareness about medical errors and the need to change. However, the IOM has also addressed safety in a number of areas including:

- identifying six goals of patient care in *Crossing the Quality Chasm: A New Health System for the 21st Century* (2001)
- proposing a national quality report in *Envisioning the National Health Care Quality Report* (2001) and leadership for quality in *Leadership*

by Example: Coordinating Government Roles in Improving Health Care Quality (2002)
- identifying 20 priority areas for action in Priority Areas for National Action: Transforming Health Care Quality (2003)
- addressing immunization safety in Immunization Safety Review: Multiple Immunizations and Immune Dysfunction (2002)
- addressing dietary and other supplement safety in Proposed Framework for Evaluating the Safety of Dietary Supplements (2002)
- responding to safety related to bioterrorism in Making the Nation Safer: The Role of Science and Technology in Countering Terrorism (2002)
- protecting research subjects in Responsible Research: A Systems Approach to Protecting Research Participants (2002) (IOM, n.d.b).

Quality Interagency Coordinating Task Force (QuIC)

The Federal Government is the largest purchaser and provider of health care services in the United States (QuIC, 1999), therefore the federal government plays an important role in the quality of health care for Americans. This includes programs such as Medicare, Medicaid, the Federal Employee's Health Benefits Plan (FEHBA) and the networks of hospitals and facilities providing care to the armed forces and veterans. Additionally, the federal government oversees employer based health coverage and ensures competition in the market. The QuIC was established in 1998 to "ensure that all federal agencies involved in purchasing, providing, studying, or regulating health care services are working in a coordinated way toward the common goal of improving quality of care" (QuIC, 1999). When QuIC was formed, two additional councils were created: the Advisory Council for Health Care Quality and the Forum for Health Care Quality Measurement and Reporting, which is now the National Quality Forum (NQF).

The impetus to development of QuIC came from the President's Advisory Commission (1998), which identified the lack of coordination and uniform quality standards in the public and private sectors that are duplicative and burdensome on health care providers. The QuIC was formed to fulfill the Commission's aims to: reduce the underlying causes of illness, injury, and disability; reduce health care errors; ensure appropriate use of health care service; expand research on effectiveness of treatments; address oversupply and undersupply of health care resources; and increase patient participation in their own care (QuIC, 1999).

QuIC is chaired by the Secretary of Health and Human Services (HHS), with the director of the AHRQ as operations chairperson, and consists of the following agencies:

- The Departments of Defense, Veterans Affairs (VA), Labor, and Commerce
- The Office of Personnel Management
- The Office of Management and Budget
- The U.S. Coast Guard
- The Federal Bureau of Prisons
- The National Highway Transportation and Safety Administration
- The Federal Trade Commission.

The following major topics with corresponding work groups were developed (see Table 2.1 for more details):

- Improve patient and consumer information on health care quality
- Identify key opportunities for improving clinical quality
- Improve efforts to measure quality of care
- Develop the health care work force
- Improve information systems
- Reduce hazards in patient care
- Improve safety and quality through value-based purchasing.

The QuIC was created to address broad issues of quality improvement in health care, but the specific problem of medical errors has been a major focus of activity. The QuIC responded to the IOM report *To Err is Human: Building a Safer Health System,* since it included a number of recommendations for federal action. The QuIC's response was summarized in *Doing What Counts for Patient Safety: Federal Actions to Reduce Medical Errors and Their Impact* (QuIC, 1999, n.d.b).

This report describes more than 100 actions that the QuIC and its participating agencies will take regarding patient safety. While the full list of work group topics (QuIC, n.d.c) are listed in Table 2.2, several will be further highlighted because of their focus on patient safety and medical errors.

One work group specifically targets "reducing medical errors" in which QuIC is working with the Institute for Healthcare Improvement (IHI) to test strategies for reducing the medical errors in "high-hazard" health care settings. The high hazard areas match those identified in chapters 1 and

TABLE 2.2 QuIC Workgroups

Workgroup Topic	Agencies	Summary
Patient and Consumer Information	CMS and OPM	This group is addressing critical barriers to effective communication with patients about quality. It will provide an opportunity for federal agencies to learn what is most effective in helping people understand quality issues and how their choices influence the quality of the services they receive. It will also develop a common vocabulary, or set of terms, for federal agencies to use in communicating with patients and consumers about quality.
Improving Quality Measurement	AHRQ and HCFA	The focus of this group will be on developing the "tool box" of quality measures and risk adjustment methods used by federal agencies, particularly those that reflect outcomes of care. The work group is developing an inventory of all of the measures and risk adjustment methods being used by federal agencies, documenting their uses, strengths and weaknesses, and examining how to institute appropriate risk adjustment methods to account for factors outside the control of the delivery system.
Developing the Workforce	DoL and HRSA	This group is determining how to expand and improve the current methods of ensuring the skills of the health care workforce and equipping health care workers to improve the care they deliver. For example, the work group has chosen to begin by improving the credentialling process for federal health care providers. This group is also looking at the relationship between the working conditions and health and safety of health care employees and the quality of care delivered. An expert panel is planned for Fall 1999 to study the issue and develop an agenda for further research.
Key Opportunities for Improving Clinical Quality	DoD and VA	This group has selected diabetes and depression as the first two areas for which it will mount an effort to improve clinical quality of care. For diabetes, the work group is focusing its efforts on having all federal programs agree to use the Diabetes Quality Indicator Project measures of care and then to improve health care provider performance based on these indicators. For depression, the work group is developing an evidence-based guideline to improve the identification and treatment of depressed individuals served by federal health care programs.

(continued)

TABLE 2.2 *(continued)*

Workgroup Topic	Agencies	Summary
Improving Information Systems	DoD and VA	This work group is exploring how its efforts can augment those of federal groups already working to develop a standardized language that will enable computerized comparisons of quality across federal agencies. The work group is also examining the potential uses of telemedicine for helping to improving quality of care, and it is in the process of developing a site for the QuIC on the World Wide Web to share information about what the QuIC is doing.
Reducing Hazards in Patient Safety	AHRQ and VA	This workgroup focuses on reducing hazard in patient care through the coordination of federal efforts to conduct research on patient safety and by piloting safety improvement strategies. Currently, it serves as a clearinghouse for the patient safety measures being implemented by each federal organization. Members currently share information on grant announcements for AHRQ and HRSA and serve as members or liaisons to the HHS Patient Safety Task Force, which seeks to develop a common reporting interface and data structure on end-stage renal disease for all HHS agencies. In addition the group is working to develop a validated Patient Safety Culture Assessment.
Improving Safety and Quality through Value-Based Purchasing	CMS and DoD	This group assists the federal government in enhancing its ability to purchase health care based on quality as well as cost, and to advocate for quality of care on behalf of its constituents. The concept of value-based purchasing is that buyers should hold providers of health care accountable for cost and quality, balancing regulatory approaches with purchasing mechanisms. It focuses on managing the use of the health care system to reduce inappropriate care and to identify and reward the best-performing providers.

QuIC, n.d.c

2 based on the acuity of patients, rapid decision making (tight time constraints and tight coupling), and the complex processes. They include emergency rooms, intensive care units, and on-site rescue operations. QuIC anticipates that some sites will be able to achieve reductions of 25% to 30% in the number of errors within 12 to 15 months (QuIC, n.d.a). The other work group focuses on "reducing hazards in patient safety" and plans to achieve its aim through research on patient safety and piloting safety improvement strategies. The QuIC is serving as a clearinghouse for the patient safety measures being implemented by each federal organization. In addition, development of a validated Patient Safety Culture Assessment tool is underway (QuIC, n.d.a).

NATIONAL INITIATIVES

Partnerships and collaboratives have become common as organizations recognize the need to bring together a variety of experts and resources and to increase dissemination across multiple settings, groups, and healthcare professionals. Many organizations have their own initiatives, but most have created partnerships and collaboratives.

American Hospital Association (AHA)

The AHA provides leadership to the hospital industry in quality and patient safety through quality advisories, tools, and advocacy on potential legislation. One of the first actions after the IOM report by the AHA was posting of medication safety practices and a partnership with the ISMP on distribution of a self-assessment survey on medication practices. After the surveys were aggregated and analyzed, AHA, the Health Research and Educational Trust and the ISMP, with support from The Commonwealth Fund, proceeded with the next phase to develop and pilot test three tools, *Pathways for Medication Safety* (AHA, 2002).

The AHA also partnered with Bridge Medical to distribute the *Beyond Blame* video to all hospitals in its efforts to support a nonpunitive culture related to medical errors (AHA, 2002). *Strategies for Leadership: Hospital Executives and Their Role in Patient Safety* was a tool developed by James B. Conway, chief operations officer at the Dana-Farber Cancer Institute in Boston. This tool was developed specifically for executives' personal use assessing their efforts to develop a culture of safety. It was mailed to all chief executive officers in early March 2001.

Recognizing the importance of leadership and culture change to improve patient safety, the AHA also partnered with the Voluntary Hospitals of America (VHA) to disseminate a tool developed by Dr. Nancy Wilson, called *Strategies for Leadership: An Organizational Approach to Patient Safety*. The tool "provides a systematic method to evaluate current processes and systems and to measure ongoing progress in establishing a safer organization" (AHA, 2002).

Strategies for Leadership: An Invitation for Conversation Workbook was developed collaboratively by the AHA and the IHI. This quality-of-care workbook is a three-part video series, *Strategies for Leadership Video Series*, which was especially designed for hospital trustees on the key issues in improving quality. This series provides a framework to help hospital boards understand their role in quality patient care. The workbook and the first videotape were sent to all AHA members (AHA, 2002).

Providing executive leadership resources is a major role for the AHA and the tool kit *Strategies for Leadership: Evidence-Based Medicine for Effective Patient Care* was developed jointly with the United Healthcare Foundation in 2003. Patient safety requires using evidence-based practice (chapter 5) to reduce errors in planning and provide consistent approaches to health conditions. This tool kit, sent to every AHA hospital, provides assistance to leaders to create the environment to translate research into daily practice (AHA, 2003b).

Having tools to analyze systems and processes for safety issues is necessary for health care practitioners. The introduction of failure mode and effects analysis (FMEA) into healthcare, primarily by the Joint Commission on the Accreditation of Healthcare Organizations (JCAHO), created a learning opportunity for practitioners. The VA developed their own version of HFMEA™ including a video, forms, and instructional materials. Through partnership between VA and AHA, these tools were sent to all hospitals in 2002 (AHA, 2002).

Computerized Physician Order Entry: Costs, Benefits and Challenges was prepared by First Consulting Group in 2003 for AHA and the Federation of American Hospitals to assist hospitals in evaluating this technology for reducing medical errors and adverse events. This technology is expensive and difficult to implement. Many hospitals are now embracing this technology (see chapter 8). This report provided hospital leaders with information on costs, benefits, and challenges as they move forward with technology plans.

The most recent effort by the AHA is *The Quality Initiative: A Public Resource on Hospital Performance*. While this initiative does not specifically focus on medical errors, it addresses patient safety within a larger framework of improving care. This initiative is a joint effort between the AHA, the Association of American Medical Colleges, and the Federation of American Hospitals to help hospitals share useful information about quality to the public. The initiative compares hospital performance in ten measures for acute myocardial infarction, heart failure, and pneumonia. These measures are already used by the JCAHO and CMS so data collection is not overly burdensome. The initial phase is voluntary with hospitals agreeing to post data already collected with accompanying information on a public Web site (AHA, 2003c).

American Organization of Nurse Executives (AONE)

The AONE is an affiliate of the American Hospital Association, representing nearly 4,000 nurse leaders. The organization "provides leadership, professional development, advocacy, and research in order to advance nursing practice and patient care, promote nursing leadership excellence, and shape healthcare public policy" (AONE, n.d.). The AONE is often an active member in supporting the AHA's safety initiatives of "bringing the issue of patient safety to the forefront, and is committed to continued work to improve patient safety" (AONE, 2002a). Participation in patient safety is evident in attendance at the first Annenberg Conference on Patient Safety in 1996, presenting the organization's position, and again in 1997. In 1997, AONE developed a monograph on quality describing the organization's position on quality management, tools and resources, and improvement in quality care, which was presented at the December IHI conference. Focus groups for nurse leaders were held at this conference to gain insight into the changing roles of nurse leaders related to quality improvement. Similar focus groups were held for nurse leaders in partnership with the American Association of Health System Pharmacists (ASHP) to learn more about how nurses and pharmacists could work together to prevent errors and improve quality (AONE, 2002a; *American Journal of Health-System Pharmacy*, 2002).

Nurse leaders have demonstrated concern about the need for culture change from blaming individuals to fixing system defects. This has translated into educational programs in many settings including a session on medication error at the AONE Annual Meeting in collaboration with the

National Patient Safety Foundation (1999). AONE also participated in the Nurse Leader Symposium on Managing the Inherent Risks of Evolving Patient Care Delivery Models and identified issues and solutions to patient safety issues in the changing health care organizations (AONE, 2002a, 2002b).

AONE also participated in the AHA Medication Error Briefing and Media Training by providing nursing's unique perspective on patient safety and the importance of quality improvement. Other actions have included the development of *Talking Points on Patient Safety: Medication Error and a Guide to Action*, collaboration with the American Society for Health System Pharmacists (ASHP) on medication error reduction (1999), and presentation of *End Page in Nursing Management on Medication Error* with steps for nurse managers to get involved in improving patient safety.

The AONE participates in advocacy efforts with regulatory and accreditation agencies. For example, the organization presented testimony at the JCAHO's hearings on restraint and seclusion in 1998 and participated in discussions and policy development on disposable equipment/supplies and latex issues in 1999. In partnership with the AHA, AONE posted the *Quality Advisory on Medical Error* on their Web site and participated in review and comment of the ISMP self assessment tool (AONE, 2002a; AONE, 2002b).

American Society of Health-System Pharmacists (ASHP)

The ASHP is a professional organization for pharmacists with 30,000 members representing pharmacists in hospitals, health maintenance organizations, long-term care facilities, home care, and other components of health care systems. Its patient safety initiatives focus exclusively on medication safety. The ASHP established a Center on Patient Safety in 2000 using advocacy, education and research to foster fail-safe medication use through pharmacists' leadership (ASHP, n.d.). The center helps health care professionals understand why medication errors occur, devises approaches to prevent them, and pursues best practices in health care. The center advocates for effective safety roles for pharmacists in health system, develops tools for medication use, develops partnerships to improve medication use, and performs research to explore issues of medication safety. Partnerships include a variety of groups such as:

- Health care professional organizations
- Consumer groups

- Pharmaceutical manufacturers
- Government agencies
- Drug-related device manufacturers
- Technology industries
- Employers and insurers.

For example, ASHP and nursing organizations, including the American Association of Colleges of Nursing (AACN), the American Association of Colleges of Pharmacy (AACP), the American Nurses Association (ANA), and AONE, partnered to "develop a shared vision of ideal medication distribution and administration in hospitals, including the best utilization of nursing and pharmacy workforces, and recommend approaches to improve medication use in hospitals with an aim toward ensuring patient safety and therapy effectiveness" (AHA, 2003a; ASHP, 2003b).

Other AHSP activities that have an impact on patient safety include the ASHP drug product shortages management resource center. If specific drugs are in short supply then substitutions or alternate forms may increase the potential for a medication error. This center provides information on drug shortages and guidance in drug shortage management. ASHP also has computerized prescriber order entry (CPOE) resource materials posted from the pharmacy perspective that identify implementation issues and considerations.

Since most medications are actually dispensed within the community, the patient's role in taking medications safely is paramount. The ASHP has a consumer education focus with a special Web site to respond to this community need (ASHP, n.d.) (see also chapter 9).

The most recent ASHP initiative is to improve the practice of pharmacy in health systems by 2015, modeled after Healthy People 2010. One goal is that "By 2015, 75% of hospital in-patients discharged with highly complex and high-risk medication regimens will receive discharge medication counseling by a pharmacist" (AHSP, 2003a).

Anesthesia Patient Safety Foundation (APSF)

The purpose of the APSF is to "ensure that no patient shall be harmed by anesthesia" (APSF, n.d.) by fostering investigations to provide a better understanding of preventable anesthetic injuries, encouraging programs that will reduce the number of anesthetic injuries, and promoting communication about the causes and prevention of anesthetic injuries. The APSF is the oldest medical organization dedicated solely to improving the safe care of patients during surgery and anesthesia. It was founded in 1985. Members include anesthesiologists and physicians, nurses and technologists, manufacturers of drugs, equipment, and supplies, insurers, legal professionals, hospital administrators and risk managers, and governmental regulators (APSF, n.dd; APSF, n.d.a).

The IOM report specifically noted the accomplishments of improved patient safety in anesthesia. The APSF has been instrumental in setting standards and guidelines for anesthesia care. Many standards are available on their Web site such as standards for patient monitoring and difficult airway (APSF, n.d.a; APSF, n.d.b; APSF, n.d.c). The APSF and its members have been leaders in the use of anesthesia simulation training, which allows education without risking harm to real patients. The improvement in anesthesia care with reduction of complications and mortalities demonstrates the application of research, standardization, and consistency in practice.

Association for Professionals in Infection Control and Epidemiology (APIC)

The APIC was organized in 1972 to address nosocomial infections through surveillance and control programs. APIC and infection control professionals work closely with the CDC and base their programs on the CDC's guidelines, nosocomial infection surveillance methodology, outbreak investigations, and laboratory studies. Infection control has been recognized as an important aspect of patient care for many years but the primary impetus for formalization came from the JCAHO in the 1960s. The role of infection is evident since over 5% of hospital patients have a hospital-acquired infection. In 2004 the JCAHO's national patient safety goals will include reducing the risk of health care-acquired infections. APIC has developed an active role in the patient safety movement through educational programs and development of resources. Infection control practitioners are key members of a patient safety team in monitoring nosocomial infections, surgical site infections, resistance trends and outbreaks. These professionals are critical to ensure safety goals are in place to reduce risk of infections and minimize patient harm.

Institute for Healthcare Improvement (IHI)

The IHI is a not-for-profit organization "driving the improvement of health by advancing the quality and value of health care" (IHI, n.d.c). The IHI has many initiatives, collaboratives, and resources on improving the quality of patient care. Many of these initiatives focus on patient safety. The IHI has led health care improvement since 1990 including medication error reduction and improvement of prescribing practices. For example, one of the first breakthrough series was on reducing adverse drug events and medication errors from 1996–1997, led by Dr. Lucian Leape (IHI, n.d.). Through additional breakthrough series, IHI teams addressed improvement in the intensive care unit, delays in the emergency department, and clinical conditions such as asthma. Lessons learned from these series are routinely shared in educational forums, publications, and online reports. In medication safety, the IHI has resources to address changes for reducing adverse drug events, changes and strategies for high-hazard drugs, and characteristics of a safe medication process (IHI, n.d.).

In keeping with its philosophy to continually improve, the IHI developed an initiative in partnership with the Robert Wood Johnson Foundation to provide grants to 13 health care organizations to redesign health care for "system redesign and organizational transformation" with new benchmarks for quality and safety. The *Pursuing Perfection: Raising the Bar for Health Care Performance* (Pursuing Perfection) initiative has worked intensively to make system changes using the IOM report, *Crossing the Quality Chasm: A New Health System for the 21st Century* (IHI, n.d.), as a framework. At least four projects focus on safety: adverse drug events (McLeod Regional Medical Center), medication safety project (Hackensack University Medical Center), medication systems (Tallahassee Memorial Healthcare), and transplant safety (Cincinnati Children's Hospital Medical Center). "To pursue perfection, organizations need to discover and apply the latest, most relevant knowledge. The application of medical science will be necessary but not sufficient to accomplish near-perfect care" (IHI, n.d.). Another goal of Pursuing Perfection is to share the learning from this initiative with the world via an electronic Learning Network (IHI, n.d.c).

Another initiative of the IHI is idealized design. The first initiative was the clinical office practice, followed by design of the medication system, the intensive care unit, and patient flow (IHI, n.d.a). Each new initiative is based on the general approach of dramatic and sustained system level changes with new models to improve performance with better outcomes, lower costs and higher satisfaction.

Project IMPACT is an IHI initiative that also addresses improvement. "Project IMPACT is a network of change-oriented health care organizations that are ready to join the improvement movement at a new level of ambition, scale, persistence, and transparency" (IHI, n.d.d). The goals are to impact patient outcomes, assess impact on patient, provider, and staff satisfaction and the bottom line (IHI, n.d.d). Improvement is based on two levels: leadership community and action teams. An IMPACT action team is a front-line, cross-functional group, formed to make dramatic change in a specific domain. The five domains of focus include office practice and outpatient settings, critical care settings, workforce development, flow in acute care, and patient safety (IHI, n.d.d).

One of the most recent efforts of the IHI is an online journal and tracking resource called *Quality Healthcare* which enables health care professionals around the world to collaborate on health care improvement. "Quality-HealthCare.org is a global knowledge environment" with the latest improvement ideas, access to experts, and a tracker tool to monitor progress over time of individual projects (IHI, n.d.b). The journal will focus on different content areas and the first will include patient safety.

Institute for Safe Medication Practices (ISMP)

The ISMP is a nonprofit organization that provides education about adverse drug events (ADE) and their prevention through the *Medication Safety Alert* and other publications, educational programs, and consultation with health care organizations.

A key role of the ISMP is the analysis and dissemination of lessons learned about adverse drug events and medication errors through two mechanisms. The first mechanism is via the FDA. The ISMP is an FDA MedWatch partner and regularly communicates with the FDA to help prevent medication errors. The ISMP encourages reporting of medication errors to the MedWatch Program and also promotes the FDA's initiatives to reduce adverse drug reactions. ISMP reviews all FDA MedWatch reports of medication errors (ISMP, n.d.).

The second mechanism in which ISMP analyzes ADEs and medication errors is through the United States Pharmacopeia (USP) Medication Errors Reporting Program (MERP) program. The USP operates a national system, MERP, in the U.S. The Institute provides an independent review of medication errors that have been voluntarily submitted by practitioners to MERP. The resources of both the USP and the ISMP are utilized to analyze reports and agree on solutions to error problems. Information from the reports may be used by the USP to impact drug standards. All information derived from the MERP is also shared with the FDA and pharmaceutical companies whose products are mentioned in reports. An FDA Medication Error Committee then reviews all reports submitted to the MERP (ISMP, n.d.c)

The ISMP works with numerous healthcare practitioners, organizations, regulatory agencies, professional organizations and the pharmaceutical industry to provide education about adverse drug events and prevention. For example the ISMP and AHA have a strategic partnership in which ISMP provides leadership and technical expertise in AHA's *Prescriptions for Safety* initiative. The AHA initiative is to help hospitals identify potential opportunities for improving medication delivery process. The partnership aims to:

- Share successful practices with every hospital and health system
- Develop for use by hospitals a "medication safety awareness test" that surveys hospitals' current status and future progress on medication error prevention
- Track implementation of the practices for reducing and preventing errors with the hospital and health system field
- Work with national experts to develop a non-punitive model medication error reporting process
- Serve as a clearinghouse of information and resources for the hospital field on medication errors

The ISMP collaborates with the U.S. Pharmaceutical Research and Manufacturer's Association (PhRMA) by serving on their Committee to Reduce Medication Errors, which examines the relationship between parenteral container labeling and medication errors. A report on suggested improvements to assure label clarity was subsequently submitted to the USP and the FDA. The ISMP is also collaborating with PhRMA's Pharmaceutical Trade Mark Group (PTMG) in their efforts to impact trademarks and medication errors. The ISMP actively pursues initiatives on the safe use of medications through improvements in drug distribution, naming, packaging, labeling, and delivery system design. In this effort, the ISMP provides consultation to pharmaceutical companies where safety and clarity of product labeling and packaging may be an issue. The ISMP also communicates with United States Adopted Names (USAN) on issues related to look-alike, or sound-alike drug names (ISMP, n.d.c).

Joint Commission on Accreditation of Healthcare Organizations (JCAHO)

The JCAHO is a nationally recognized accreditation agency for almost 17,000 healthcare organizations in the United States. JCAHO is an independent, not-for-profit organization created in 1951. JCAHO develops standards and evaluates the compliance of health care organizations against these standards through a survey process. The JCAHO has published patient safety standards that accredited organizations, are required to comply with. Prior to the development of specific standards, the JCAHO developed a sentinel event policy (JCAHO, 2002c) with four reporting options. As part of the sentinel event policy, JCAHO requires a root cause analysis (RCA) to be conducted of sentinel events. A RCA is a reactive approach to an event that has already occurred. The JCAHO later required a preventive approach to a high-risk process. In many organizations the FMEA tool has been used for this purpose. To assist organizations in learning from sentinel events that are reported, the JCAHO analyzes patterns and then publishes recommendations in its *Sentinel Event Alerts*. The amount of information and recommendations in the *Alerts* has continued to grow, often making it difficult for organizations to assign resources to multiple projects. The Sentinel Event Advisory Board (JCAHO, 2002a) was established to create a focus on specific patient safety areas. The result was the development of six national patient safety goals, which were to be implemented January 2003 (see chapter 11). As health care organizations implement these six goals, JCAHO continues to evaluate new goals for the future (JCAHO, 2002b).

The *Speak Up* campaign was created by the JCAHO in 2002 to educate patients and consumers about patient safety issues. The campaign identifies key areas that patients should be knowledgeable about and questions they should ask to be informed about and involved in their care (JCAHO, 2003b).

The Leapfrog Group (Leapfrog)

The Leapfrog Group is a voluntary coalition of over 134 public and private organizations that provide health care benefits. Leapfrog was created to reduce preventable medical mistakes by mobilizing employer purchasing power. It enlists large purchasers to apply pressure to the healthcare industry to engage in three major goals designed to improve patient safety. Leapfrog was founded by The Business Roundtable, a national association of Fortune 500 companies that provide health benefits to approximately 33 million Americans and spend more than $56 billion on health care annually (Leapfrog, n.d.a). Leapfrog members agree to specific purchasing principles. These six principles include (1) informing and educating employees, (2) using comparative ratings, (3) using substantial incentives,

(4) focusing on discrete goals in patient safety, (5) holding health plans accountable for Leapfrog implementation, and (6) encouraging support of consultants and brokers (Leapfrog, n.d.a).

The three goals established by Leapfrog include: implementation of computerized physician order entry; evidence-based hospital referral (EHR); and ICU physician staffing (IPS) (see chapter 11). The rationale for these three goals was that implementation of these goals could save up to 58,300 lives per year and prevent 522,000 medication errors (Leapfrog, n.d.b). In spring 2003 Leapfrog changed its voluntary Hospital Patient Safety Survey and recommended safety practices to allow more time for hospitals to adopt CPOE, and it broadened the definition of "intensivist" and included clinical process and outcome measures of quality. Leapfrog has eased some of its recommended practices, which now include:

- providing hospitals partial credit for implementing CPOE
- providing partial credit for hospitals that take intermediate-level risk reduction strategies
- expanding the definition of a physician "certified in Critical Care Medicine" to include physicians with a long history of experience in intensive care medicine
- giving partial credit for hospitals where intensive care practitioners lead multidisciplinary team rounds each day or make admissions and discharge decisions during the weekday (Leapfrog, 2003).

However, some of Leapfrog's standards have changed with new requirements. For instance, in addition to the adult ICUs, hospitals must now staff pediatric ICUs with intensive care practitioners (Leapfrog, 2003).

Leapfrog's initial efforts were focused on seven regions around the country: Atlanta, California, East Tennessee, Michigan, Minnesota, Seattle-Tacoma-Everett, and St. Louis. In April 2002, 12 new regions were announced: Central Florida, Colorado, Dallas-Forth Worth, Kansas City, Missouri, Massachusetts, Memphis, Metro New York, New Jersey, Rochester, Savannah, South Central Wisconsin, and Wichita. Then in April 2003, Leapfrog launched the following three new regions: Hampton Roads, Virginia, Illinois, and Maine (Leapfrog, n.d.c).

National Coordinating Council for Medication Error Reporting and Prevention (NCCMERP)

In 1995, the United States Pharmacopeia led the formation of NCCMERP with numerous national health care organizations to address the interdisciplinary causes of errors and to promote the safe use of medications. NCCMERP is an independent body comprising 24 organizations. Its major activities include: medication error reporting, medication error understanding, and medication error prevention. NCCMERP has issued a variety of recommendations for the management of medications and the reporting and investigation of error. The council plans to promote its recommendations to colleges, schools, state associations of medicine, pharmacy, and nursing; national professional associations; managed care organizations; and third-party payers (NCCMERP, n.d.b).

NCCMERP has also provided two useful tools related to medication safety. First it has defined medication error that could provide a standard definition for researchers, software developers and organizations:

> A medication error is any preventable event that may cause or lead to inappropriate medication use or patient harm while the medication is in the control of the health care professional, patient, or consumer. Such events may be related to professional practice, health care products, procedures, and systems, including prescribing; order communication; product labeling, packaging, and nomenclature; compounding; dispensing; distribution; administration; education; monitoring; and use (NCCMERP, n.d.b).

Second, NCCMERP has developed a taxonomy of medication errors which identifies errors that cause potential harm and actual harm (NCCMERP, n.d.a).

National Coalition on Health Care (NCHC)

The NCHC, which was founded in 1990, is "an alliance of businesses, labor unions, health care providers, consumer groups and religious organizations to work on affordable health care" (NCHC, 2002). It is nonprofit, nonpartisan and comprises 94 organizations, employing or representing approximately 100 million Americans. NCHC is united in its support of five guiding principles: (1) health insurance for all; (2) improved quality of care; (3) cost containment; (4) equitable financing; and (5) simplified administration (NCHC, 2002).

The NCHC and the IHI have created the Accelerating Change Today (ACT) initiative. Patient safety is not the primary mission of this organization but it has produced an important report *Reducing Medical Errors and Improving Patient Safety: Success Stories from the Front Lines of Medicine* (March 2000). The report features health care facilities that are leaders in patient safety and innovation. Two additional reports were published in 2002, *Care in the ICU: Teaming up to Improve Quality* and *Curing the System: Stories of Change in Chronic Care* (NCHC, 2002).

National Patient Safety Foundation (NPSF)

The NPSF is a nonprofit organization founded by the American Medical Association to "improve the safety of patients" (NPSF, 2003). The NPSF is one of the most comprehensive sources on patient safety. The NPSF provides multiple educational programs, seminars and other patient safety events. It has developed a literature summary of over 3,000 books, articles and reports that is updated regularly with the most current research. NPSF coordinates an e-mail discussion forum with over 2,000 people to share information. Its patient safety site contains resources and information, with online fact sheets, brochures, and newsletters. Other resources include information on patient safety officers with job descriptions and a bibliography. There are four Councils of the NPSF to coordinate initiatives: Consumer Council, Purchaser Council, Provider and Health Plan Council, and Research and Quality Improvement Council (NPSF, 2003).

The NPSF has a program to promote research on human and organizational error and prevention of accidents in health care. The NPSF also plans to catalog the current status of patient safety and medical error research in the US (NPSF, n.d.b) to build a foundation on which to base clinical practice.

With a strong focus on consumers, the NPSF has a number of projects addressing patient participation including a Patient and Family Advisory Council (PFAC) with downloadable resources. Through the PFAC, additional input is received regarding medical errors. For example, *Preventing Infections in the Hospital—What You as a Patient Can Do* published in 2002 is a consumer-based brochure. This brochure is designed to provide patients with helpful principles for managing their health care and becoming an active partner in their health care team. The NPSF enlists health care organizations to demonstrate their commitment to patient safety and the *Stand UP for Patient Safety* campaign for hospitals and health systems is an initiative to achieve this (NPSF, n.d.c).

National Quality Forum (NQF)

The NQF is a public private partnership with 173 member organizations representing all sectors of the health care industry, and focusing on improving patient care. The NQF was created in 1999 in response to the President's Advisory Commission on Consumer Protection and Quality in the Health Care Industry (NQF, 2002). NQF was created as one part of an integrated national quality improvement agenda. It "has broad participation from all parts of the health care system, including national, state, regional, and local groups representing consumers, public and private purchasers, employers, health care professionals, provider organizations, health plans, accrediting bodies, labor unions, supporting industries, and organizations involved in health care research or quality improvement" (NQF, 2002). Members include the American Association of Retired Persons (AARP), AFL-CIO, AHA, the American Medical Association, the American Nurses Association, the American Society of Health-System Pharmacists, the Ford Motor Company, and General Motors.

A 19-member board governs the NQF. Although NQF does not have regulatory authority, two federal agencies, the CMS and the AHRQ are on the board with the potential ability to transfer NQF recommendations into requirements. The board has four nonvoting members including the American Medical Accreditation Program (AMAP), JCAHO, the National Committee for Quality Assurance (NCQA), and the IOM (NQF, 2002).

The members have nine improvement projects currently underway including:

- Mammography center quality project
- Cancer project
- Diabetes measures project
- Hospital performance measures project
- Information management/technology summit
- Minority health project
- Never events project
- Nursing home measures project
- Safe practices project (NQF, n.d.).

The two projects related to safety include the "never events" project and the "safe practices" project. In May 2003 NQF issued a new report *Safe Practices for Better Healthcare: A Consensus Report. Safe Practices for Better Healthcare: It's Time to Act* (NQF, n.d.). Thirty best safety practices "that should be universally used in health care settings to reduce the risk of harm resulting from processes, systems, or environments of care" (NQF, n.d.) were published in this report. The report is based on work by researchers at AHRQ's Evidence-based Practice Center at Stanford University/University of California at San Francisco (Shojania, Duncan, McDonald, & Wachter, 2001). This team identified 73 patient safety practices from the literature in which there were varying levels of scientific evidence. The 30 NQF consensus standards were culled from a list of 220 practices based on each practice's specificity, effectiveness, potential benefit, generalizability, and readiness for implementation. This report also identified 27 practices that have great potential for reducing adverse events (see also chapter 11).

Some examples of the 30 patient safety practices in the report include:

- Informing patients that they are likely to fare better if they have certain high-risk, elective surgeries at facilities that have demonstrated superior outcomes
- specifying explicit protocols for hospitals and nursing homes to ensure adequate nurse staffing
- hiring critical care medicine specialists to manage all patients in hospital intensive care units
- making sure hospital pharmacists are more actively involved in the medication use process
- creating a culture of safety in all health care settings (NQF, n.d.)

"By achieving consensus on this set of evidence-based, high-priority safe practices, NQF seeks to stimulate their universal implementation in applicable health care settings and, in turn, achieve substantial improvements in patient safety" (NQF, n.d.).

Partners for Patient Safety (P4PS)

P4PS is a "is a patient-centered initiative to advance the reliability of health care systems worldwide. The mission of P4PS is to initiate focused partnerships and joint ventures with organizations and individuals that share its core values and objectives of achieving a healthcare system that is authentically patient-centered and systems-based" (P4PS, 2003). While many organizations have focused on practitioners and the use of evidence-based practice for patient safety improvement, P4PS is focused on the consumer's role as partner in advancing the safety of the healthcare system" (P4PS, 2003) (see chapter 9). Currently, P4PS is participating in a grant awarded in 2002 by AHRQ to facilitate consumer participation to advance patient safety. The grant monies will fund a workshop to build on actual consumer experiences with the healthcare system to envision partnership roles for patients. The grant is based on the perspective that consumers have a role and a responsibility in ensuring their own safety in the health care system, and other stakeholders have a responsibility to make health care systems more patient-centered and systems-based. Specific goals include:

- Engage stakeholders in the consumer, regulatory, legal, and political arenas
- Experience interactive learning through simulation
- Explore the latest smart designs to reduce adverse events and improve care

P4PS cosponsored conferences on *Patient Safety: Stories of Success 2001*, and *Smart Designs for Patient Safety 2002.* Convening partners included Premier Inc., VHA Inc., and VHA Health Foundation, The conference embodies the P4PS philosophy to articulate ways for consumers to contribute to safety; identify obstacles in the environment that consumers encounter to advance patient safety; identify additional action to be taken; and make recommendations. "Healthcare consumers are the least represented stakeholder group in deliberation on healthcare safety and quality issues, and when we do hear from them it's usually in the roles of adversary or passive victim," according to Martin J. Hatlie, JD, President of P4PS (P4PS, n.d.). "In fact patients, their families and friends often see rips in the safety net the healthcare system doesn't, and have suggestions for improvement the system doesn't capture". The P4PS is ensuring that patients and their families have a voice in patient safety (P4PS, n.d.).

United States Pharmacopeia (USP)

The USP is a private, not-for-profit public service organization that develops standards and disseminates authoritative information for health care professionals, patients, and consumers about medicines and other health care technologies. A key function of the USP for patient safety is the system for managing, reporting, and benchmarking medication errors called MedMarx™. This comprehensive, Internet-accessible, anonymous database is designed to help hospitals and other health care organizations document, track, and prevent medication errors. MedMarx™ helps to improve the standard of patient care, ensure patient safety, and reduce morbidity and mortality due to medication errors. The USP is also an FDA MedWatch partner which collaborates with ISMP for error analysis and promotes changes for improvement (USP, 2003; n.d).

CONCLUSION

Multiple, overlapping resources and initiatives exist related to patient safety at the federal and national levels. Some of the initiatives create regulations or standards that health care organizations must adhere to; others are recommendations only and may be later translated into regulations. The collective goal of these many activities is to improve patient safety.

WEB RESOURCES

Name of Resource/URL	Description
AHRQ Agency for Healthcare Research and Quality www.ahrq.gov	Federal agency providing patient safety grants; resources; online journal
AHA American Hospital Association www.aha.org	National association representing hospitals and leading patient safety actions, especially for executives
AONE American Organization of Nurse Executives www.aone.org	National association representing nurse leaders with active participation in supporting patient safety initiatives
APIC Association of Practitioners in Infection Control www.apic.org	National association representing infection control practitioners focusing on reducing risk of nosocomial infections and monitoring antimicrobial resistance.
ASHP American Society of Health System Pharmacists www.ashp.org www.safemedications.org	National association representing pharmacists focusing on medication safety; includes a consumer Web site

APSF Anesthesia Patient Safety Foundation www.apsf.org	National association providing resources for anesthesia safety
Aviation Safety Reporting System (the PSRS system model) http://asrs.arc.nasa.gov	ASRS system for the aviation industry
CDC Centers for Disease Control and Prevention www.cdc.gov	Federal agency for disease control and prevention; provides current information, guidelines, and recommendations on infection control issues
CMS Centers for Medicare and Medicaid Services www.cms.gov	Federal agency that manages care for Medicare: information about quality improvement projects and conditions of participation
FDA Food and Drug Administration http://www.fda.gov/medwatch	Federal agency that approves drug use and labeling; also has medication error reporting system
IHI Institute for Healthcare Improvement www.ihi.org	National organization with multiple quality and patient initiatives
Institute of Medicine www.national-academies.org	National organization that produces reports on key issues
ISMP Institute for Safe Medication Practices www.ismp.org	National organization that targets medication safety; multiple resources on medication errors and prevention
JCAHO Joint Commission for the Accreditation of Healthcare Organizations www.jcaho.org	National accreditation organization that provides standards, sentinel events statistics, sentinel event alerts, and tools
Leapfrog The Leapfrog Group www.leapfroggroup.org	National organization serving employers with hospital survey; hospital results, and three safety goals
NCCMERP National Coordinating Council for Medication Error Reporting and Prevention www.nccmerp.org	National organization with definition and taxonomy of medication errors

NCHC
National Coalition for Health Care
www.nchc.org

National organization united to make health care affordable; three health care reports online

NPSF
National Patient Safety Foundation
www.npsf.org

National organization with numerous safety resources including library, brochures, education, and other programs

National Quality Forum
www.qualityforum.org

National organization focusing on quality and patient safety recommendations

P4PS
Partners for Patient Safety
www.p4ps.com

National organization focusing on the consumer role in patient safety

QuIC
Quality Interagency Coordinating Council
www.quic.gov

Federal organization coordinating activities of quality and patient safety for federal government

VA
Veterans Administration Patient Safety Initiative
www.patientsafety.gov

Federal organization serving veterans; site includes safety handbook, tools, and definitions

REFERENCES

Agency for Healthcare Research and Quality (AHRQ). (n.d.a). *Agency for healthcare research and quality: Reauthorization fact sheet.* Retrieved May 21, 2003, from www.ahrq.gov/about/ahrqfact.htm

Agency for Healthcare Research and Quality (AHRQ). (n.d.b). *Medical errors & patient safety.* Retrieved May 21, 2003, from www.ahrq.gov/qual/errorsix.htm

Agency for Healthcare Research and Quality (AHRQ). (2003). *National quality forum finds consensus on 30 patient safety practices.* Retrieved May 21, 2003, from www.ahrq.gov/news/press/pr2003/forumpr.htm

Agency for Healthcare Research and Quality (AHRQ). (n.d.c). *Web M&M.* Retrieved May 23, 2003, from www.webmm.ahrq.gov/

Agency for Healthcare Research and Quality (AHRQ). (n.d.d). *What is AHRQ?* Retrieved May 21, 2003, from www.ahrq.gov/about/whatis.htm

American Hospital Association (AHA). (2002). *Tools & resources patient safety.* Retrieved May 23, 2003, from www.hospitalconnect.com/aha/key_issues/patient_safety/resources/index.html#patientsafety

American Hospital Association (AHA). (2003a). *Nurse, pharmacist leaders build shared vision for safe medication use.* Retrieved May 23, 2003, from www.hospitalconnect.

com/ahanews/jsp/display.jsp?dcrpath=AHA/NewsStory_Article/data/ann_030514_ASHPjournal&domain=AHANEWS

American Hospital Association (AHA). (2003b). *Strategies for leadership toolkit*. Retrieved May 31, 2003, from http://www.hospitalconnect.com/aha/key_issues/patient_safety/whatsnew/strategiesforleadership.html

American Hospital Association (AHA). (2003c). *The quality initiative: A public resource on hospital performance*. Retrieved May 23, 2003, from www.hospitalconnect.com/aha/key_issues/patient_safety/advocacy/030502qualinitiate.html

American Journal of Health-System Pharmacy. (2002). Pharmacy-Nursing shared vision for safe medication use in hospitals: Executive session summary. *American Journal of Health-System Pharmacy, 60*, 1046–1052.

American Organization of Nurse Executives (AONE). (n.d.). *About AONE*. Retrieved May 23, 2003, from www.hospitalconnect.com/aone/about/home.html

American Organization of Nurse Executives (AONE). (2002a). *AONE on patient safety*. Retrieved May 23, 2003, from www.hospitalconnect.com/aone/keyissues/patient_safety.html

American Organization of Nurse Executives (AONE). (2002b). *Key issues: Patient safety*. Retrieved May 23, 2003, from www.hospitalconnect.com/aone/keyissues/patient_safety_home.html

American Society of Health System Pharmacists (ASHP). (2003a). *ASHP proposes to significantly improve health-system pharmacy practice by 2015*. Retrieved May 21, 2003, from www.ashp.org/news/ShowArticle.cfm?cfid=4945880&CFToken=12049441&i d=3392

American Society of Health System Pharmacists (ASHP). (2003b). *Pharmacists, nurses meet to improve medication safety in hospitals. National organizations join forces to devise ideal medication administration system*. Retrieved May 22, 2003, from www.ashp.org/news/ShowArticle.cfm?cfid=4945880&CFToken=12049441&id=3396

American Society of Health System Pharmacists (ASHP). (n.d.). *About ASHP*. Retrieved May 24, 2003, from www.ashp.org/aboutashp/ashpmission.cfm?cfid=4945880&CFToken=12049441

Anesthesia Patient Safety Foundation (APSF). (n.d.a). *APSF: Clinical safety net*. Retrieved May 23, 2003, from www.apsf.org/safetynet/safetynet.html

Anesthesia Patient Safety Foundation (APSF). (n.d.b). *Anesthesia Patient Safety Foundation grant program*. Retrieved May 24, 2003, from www.apsf.org/guidelines/guidelines.html

Anesthesia Patient Safety Foundation (APSF). (n.d.c). *APSF. Safety links*. Retrieved May 23, 2003, from www.apsf.org/links/links.html

Anesthesia Patient Safety Foundation (APSF). (n.d.). *Our mission*. Retrieved May 24, 2003, from www.apsf.org/foundation/foundation.html

Authier, P. (2002). *Testimony of the American Organization of Nurse Executives before the work environment for nurses and patient safety committee of the Institute of Medicine*. Retrieved May 21, 2003, from www.hospitalconnect.com/aone/advocacy/iom_testimony20020924.html

Aviation Safety Reporting System. (n.d.). *Aviation safety reporting system*. Retrieved May 23, 2003, from http://asrs.arc.nasa.gov

California HealthCare Foundation. (2001). *Addressing medication errors in hospitals: A practical toolkit.* Retrieved May 23, 2003, from www.chcf.org/topics/view.cfm? itemID=12682.

Centers for Disease Control and Prevention (CDC). (n.d.a). *About CDC.* Retrieved May 21, 2003, from www.cdc.gov/aboutcdc.htm

Centers for Disease Control and Prevention (CDC). (n.d.b). *National nosocomial infections surveillance system.* Retrieved May 24, 2003, from www.cdc.gov/ncidod/hip/ SURVEILL/NNIS.HTM

Centers for Disease Control and Prevention (CDC). (2002). *Feasibility of national surveillance of health-care-associated infections in home-care settings* (Vol. 8, No. 3). Retrieved May 23, 2003, from www.cdc.gov/ncidod/EID/vol8no3/01-0098.htm

Centers for Disease Control and Prevention (CDC). (2002, May). Life after NNIS. Lecture given at the APIC National Conference.

Centers for Medicare and Medicaid Services (CMS). (n.d.a). *CMS/HCFA history.* Retrieved May 21, 2003, from www.cms.gov/about/history/default.asp

Centers for Medicare and Medicaid Services (CMS). (n.d.b). *Introducing CMS.* Retrieved May 21, 2003, from www.cms.gov/about/reorg.asp

Clinton, W. J. (1998). *Establishment of the QuIC task force.* Retrieved May 21, 2003, from www.quic.gov/about/clintonestablish.htm

Federal Register. (1999). *Federal Register Online* (volume 64, number 127, pp. 36069–36089). Retrieved from wais.access.gpo.gov

Federal Register. (2003). *Federal Register Online,* (volume 68, number 16, pp. 3435–3455). Retrieved from wais.access.gpo.gov

Food and Drug Administration (FDA). (2002). *FDA announces new framework for 21st century patient safety programs.* Retrieved May 21, 2003, from www.fda.gov/oc/ initiatives/barcode-sadr/fs-future.html

Food and Drug Administration (FDA). (n.d.). *FDA proposes bar codes on drugs, blood, vaccines.* Retrieved May 21, 2003, from www.accessdata.fda.gov/scripts/cdrh/ cfdocs/psn/transcript.cfm?show=19#6

Food and Drug Administration (FDA). (2003). *FDA proposes drug bar code regulation.* Retrieved May 21, 2003, from www.fda.gov/oc/initiatives/barcode-sadr/fs-barcode.html

Institute for Healthcare Improvement (IHI). (n.d.a). *Idealized design.* Retrieved May 23, 2003, from www.ihi.org/idealized/

Institute for Healthcare Improvement (IHI). (n.d.b). *IHI patient safety resources.* Retrieved May 23, 2003, from www.ihi.org/resources/patientsafety/

Institute for Healthcare Improvement (IHI). (n.d.c). *Pursuing perfection.* Retrieved May 23, 2003, from www.ihi.org/pursuingperfection/

Institute for Healthcare Improvement (IHI). (n.d.d). *What is IMPACT?* Retrieved May 23, 2003, from www.ihi.org/impact/

Institute of Medicine (IOM) (n.d.a). *About the IOM.* Retrieved May 23, 2003, from www.iom.edu/iom/iomhome.nsf/Pages/About+the+IOM

Institute of Medicine (IOM). (n.d.b). *Recent reports.* Retrieved May 23, 2003, from www.iom.edu/iom/iomhome.nsf/Pages/Recently+Released+Reports

Institute for Safe Medical Practices (ISMP). (n.d.a). *About ISMP.* Retrieved May 22, 2003, from www.ismp.org/Pages/about_ismp.html

Institute for Safe Medical Practices (ISMP). (n.d.b). *ISMP medication safety self assessment*. Retrieved May 22, 2003, from www.ismp.org/Survey/

Institute for Safe Medical Practices (ISMP). (n.d.c). *USP-ISMP medical error reporting system (MERP)*. Retrieved May 22, 2003, from www.ismp.org/Pages/mederr_usa.html

Joint Commission for Accreditation of Healthcare Organizations (JCAHO). (2003a). *Facts about the Joint Commission on Accreditation of Healthcare Organizations*. Retrieved May 23, 2003, from www.jcaho.org/about+us/index.htm

Joint Commission for Accreditation of Healthcare Organizations (JCAHO). (2002a). *Facts about the Sentinel Event Advisory Group*. Retrieved May 23, 2003, from www.jcaho.org/accredited+organizations/hospitals/sentinel+events/se_advisory.htm

Joint Commission for Accreditation of Healthcare Organizations (JCAHO). (2002b). *Facts about the Speak Up program*. Retrieved May 23, 2003, from www.jcaho.org/accredited+organizations/speak+up/facts+about+the+speak+up+program.htm

Joint Commission for Accreditation of Healthcare Organizations (JCAHO). (2002c). *Sentinel event policy and procedures*. Retrieved May 23, 2003, from www.jcaho.org/accredited+organizations/hospitals/sentinel+events/se_pp.htm

Joint Commission for Accreditation of Healthcare Organizations (JCAHO). (2003b). *2003 national patient safety goals*. Retrieved May 23, 2003, from www.jcaho.org/accredited+organizations/hospitals/standards/npsg_03.htm

Kohn, L. T., Corrigan, J. M., & Donaldson, M. S. (Eds.). (2000). *To err is human. Building a safer health system*. Washington, DC: National Academy Press.

The Leapfrog Group. (n.d.a). *About us*. Retrieved May 24, 2003, from www.leapfroggroup.org/about.htm

The Leapfrog Group (n.d.b). *Leapfrog initiatives to drive great leaps in patient safety*. Retrieved May 24, 2003, from www.leapfroggroup.org/safety1.htm

The Leapfrog Group. (n.d.c). *Patient safety*. Retrieved May 24, 2003, from www.leapfroggroup.org/safety.htm

The Leapfrog Group. (2003). *NEW survey version online*. Retrieved May 22, 2003, from https://leapfrog.medstat.com/new.html

National Coalition on Health Care (NCHC). (2002). *National Coalition on Health Care provides hospitals with two reports*. Retrieved May 23, 2003, from www.nchc.org

National Coordinating Council for Medication Error Reporting and Prevention (NCCMERP). (n.d.a). *About medication errors*. Retrieved May 23, 2003, from www.nccmerp.org/index.htm?http://www.nccmerp.org/sidebar.htm

National Coordinating Council for Medication Error Reporting and Prevention (NCCMERP). (n.d.b). *About NCCMERP*. Retrieved May 23, 2003, from www.nccmerp.org/index.htm?http://www.nccmerp.org/sidebar.htm

National Patient Safety Foundation (NPSF). (2003). *About the foundation*. Retrieved May 23, 2003, from www.npsf.org/html/about_npsf.html NPSF

National Patient Safety Foundation (NPSF). (n.d.a). *Impact of staffing shortages on patient safety*. Retrieved May 23, 2003, from www.npsf.org/html/staffshortage.html

National Patient Safety Foundation (NPSF). (n.d.b). *Patient safety resources*. Retrieved May 23, 2003, from www.npsf.org/html/resources.html

National Patient Safety Foundation (NPSF). (n.d.c). *Stand up for patient safety*. Retrieved May 24, 2003, from www.npsf.org/html/StandUp/standup.html

National Quality Forum (NQF). (n.d.). National Quality Forum. *Current activities and consensus reports*. Retrieved May 23, 2003, from www.qualityforum.org/news/qfacrnew2.htm

National Quality Forum (NQF) (2002). *About the National Quality Forum*. Retrieved May 23, 2003, from www.qualityforum.org/about/home.htm

National Quality Measures Clearinghouse™ (2003). *National Quality Measures Clearinghouse™*. Retrieved May 23, 2003, from www.qualitymeasures.ahrq.gov/

Partners for Patient Safety (P4PS). (n.d.). *About P4PS*. Retrieved May 23, 2003, from www.p4ps.org/frame.html

Partners for Patient Safety (P4PS). (2003). *News and events*. Retrieved May 23, 2003, from www.p4ps.org/frame.html

Patient Safety Reporting System (PSRP). (2003). *Patient safety reporting system*. Retrieved May 24, 2003, from http://psrs.arc.nasa.gov/

President's Advisory Commission on Consumer Protection and Quality in the Health Care Industry. (1998). Retrieved May 23, 2003, from www.hcqualitycommission.gov/final/stablis

Quality Interagency Coordinating Council (QuIC). (1999). *About QuIC*. Retrieved May 23, 2003, from www.quic.gov/about/index.htm

Quality Interagency Coordinating Council (QuIC). (2002). *About the National Quality Forum*. Retrieved May 23, 2003, from www.qualityforum.org/about/home.htm

Quality Interagency Coordinating Council (QuIC). (n.d.a). *Improving safety and quality through valued based purchasing*. Retrieved May 24, 2003, from www.quic.gov/safety/charter.htm

Quality Interagency Coordinating Council (QuIC). (n.d.b). *Reducing hazards in patient care workgroup overview*. Retrieved May 23, 2003, from www.quic.gov/hazards/charter.htm

Quality Interagency Coordinating Council (QuIC). (n.d.c). *Workgroups*. Retrieved May 23, 2003, from www.quic.gov/workgroups/index.htm

Shojania, K. G., Duncan, B. W., McDonald, K. M., & Wachter, R. M. (2001). *Making health care safer: A critical analysis of patient safety practices* (Publication 01-E058). Rockville, MD: Agency for Healthcare Research and Quality.

United States Pharmacopeia (USP). (2003). *About USP*. Retrieved May 23, 2003, from www.usp.org/frameset.htm?http://www.usp.org/body.htm

United States Pharmacopeia (USP). (n.d.). *Medication error reporting program*. Retrieved May 23, 2003, from www.usp.org/reporting/merform.htm

Veterans Affairs (VA). (2002). *Healthcare failure mode and effects analysis course materials*. Retrieved May 23, 2003, from www.patientsafety.gov/HFMEA.html

Veterans Affairs. (2001). *National patient safety improvement handbook*. Retrieved May 23, 2003, from www.patientsafety.gov/NCPShb.pdf

Veterans Affairs. (2002). *Root cause analysis*. Retrieved May 24, 2003, from www.patientsafety.gov/tools.html

Veterans Affairs. (n.d.). *VA National Center for Patient Safety*. Retrieved May 23, 2003, from www.patientsafety.gov

Part **II**

Putting Patient Safety Into Practice

Chapter **3**

Improving Patient Safety Using Quality Tools and Techniques

Susan V. White

INTRODUCTION

In chapter 1 an overview of medical errors was presented, including types of errors, characteristics of error-prone processes, and traits of humans that may contribute to errors. This chapter applies an understanding of errors, error-prone situations, and a comprehensive approach to create an organized method of assessing each of the six areas in the comprehensive approach cited in chapter 1. The focus is on improving patient safety and reducing the risk of errors with the ultimate goal to reduce harm to patients.

UNDERSTANDING SYSTEMS AND PROCESSES

First, a description of systems and processes is provided since they are the foundation for much of the work performed in health care organizations. Systemic failures and process failures are often the cause of undesirable outcomes in patient care. Next, a model for clinical care improvement will be described with the specific dimension of patient safety addressed. This chapter describes the improvement model with specific tools, general concepts that can be applied across multiple areas, applications using our

87

comprehensive approach, and finally specific applications common to many nurses.

PROCESS AND OUTCOME MEASURES

A system is an integrated set of processes designed to achieve specific outcomes (Figure 3.1). A system consists of inputs and outputs with the "work" accomplished by throughput. The throughput may involve a number of different processes and subprocesses. Each process is a series of steps to achieve specific action. The only way to know if the correct outcome has been achieved is to measure. There are several key points within a process cycle that must be measured. The process itself is measured by "in-process" measures and the outcome of the process is measured as "end-process" measures. There are several reasons this distinction in types of measures is important.

If only the final outcome of the system were measured then we would not know how the desired outcome was achieved. There would not be a way of ensuring a repeatable, systematic process to achieve the same outcome, especially if it is good. If the outcome is not what was intended, then we would not know how to change the process to achieve a different outcome. We would not know key process aspects such as the costs to achieve the outcome; the amount of time to achieve the outcome; the amount and type of resources required to achieve the outcome; the level of safety of

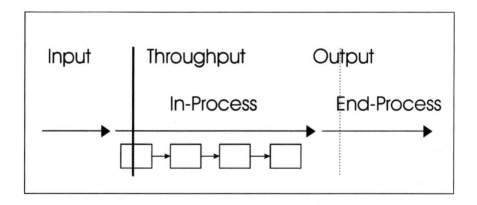

FIGURE 3.1   Systems and outcomes.

the process; or the level of satisfaction of the patient, family, and staff with the process. Now you see the types of process measures that we might consider and the importance of distinguishing process and outcome measures.

Having in-process measures provide a constant, up-to-date picture of what is taking place during the process. The end-process measure provides a picture of the outcome of each process (or subprocess) and provides an opportunity for correction before the final outcome. A review of a few process examples will illustrate this concept. In the medication delivery process there are many subprocesses such as (1) the ordering process, (2) the dispensing process, (3) the administration process, and (4) the monitoring process. Now consider only the administration process, which is primarily performed by nurses. The end-process measure of medication administration is the administration of the correct medication, to the correct patient, by the correct route, at the correct time, and in the correct form and dose. The in-process measures to monitor this might include verification of the medication label against the patient's chart and identification band, drug name in generic and brand form, dosage, route for administration, and purpose of the medication. Another measure might be the identification of the patient using two identifiers, as well as active identification rather than passively checking identification bands. And still another measure might be the time of arrival of the medication to the unit from the pharmacy to ensure timely administration.

In summary, systems and processes are important in the delivery of healthcare. Performance must be measured at different points in the process (in-process and end-process). Understanding characteristics of systems, processes and people that may contribute to errors is critical to redesigning systems of safe care.

USE OF PDSA CYCLES AND IMPROVEMENT PROCESS

Our next step is to identify an improvement model for quality and safety. The most widely used model for improvement across industries, not just healthcare, is the Plan–Do–Study–Act (PDSA) model (Langley, Nolan, Nolan, Norman, & Provost, 1996) (Figure 3.2). This model includes a number of steps and is often called different names within an organization or a name coined for a specific health care organization. The steps are generally the same, so if your organization is using a different name for this model, you will likely find similar steps. Before applying the PDSA model, there

What are we trying to accomplish?

How will we know that a change is an improvement?

What change can we make that will result in an improvement?

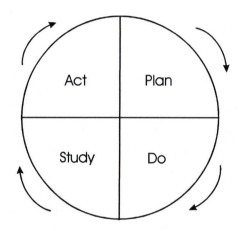

FIGURE 3.2   Performance improvement model.

Langley, Nolan, Nolan, Norman, & Provost, 1996. *The improvement guide.* San Francisco: Jossey-Bass. Used with permission of John Wiley & Sons, Inc.

are three questions to guide its l: (1) "What are we trying to accomplish? (2) How will we know that a change is an improvement? (3) What change(s) can we make that will result in improvement?" (Langley, Nolan, Nolan, Norman, & Provost, 1996, p. 10).

These three questions may seem simple on the surface, but each one is critical to the success of the improvement project. The first question, "What are we trying to accomplish?" will create a clear focus for the team with a desired outcome. Answering this question will guide the improvement project and keep all team members working toward the same goal. It is essential that the aim be specific or the scope of the improvement project will be too large and without clear direction. Once the aim has been established, the team will then know when the project has been completed and if the desired outcome was achieved. There are tools and techniques that will be described later in this chapter that are useful for this step of idea generation.

The second question, "How will we know that a change is an improvement?" requires the identification of measures to determine improvement has taken place. While all improvement involves change, not all changes are improvements, so measures of success are critical to identify actual improvement (Langley, Nolan, Nolan, Norman, & Provost, 1996). In-process and end-process measures should be considered depending on the improvement project. There are sample measures specifically related to patient safety initiatives found in a variety of resources. For example the Institute for Safe Medication Practices (ISMP), the Institute for Healthcare Improvement (IHI), and others have developed breakthrough collabora-tives for organizations to demonstrate improvement in medication safety, intensive care, and delays in emergency care. Additional models are also recognized by the NPSF and the ISMP through various awards. The Agency for Healthcare Research and Quality (AHRQ) has developed a specific list of patient safety indicators, as has the National Quality Forum (NQF). And multiple state collaboratives such as those reported by the Massachusetts Coalition (www.mhalink.org), Minnesota (www.mnpatientsafety.org), Vir-ginia (www.vipcs.org), and California (http://quality.chcf.org) provide ad-ditional examples and resources. These models provide organizations with tested practices as they embark on projects to use these best practices for patient safety improvement (Findlay, 2000; IHI, n.d.; NPSF, 2002).

Measurements should focus on the few critical aspects of the process rather than providing excessive work for data capture and information glut. While measurement should include error rates, one should measure positive outcomes as well. Here are sample measures for medication deliv-ery to illustrate different types of measures: (1) the medication error rate in which medication was administered to the wrong patient, which presents a negative outcome measure, (2) the rate at which a "trigger" or "marker" of an adverse drug event occurs, such as administration of protamine; this identifies potential preventable adverse events (adverse event with anticoagulation), and (3) the percentage of first doses of antibiotics admin-istered within two hours of order; this represents a positive process measure in patient care since early administration of antibiotics can improve recov-ery time and shorten length of stay.

In order to have comparative data, look for standard definitions where possible such as the National Coordinating Council for Medication Error Reporting and Prevention (NCCMERP) (2001) definitions of medication error, the Institute of Medicine (IOM) definition of adverse event (Kohn, Corrigan, & Donaldson, 2000) or the Centers for Disease Control's (CDC, n.d.) definition of nosocomial infections for the national nosocomial infection surveillance system (See Glossary of Terms).

The ISMP (1998) recommends that organizations not compare or benchmark medication error rates for several reasons. The true incidence of medication errors varies, depending on the controls applied for identifying and reporting errors. One cannot assess the quality and safety of the medication process by simply comparing error rates. Currently, there is no single standardized process among health care organizations for identifying and reporting errors. Since many medication errors cause no harm to patients, they are often not reported, yet organizations depend on voluntary reports to determine medication error rates. A high error rate may indicate either unsafe medication practices or an organizational culture that promotes error reporting. Conversely, a low error rate may suggest either successful error prevention strategies or a punitive culture that inhibits error reporting. Although not meaningful, health care organizations have embraced the practice of comparing medication error rates for years.

The definition of a medication error may not be consistent among organizations or even between individual practitioners in the same organization. Organizations focus undue attention on maintaining a low error rate, giving the errors, rather than their correction, misguided importance. Low error rates can result in a false sense of security. Benchmarking for the medication use process can be effective only if a system of objective measurement is used to identify best practices. The ISMP urges organizations to place less emphasis on error rates based on voluntary reporting programs and encourages error reporting to identify and remedy problems, not to provide statistics for comparison (ISMP, 1998).

While different tools or techniques may be useful to evaluate whether improvement has taken place, the statistical process control chart is often used to determine change in performance over time including type of variation and maintenance of the improvement.

The last question, "What change(s) can we make that will result in improvement?" will require a plan to test the change. The team determines what improvement change is to be tested, which now moves into using the PDSA model.

The Plan phase identifies the specific change or test to be implemented. In the Plan phase, the specific components of who, what, when, and where are outlined. The Do phase is the actual implementation of the plan. To implement improvement projects, organizations often select a change concept and then brainstorm specific ways to apply the concept. A complete list of 70 change concepts is found in *The Improvement Guide* (Langley, Nolan, Nolan, Norman, & Provost, 1996, p. 295), but the nine major change categories include:

- Eliminate waste
- Improve work flow
- Optimize inventory
- Change the work environment
- Enhance the producer/customer relationship
- Manage time
- Manage variation
- Design systems to avoid mistakes
- Focus on product or service

In the Do phase, the team will document any problems and begin to analyze the findings. The Study phase is a complete analysis and summary of what was learned during the implementation.

Finally, the Act phase determines what changes are to be made based on the analysis. The cycle is then repeated for continuous improvement. One of the most difficult tasks of an improvement project is to sustain the change over time. An implementation project is fairly structured from start to finish, but strategies are needed to make it easy to continue practicing the new change and hard to revert back to the old routine. An organization may have many teams conducting PDSA cycles on different topics with improvement gains from each cycle so periodic monitoring is necessary for maintaining the changes and continuing improvement.

While continuous performance or quality improvement is the right thing to do for patients, it is also a requirement of many regulatory and accreditation bodies. Both the Joint Commission on Accreditation of Healthcare Organizations (JCAHO) (2002) and the National Committee on Quality Assurance (NCQA) (2002) have standards that require organizations to have systems and processes in place to assess, implement and evaluate care for continuous improvement. Additionally, the JCAHO established specific safety standards and national patient safety goals (2002d). Most state agencies that regulate health care agencies require quality monitoring programs. The federal Centers for Medicare and Medicaid Services (CMS) have long had requirements for quality programs, and in 2003 issued new conditions of participation that require a quality program including aspects of patient safety and reducing medical errors (CMS, 2003).

GETTING STARTED ON THE RIGHT PROJECT

While most organizations have performance improvement programs in place there are varying degrees of implementation of safety initiatives. Many organizations that have encountered a significant sentinel event, such as one of the celebrity cases described in chapter 1, have embarked on leading the way and providing exemplars of safety practice (Findlay, 2000). Other organizations are only meeting the basic requirements of the JCAHO, the CMS and/or state regulations. Recognizing that there is a wide range of experiences in patient safety initiatives, this chapter provides guidance that should be tailored to individual organization needs.

Organizations frequently want to know where to get started, which projects to implement, and the order of implementation. Every organization must begin where it is appropriate based on the level of leadership support, resources available, existing problems, key strategies, and major types of patients and care associated with these patients. The key steps to improving safety using quality management tools and techniques are identified in Table 3.1.

TABLE 3.1 Key Steps to Improving Safety Using Quality Management Tools

Step 1	Ensure leadership support and commitment for patient safety initiative
Step 2	Assess priority and feasibility of patient safety initiative based on risk, resources, leadership support, and organizational strategies
Step 3	Identify the aim of the initiative and include the topic, process, or problem for improvement (have a good rationale for the topic)
Step 4	Convene an interdisciplinary team of content and process experts with all key disciplines as participants (involve all of the right people and have a champion for the change)
Step 5	Utilize tools and techniques to analyze processes, best practices, research, and consensus-based evidence for the desired change
Step 6	Develop the change to be implemented
Step 7	Identify the measure(s) to know that the change has resulted in improvement
Step 8	Educate staff on the desired change
Step 9	Implement and test the change via redesigned processes
Step 10	Collect, analyze, and evaluate data on the redesigned process
Step 11	Make additional changes based on findings and disseminate to all areas
Step 12	Report and display results to reward staff on improvements
Step 13	Continue to monitor performance that the change is sustained
Step 14	Compare performance internally and externally

For example, a rehabilitation hospital, a behavioral health facility and a pediatric hospital will have different plans even though they may use many of the same safety concepts. Organizations should align their performance improvement plans and safety initiatives with regulations and other requirements. The organization should implement initiatives that are important to the organization but also meet standards for the JCAHO, the state, and the CMS to reduce unnecessary work. In most cases the initiatives selected will focus on core processes, high-risk processes, high-risk patients, high-risk medications, or high-risk actions. The level of risk is based on the consequences of injury or harm to patients. Managing high-risk patients and processes will significantly impact morbidity and mortality. Examples of high-risk processes include:

Core processes:	Admission, transfer, discharge
High-risk processes:	Medication delivery, surgery
High-risk patients:	Patients with reduced renal function, patients who are immunocompromised, neonates, patients in critical care units
High-risk medications:	Heparin, insulin, chemotherapy, opiates
High-risk actions:	Blood transfusions, applying restraints, extracorporeal circulation.

PRINCIPLES TO REDUCE MEDICAL ERRORS

The next section will present key concepts to reduce the risk of medical errors. These concepts can be applied across all areas of the comprehensive patient safety approach presented in chapter 1 that includes (1) structure (Table 3.2), (2) environment (Table 3.3), (3) equipment/technology (Table 3.4), (4) processes (Table 3.5), (5) people (Table 3.6), and (6) leadership/culture (Table 3.7). Related patient safety principles will be briefly described.

Simplify

The first concept of simplification is designed to overcome complexity, whether the complexity is in a process, equipment functioning, or policies and procedures. Each additional step in a process has a statistical chance for an error to occur or for the right action to be made so simplification

TABLE 3.2   Structure Assessment

a. Policies and Procedures	b. Facilities	c. Supplies
Policy assessment	Physical assessment	Limit number of brands of same products
Implementation of recommendations such as CDC, FDA, ISMP and others	Safety rounds	Users to review and trial use of products
	Use established checklist for current and future design	Standardize location of supplies and room layout
	Use FMEA on design	Assess access and distribution of supplies so the right item is available when needed
	Engage a wide representation of stakeholders on design	
	Design around vulnerable populations	
	Provide accessible information systems at point of service	
	Provide sufficient handwashing facilities	
	Assess signage and warnings (e.g,. to MRI)	
	Assess standardization and location for electrical outlets, emergency outlets, and gas outlets	

or reduction in the number of steps in a process will increase the statistical odds of reducing risk of error (Langley, Nolan, Nolan, Norman, & Provost, 1996; Merry & Brown, 2002; Turnbull, 2002). For instance, medication delivery often encompasses a large number of steps, so reducing the number of steps can reduce the medication errors.

Standardization

The next concept is standardization to overcome inconsistency. Inconsistent or variable input occurs with patients and all of the people who work

TABLE 3.3 Environment

a. Lighting	b. Surfaces	c. Temperature	d. Noise	e. Space	f. Design	g. Functionality	h. Ergonomics
Assess visibility for staff	Assess floor types for slippage	Assess temperature for staff comfort	Monitor decibel levels and excess noise	Assess access to patient by staff and by others	Assess visibility of patients while ensuring privacy	Assess grab bars in rooms and bathrooms. Assess location of other items that are often "grabbed"	Assess location, portability, weight of computers
Assess visibility for patients	Assess floor types for mitigation of injury during falls (e.g., floor mats)	Assess temperature for patient homeostasis	Reduce noise of phones, pagers, overhead paging	Assess access to equipment, supplies	Assess entrance and exits	Evaluate breakaway bars in mental health units	Assess portability and weight of other equipment
Add auto lighting or night lights for bathroom		Assess temperature of foods and fluids	Assess alarm levels and distinctive tones	Assess ability of patient to move freely in room when ambulating	Monitor walking distance for patients and staff	Assess corridor railing	Assess repetitive motion activities for staff

(continued)

TABLE 3.3 (continued)

a. Lighting	b. Surfaces	c. Temperature	d. Noise	e. Space	f. Design	g. Functionality	h. Ergonomics
		Assess temperature of equipment (e.g., cooling blanket)	Consider music, white noise to reduce stress	Assess ability to move and not contaminate	Assess access to proper outlets	Assess call systems for use by all patients	
		Assess temperature of hot water in sinks and special hot water dispensers		Assess elevator space for transport	Conduct safety rounds with a team	Assess transport mechanisms (e.g., dumb-waiter, pneumatic tube)	
				Assess availability of cues for orientation	Perform physical assessment and do mock-ups of new construction	Assess stability of furniture and beds for tipping or sliding	
					Assess air filtration and positive and negative pressure	Assess walking distances to key areas (especially for those with limitations or at risk for falls)	

TABLE 3.4 Equipment/Technology

a. Design features	b. Functionality	c. Safety features	d. Override features	e. Default modes	f. Instructions/labels	g. Alarms
Assess ease of use	Assess effectiveness of the equipment to achieve its purpose	Assess visibility of on/off	Assess if override features exist	Assess if default mode is the safest mode	Assess visibility, clarity of instructions for use	Assess audibility
Assess intuitiveness and features of design so that there is no need to explain how something is to be used (especially with minimal training)	Assess "lag time" to start up equipment prior to use	Assess preventive maintenance schedule	Assess circumstances under which an override can be used	Assess if default mode must be identified or is pre-programmed	Assess any special warnings and their visibility	Assess distinctiveness from other alarms and noises

(continued)

TABLE 3.4 *(continued)*

a. Design features	b. Functionality	c. Safety features	d. Override features	e. Default modes	f. Instructions/ labels	g. Alarms
Assess input on design by key types of users	Assess accuracy and calibration methods	Assess "poke-yoke"—the ability to use only correct item and connectors (e.g., interchangeability of syringes into multiple ports; pin indexing on gases)	Assess staff training on features			Assess mechanism to ensure alarms are active
Are controls visual and tactile						Assess preventive maintenance schedule for equipment alarms
Assess reliability of item						
Assess durability of item and ability to be cleaned, sterilized						

TABLE 3.5   Processes

a. Design	b. High-risk features	c. Cycle time	d. Efficiency	e. Effectiveness
Assess ideal and actual process for gaps	Assess complexity of process and ways to simplify (number of steps, sequencing, and decision choices)	Assess time intervals for each step "in process" and for "end process"	Assess number of handoffs in a process and determine ways to reduce	Assess process for desired outcome results
Conduct FMEA on high-risk processes to design out failures	Assess level of variable input for standardization and methods to reduce variation	Monitor cycle time for delays	Assess number of same items of different brands and limit	Assess contingency plans when outcome does not result
Assess redundancies and back-up systems to reduce error	Assess use of human intervention and reduce reliance on memory with checklists, protocols, and automated alerts	Assess impact of delays in cycle time on delivery of care and safety issues (e.g., delay in diagnostic reports)	Assess for redundancies that create a safety check without increased documentation or rework	Assess feedback loops that ensure desired outcome was attained
Assess access to information and ensure availability (e.g., drug information)	Assess common errors and apply constraints, and forcing functions to error-proof the process		Assess processes for ability to synchronize steps. Assess parallel and sequential steps	
Assess barriers and bottlenecks and design steps to remove	Eliminate look-alike and sound-alike products and differentiate products and medications		Assess "read back" or "call back" methods to ensure accuracy of activities	

(continued)

TABLE 3.5 *(continued)*

a. Design	b. High-risk features	c. Cycle time	d. Efficiency	e. Effectiveness
	Reduce reliance on memory by adding check-lists, proto-cols, and automated re-minders			
	Increase access to information at the point of care (e.g., drug information)			
	Reduce number of handoffs per step			

within the organization. Standardization will increase the likelihood of steps in a process being performed correctly each time. Standardization should be implemented based on the best-known practices. While standardization is critical, it should be combined with customization so that individual patient characteristics and unique organization factors are addressed. While standardization of processes creates visible patient safety results, standardization in other areas such as room layout or supplies can also improve staff efficiency and safety, especially when traveler, per diem, or other floating staff is used.

Constraints and Forcing Functions

Constraints to limit the wrong action and the use of forcing functions to make the wrong action impossible can be used for processes as well as with equipment and technology. A common example is the interchangeability of syringes for oral use, intravenous use, or intramuscular use. The use of syringes designated strictly for oral use will "force" the nurse to administer the medication correctly. In health care there are few applications of con-

TABLE 3.6 People

a. Attitude	b. Physical health	c. Mental health	d. Human factors	e. Cognitive factors	f. Education	g. Communication
Managers assess staff attitude and general morale	Assess work stressors and ways to reduce	Assess work stressors and ways to reduce	Reduce reliance on memory using checklists and reminders	Assess processes and reduce reliance on memory with checklists, protocols, and automated reminders	Assess use of best practices and practice guidelines; implement	Assess policies on verbal orders and reduce reliance on oral communication of orders. Use read-back for verbal order
	Assess work patterns for fatigue and sleep deprivation and strategies to minimize	Educate staff about EPA programs to assist staff	Reduce reliance on vigilance with work design and supporting equipment and technology		Assess access to information such as drug resources, policies and procedures, research and best practices	Assess policies on ordering and reduce risks posed by illegibility and abbreviations by placing limits on abbreviations, and using CPOE and bar coding

(continued)

TABLE 3.6 (*continued*)

a. Attitude	b. Physical health	c. Mental health	d. Human factors	e. Cognitive factors	f. Education	g. Communication
	Assess "outbreaks" such as flu and adjust work schedules	Educate staff about intervention projects to assist staff	Limit cognitive bias with tight process control			Assess team processes and walking rounds involving patients
			Reduce distractions and interruptions			
			Ensure methods of clear direct communication and reduce illegibility in documentation			
			Provide resources and tools that will aid staff when "working memory" is overloaded			

TABLE 3.7 Leadership/Culture

a. Philosophy	b. Communication	c. Reporting	d. Staffing	e. Teams	f. Hierarchy
Assess policy on safety and error reporting	Assess policies on communication channels for both operational and medical staff	Assess policy on safety and error reporting (e.g., non-punitive with rewards for reporting)	Assess staffing patterns to meet patient population	Assess team structure for membership, goals and activities (e.g., MedTeams and Crew Resource Management approaches)	Assess ability to move against the higher authority without penalty
Assess leadership knowledge and attitudes about safety and medical errors	Reduce communication handouts to increase direct communication	Assess ease of reporting (e.g. hotline, online report)	Assess fatigue and performance concerns especially on 12-hour shifts, double shifts, and night shifts	Assess team responsibilities for identifying and reporting safety issues	Assess "stop" or "hold the line" procedures when safety issue encountered
		Assess impact to staff on reporting errors	Assess rest times between shifts	Assess team communication methods such as "readback"	Assess "challenges" to action without punishment

(continued)

TABLE 3.7 *(continued)*

a. Philosophy	b. Communication	c. Reporting	d. Staffing	e. Teams	f. Hierarchy
		Assess lessons learned by reenactments, story telling, or videos	Assess strategies that minimize sleepiness and fatigue (e.g., caffeine, chewing)	Assess team training on RCA and FMEA	
		Display improvements in reports	Assess job activities to maintain vigilance (e.g., watching monitors for long periods without break)		
		Conduct RCA of sentinel events and FMEA of high-risk processes	Assess work hours and shift scheduling, including direction of shift rotation		

straints and forcing functions, but these yield untapped opportunities to promote patient safety.

Reduce Reliance on Memory and Vigilance

To address memory lapses of humans there are several concepts that will reduce reliance on memory and reduce error risk. Checklists, protocols, and algorithms are useful tools to readily provide all critical items in a single location for a particular process so that nurses do not have to remember or perform research each time they encounter a particular process, condition, or disease (see chapter 4). Another way to reduce reliance on memory is to use timers, automatic reminders, or other alerts that an action is due. The use of alerts in other systems, such as pharmacy, will remind the practitioner to check lab values before administration of certain medications, identify food-drug and drug-drug interactions, and flag contraindications. With over 17,000 medications on the market the use of technology to notify caregivers of critical alerts is a necessity.

Another human capacity issue, besides memory, is our attention span and ability to attend to certain number of items at one time. Reducing reliance on vigilance can also reduce risk of errors. For example, the use of clinical monitoring equipment allows nurses to perform multiple care activities while "allowing" pulse oximetry, cardiac monitoring, and infusion devices to provide the vigilance of noting abnormalities in oxygen saturation, rhythm, and completion of an infusion through alerts and alarms.

Cognitive bias or seeing what we expect is another human capacity limitation. The elimination of look-alike and sound-alike products can reduce errors and has been widely reported by the ISMP with many medications and also in the JCAHO (2001c) *Sentinel Event Alert* such as Axert and Antivert; Zyvox and Zovirax; Taxotere and Taxol.

Access to information is critical for patient safety and this means all patient care information, such as allergies, history, and medications. It also means access to resources such as medication resources, communicable diseases information, and other reference texts. Errors are still reported in which patients receive medications to which they have allergies; medications are given because staff do not know about interactions; and wrongsite surgery occurs because imaging studies are not available. Lack of information about other episodes of care across the health care continuum compromises patient safety. Access to information about care provided in different settings averts errors by preventing duplication of tests or medications. With few exceptions, electronic records that can be accessed in all settings for patient care are rare. Usual transfer of information requires a reliable patient to accurately report to each caregiver in each setting.

Communication and Training

Complex communication, miscommunication, or lack of communication plays an important role in medical errors. Direct communication with few handoffs will increase the reliability of communication with each transmission. Direct communication among all levels of caregivers will reduce errors associated with communication passed from higher levels of authority through multiple levels in a hierarchy. Limitation of verbal orders to written communication will reduce errors associated with language, dialects, and other factors that may create misunderstanding.

Training and education of staff is a key concept in all aspects of health care to ensure staff understands processes of care delivery and how to perform safely. A factor that contributes to risk of errors is the tendency to use past solutions to problems. If a new health care provider or "novice" does not have a large repertoire of past experiences and knowledge, then he/she is more likely to make a mistake in unfamiliar settings. The expert health care provider has more knowledge, experience and skills on which to draw and is an important resource in education and role modeling for other staff.

Teams are essential to address all perspectives of care delivery and training teams to function effectively is needed. Teams provide multiple perspectives of an issue or problem and generate many possible solutions. Teams can increase the efficiency and effectiveness of processes by reducing unnecessary work and providing safety checks or redundancies to reduce errors.

Ensure Leadership Commitment and Nonpunitive Culture

Leadership commitment and support of a philosophy of safety and nonpunitive culture is necessary for initiatives to be supported and resources provided. The culture will enable—by rewarding, or limit—by punishment, the reporting of errors. Driving out fear of reporting will reinforce a nonpunitive culture and support actual and potential error reporting. By having a database of reported errors, the organization will have many problems that can be corrected. This information can be used prospectively to design out failure modes. The next concept is that leaders must increase feedback to staff about errors, performance, and corrective action.

Additional concepts include adjusting work schedules to reduce fatigue, sleep disruptions, and stress. Environmental adjustments include reducing distractions, interruptions, and noises to make it easier and safer for staff to perform patient care.

The patient safety concepts presented in this chapter often rely on individual human actions, which are the weakest change concepts. Leveraging for the greatest patient safety impact will involve the use of technology and automation in addition to changing individual actions. Since technology is not available for all processes, or for all organizations, these concepts can be used to improve patient safety now. Technology will be discussed further in chapter 8.

TOOLS AND TECHNIQUES TO MANAGE AND IMPROVE DECISION MAKING RELATED TO PATIENT SAFETY

There are many tools that can be used in performance improvement, depending on what needs to be accomplished. These tools and techniques are basic for health care quality improvement activities. A complete reference on tools can be found in one of the reference books (Brassard & Ritter, 1994; Carey & Lloyd, 1995; Tague, 1995). The most commonly used tools and techniques that will be presented include: brainstorming, cause and effect diagrams, flow diagrams, force field analysis, histograms, pareto chart, scatter diagram, run chart, control chart, failure mode and effects analysis, and root cause analysis.

Brainstorming

Brainstorming is a technique to generate multiple ideas on any subject or problem over a short time period so it is an efficient way to be creative. Brainstorming can be used when a broad range of ideas is needed and when participation of the entire team is desired. The first step is to clearly identify the topic to be addressed with all members in agreement on the topic. Then ideas are generated. Brainstorming can be structured with a group so that each member suggests an idea in ordered sequence until all ideas are exhausted. It is more often unstructured where any member calls out ideas. During the idea generation step, ideas are recorded without discussion, critique, or evaluation of the idea. All team members should be encouraged to participate and build on ideas. In this case, more is better. When all ideas are exhausted then review for clarity and discard duplicates. There are variations of brainstorming, such as brainwriting, if verbal discussions might limit full team participation. Brainwriting is written, instead of oral, with ideas generated on paper.

Nominal group technique provides a way for all members of a group to have an equal voice in coming to consensus on prioritizing the ideas or problems generated by brainstorming. The first step is to take the list of ideas or problems generated and eliminate duplications and clarify the exact meaning of each item. Distinguish each idea by a letter such as A, B, C, and so on. Then, each team member ranks the idea with a number system, such as 1 is least important and 5 is most important. Combine the rankings of all team members for each idea and total the points to create a final ranking. This tool allows all of the team members to participate equally and rank the ideas based on team prioritization. The ideas should be worked on in the order of their ranking.

Cause and Effect Diagrams

Cause and effect diagrams (Figure 3.3) are also called fish bone diagrams and Ishikawa diagrams. This tool is used for analysis and to discover root causes. The format allows one to identify and graphically display all of the possible causes of a problem or condition. It helps teams organize multiple factors to focus attention where needed. Brainstorming is a good first step to use with cause and effect diagrams in thinking broadly about a particular problem. The cause and effect diagram then provides a technique to sort causes into major categories such as people, processes or methods, materials, and machinery or equipment. These are categories often used as a starting point but they should not be a limiting factor if other categories are more appropriate. The first step is for all of the team members to identify and agree on the problem, which is then written in a box. Next, diagram the fish bone frame with major categories per "bone." Continue to add additional bones as causes are identified. When the team runs out of ideas, review the diagram for completeness.

Flow/Process Diagram

A flow diagram (Figure 3.4) is used to analyze steps in a process. It is a graphic picture of the steps in sequential order using symbols to indicate

Major Uses:
Identify causes
Analyze causes

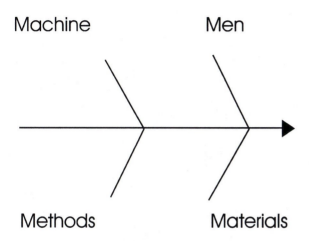

Machine   Men

Methods   Materials

FIGURE 3.3   Cause and effect diagram (Fishbone or Ishikawa).

the type of step (decision point, report, or activity) and arrows to show direction of flow. The major inputs to the process should be identified as well as the final output. This will help determine the scope of the process with starting and stopping points. Again, brainstorming may be a good place to begin by identifying the activities and decisions of a particular process. Then, diagram the process with the steps in the order in which they occur. Diagramming a process must involve those staff members most closely involved in performing the process. The process diagram can be analyzed for how work is really performed, the complexity of steps, the output of each step, and where gaps occur. This analysis can then be used to improve the process.

Force Field Analysis

Force field analysis (Figure 3.5) is used to identify driving and restraining forces for a desired change. This tool is helpful to determine if a planned

Major Uses:
Analyze processes and problems
Identify root causes
Consider alternatives or changes
Design solutions or controls

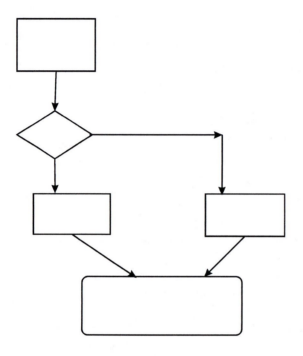

FIGURE 3.4   Flow/process.

change can succeed or what actions need to be taken to reduce restraining forces. Brainstorming may be useful in identifying the driving and restraining forces so that the team has an accurate assessment of the issues facing implementation. First, be clear about what the desired change is. Then identify all of the driving forces that will support the change and clarify the opposition to the change. To make the analysis useful, the team should prioritize the important driving forces that can be strengthened to

Major Uses:
Identify opposing aspects of change
Analyze problems and plan strategies

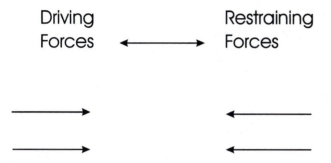

FIGURE 3.5   Force field analysis.

ensure success of the change while simultaneously discussing ways to diminish or eliminate restraining forces.

Histogram/Bar Graph

A histogram (Figure 3.6) is similar to a bar graph. It is a graphic display of data collected over a period of time (using an X and a Y axis). Data are collected and organized into a frequency table with a histogram drawn from the table. The histogram summarizes data that would be difficult to interpret in tabular form, by showing measures of central tendency, range and distribution of data, variation, shape of data, and centering.

Pareto Chart

A pareto chart (Figure 3.7) is used to help identify the most significant problem or cause in a process and helps prioritize areas for action to the critical few, or to those areas with the greatest potential for improvement. Data are displayed in a bar graph format but presented in descending order.

Major Uses:
Collect and analyze data
Identify root causes
Check performance

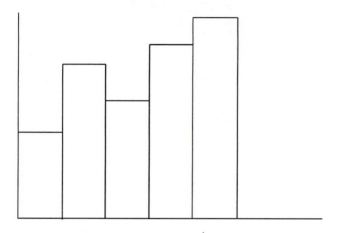

FIGURE 3.6   Histogram (bar graph).

Then a percentage is calculated for each category with cumulative values posted. This type of display often indicates that 20% of sources cause 80% of problems, known as the 80/20 rule (Brassard & Ritter, 1994).

Scatter Diagram

Data can be displayed in many different formats. The format selected should pictorially present the data in a way that will make it easy for the reader to understand the process. A scatter diagram (Figure 3.8) displays data to demonstrate relationships. Data of paired samples are collected and plotted on an X and a Y axis. Data may appear visually to demonstrate a relationship, but statistical tests must be applied to determine the strength of the relationship. One example in which this tool may be useful in assessing relationships is the JCAHO staffing effectiveness standards. An organization may plot specific clinical indicators with staffing to assess relationships and then determine improvement areas.

Major Uses:
Analyze causes
Analyze and sort categories
Prioritize
Identify root causes
Check performance

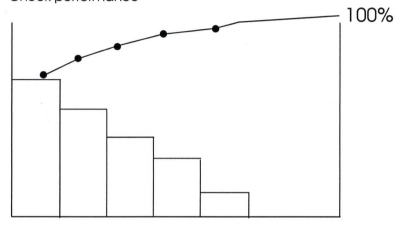

FIGURE 3.7   Pareto chart.

Run Chart

An alternative data display is a run chart (Figure 3.9). It is a display of actual data points over time to monitor performance of a process. The analysis of the run chart will help identify trends or patterns that the organization may want to address.

Statistical Process Control Chart

Statistical process control charts (Figure 3.10) are similar to run charts with data points displayed over time. There are many types of control charts and the use of the correct chart is dependent on whether attribute data (also called discrete or count data) or variable data (also called continuous data) are measured. There are several resources that provide detailed discussions of the different charts and how to select the proper one

Major Uses:
Collect data and analyze causes
Identify root causes
Identify relationships

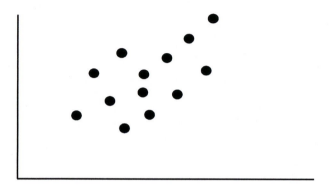

FIGURE 3.8   Scatter diagram.

Major Uses:
Collect data and analyze performance
Monitor performance over time

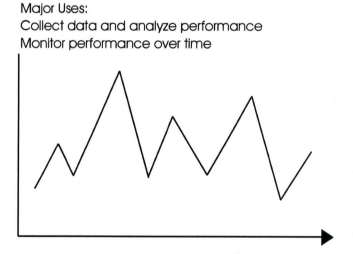

Time

FIGURE 3.9   Run chart.

Major Uses:

Collect data and
  analyze performance
Monitor performance
  over time

Identify root causes
Determine process stability
Identify causes of variation

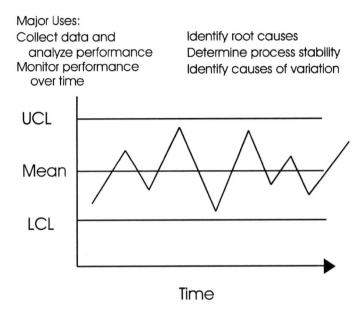

FIGURE 3.10   Control chart.

Control Chart

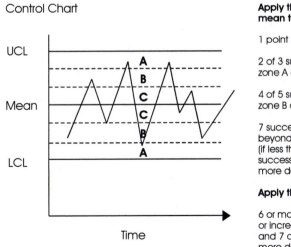

Time

FIGURE 3.11   Control chart.

Apply these rules to each side of the mean to identify special cause:

1 point is outside the 3 sigma limit

2 of 3 successive points are in zone A or beyond

4 of 5 successive points are in zone B or beyond

7 successive points are in zone C or beyond on one side of the mean (if less than 20 data points) and 8 successive points (if you have 20 or more data points)

Apply this rule to the entire chart:

6 or more points in a row are decreasing or increasing (if 20 or less data points) and 7 or more points (if you have 21 or more data points)

(Carey & Lloyd, 1995; Carey, 2003; Brassard & Ritter, 1994). Generally the steps to create a control chart are: select the process to be analyzed; determine the sampling method; identify the data type (attribute or variable data); identify the type of control chart (there are seven chart types); calculate the mean, upper control limit which is three sigma (UCL) and the lower control limit which is three sigma (LCL); and plot the data points. Specific rules have been developed to determine process stability and variation. The rules will help distinguish special cause from common cause variation. The control chart will help determine if the process is stable or out of control, but the team must determine what action needs to be taken to either improve the entire process or to address specific problems.

Failure Mode and Effects Analysis (FMEA)

FMEA (Figure 3.12) is a preventive approach to design out failures and opportunities for error. FMEA can be used for processes as well as equipment. The traditional techniques for FMEA have come from industrial models and require adaptation to health care. The Veterans Affairs (VA) National Center for Patient Safety has created HFMEA™ specifically for health care. There are six main steps to HFMEA™: (1) define a topic and process to be studied; (2) convene an interdisciplinary team with content and process experts; (3) develop a flow diagram of the process with consecutive numbering of each step and lettering of all subprocesses; (4) list all possible failure modes of each subprocess including the severity and probability of the failure mode and then number these failure modes (brainstorming may be helpful to identify failure modes); (5) after analyzing the failure modes determine the action for each failure mode to eliminate, control, or accept; and (6) identify the corresponding outcome measure to test the redesigned process. The use of a flow diagram and worksheets will facilitate FMEA. Tracking processes, sub-processes, and failure modes accurately with a numbering and lettering system will organize the work and ensure that action to eliminate failure modes is performed at the correct step (VA National Center for Patient Safety, n.d.). The JCAHO standards require analysis of high-risk processes to reduce risk for error and FMEA has been commonly used to comply with this standard (JCAHO, 2002a).

Major Uses:
Identify failures in processes or equipment
Analyze processes
Redesign processes

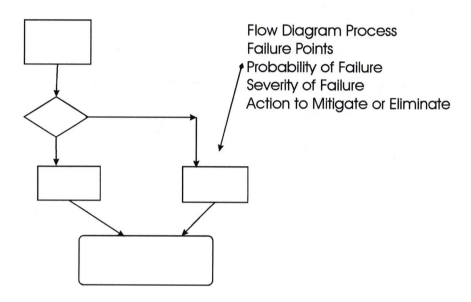

Flow Diagram Process
Failure Points
Probability of Failure
Severity of Failure
Action to Mitigate or Eliminate

FIGURE 3.12   Failure mode and effects analysis.

Root Cause Analysis (RCA)

RCA (Figure 3.13) is a tool to analyze a major error or sentinel event and identify prevention strategies. This tool gained popularity in health care when JCAHO required RCA in the investigation of a sentinel event (JCAHO, 2000b). The JCAHO has specifically defined criteria for a RCA to be thorough and credible to fulfill the standard (JCAHO, 2000b). This type of analysis or similar corrective action plan is often required with mandatory error reporting systems as well.

The purpose of RCA is to find out "what happened, why did it happen, what do you do to prevent it from happening again" (VA National Center

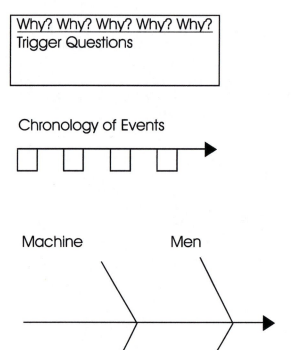

Major Uses:
Analyze serious error or event
Identify root causes
Correct causes

Why? Why? Why? Why? Why?
Trigger Questions

Chronology of Events

Machine   Men

Methods   Materials

FIGURE 3.13   Root cause analysis.

for Patient Safety, n.d.). While RCA implies a single root cause, rarely is this the case. More often there are many contributory causes with several being primary. As contributory causes are identified the goal should always be to determine ways to prevent recurrence. One simple rule is to ask "why" five times. Each "why" question should prompt a more detailed analysis of systems and processes that contributed to the event.

TABLE 3.8   General Patient Care Safety Practices

Separate patients with same or similar names
Use two identifiers for patient identification
Use active method for patient identification
Use simulation models for training
Assess culture of safety
Conduct safety rounds
Conduct team training

IHI, n.d.; JCAHO, 2002b; Turnbull, 2002

The RCA should include an interdisciplinary team and involve those most familiar with the situation. Brainstorming, flow diagram, and cause and effect diagrams are useful since an RCA may involve multiple systems. The different systems that should be analyzed include:

- human factors—communications and information management systems
- human factors—training
- human factors—fatigue/scheduling
- environment factors
- equipment factors
- rules, policies, procedures
- leadership systems and culture
  (VA National Center for Patient Safety, n.d.; JCAHO, 2000b).

After the analysis, indicate the planned action, implementation date, responsible persons, and measure of effectiveness. Improvements to reduce risk should then be implemented in all areas where applicable, not just where the event occurred.

EXAMPLES OF SAFETY ACTIONS IN PATIENT CARE PROCESSES

Common examples of actions that can be taken to improve safety in a variety of clinical areas are summarized in Tables 3.2 to 3.8. These examples are based on concepts and learnings from multiple sources. The concepts and learnings have been identified from analysis of errors; research on best practices; expert consensus, and understanding of error causation (Cohen, 1999; JCAHO, 1998a; JCAHO, 1998b; JCAHO, 1999a; JCAHO, 1999b; JCAHO, 1999c; JCAHO, 2000a; JCAHO, 2001a; JCAHO, 2001b; JCAHO, 2001c; JCAHO, 2001d; JCAHO, 2001e; JCAHO, 2002; JCAHO, 2003; Reason, 1990; Shojania, Duncan, McDonald, & Wachter, 2001). Practice examples are provided on the following topics: general patient care (Table 3.8), medications (Table 3.9), surgery (Table 3.10), falls (Table 3.11), blood transfusions (Table 3.12), restraints (Table 3.13), and nosocomial infections (Table 3.14). Additional discussion about specific patient populations will be presented in later chapters. For example, falls will be further addressed with geriatric populations, and restraints will be addressed with behavioral health.

Many practice examples identify technology, such as CPOE, electronic medical records, bar coding, and robotics. Since organizations are in various stages of implementation of technology solutions, a variety of other practices that are less dependent on technology, are provided. In the future, technology solutions will eliminate "paper solutions." For example, working with individual physicians on legibility of writing will likely result in inconsistent results but using CPOE virtually eliminates legibility issues for all physicians and eliminates many recommendations related to abbreviations which result in error primarily due to legibility and paper forms.

Training individual nurses on the five rights is much less effective than a bar coding system that will readily identify any mismatch in the five rights, and is not subject to distraction, memory lapses, or knowledge/skill issues. Therefore, these practice examples should be considered dynamic as new processes, technology, and skills are implemented. Unfortunately, many of the technology solutions will take years for implementation and strategies that can be applied now should be used to create safer systems and reduce the risk of errors.

CONCLUSION

The use of the performance improvement model (PDSA), various performance improvements, key principles, and specific health care applications will help create safer health care systems. This chapter has built on understanding errors, presented a comprehensive approach regarding the many factors which contribute to errors, and provided tools and strategies for improvement. Those organizations that tend to be more successful in this process are often termed "high reliability organizations" (HRO) and there

TABLE 3.9   Medication Patient Care Safety Practices

Purchasing	Reduce/eliminate look-alike, sound-alike packaging of products
	Limit formulary options in number of equivalent therapeutic and generic products
	Limit formulary options in number of drug concentrations and volumes
	Require approval for unusual drugs or doses
	Reduce floor stock options, including high-hazard drugs
Ordering	Have essential patient information available
	Have drug references available
	Document allergies in conspicuous way
	Standardize MAR, including times of administration
	Special protocols for high-risk drugs (e.g., heparin and insulin)
	Develop protocols to limit verbal orders
	Develop protocols for verbal orders
	Develop protocols for automatic consultations (e.g., Vancomycin)
	Avoid multiple protocols for same drug
	Include all elements in med order
	Use only metric system
	Develop list of accepted abbreviations, acronyms, and abbreviations not allowed
	Order by dose not volume
	Use dosing charts and formulas (for pediatrics, geriatrics, renal failure, etc.)
	Develop alerts for certain meds that require lab results (e.g., insulin and glucose, or heparin and INR)
	Develop alerts on dosage ranges
	Develop policy on legibility of orders and clarification method
	Use preprinted orders for legibility and limitations on certain types of orders
	Require approval of certain high-hazard drugs by senior physician when ordered by residents and interns
	Standardize method of communicating orders
	Use CPOE
Dispensing	Have drug references available
	Develop patient profile with all necessary information
	Have access to other patient information such as labs (e.g., INR, PTT, creatinine)
	Develop process for order clarification
	Develop dispensing area to minimize distractions: make sure it has adequate lighting and air flow, and includes equipment interface considerations

(continued)

TABLE 3.9 *(continued)*

	Use unit dose
	Dispense in ready to administer form
	Pharmacy intravenous admixture
	Do not mix pediatric and adult dose forms on unit
	Have process to double check calculations
	Have a process to double check chemotherapy
	Review floor stock and eliminate concentrated electrolytes
	Consider automated dispensing devices
	Label all medications with all required information in clear readable form (including purpose)
	Develop procedure to notify users of changes in packaging, labeling, concentration, etc.
	Use standard concentrations of high-risk medications
	Separate look-alike or sound-alike medications in dispensing area
	Implement pharmacy system with alerts, warnings
	Have clinical pharmacists on rounds
	Special syringes only for oral meds or epidural meds, etc., to prevent wrong route administration
	Use distinctive labels for hazardous drugs
	Develop process for investigational drugs
	Have pharmacist available 24 hours/day
	Have pharmacist on patient units for consultation and rounds
	Use robotics for dispensing
Admin- istration	Have all patient information readily available
	Have all diagnostic information readily available (e.g., labs)
	Have drug information readily available
	Ensure staff education and competency on medication administration and use of equipment such as infusion devices, PCA pumps
	Have process for order clarification (especially illegible orders)
	Have order verification process
	Administer medication that are fully and correctly labeled
	Create environment to minimize distractions and interruptions
	Use standard MAR and administration time schedule
	Have automatic reminders for timely administration
	Independent double checks on calculations
	Independent double checks on high-risk drugs (e.g., insulin) and drips (e.g., PCA pumps)
	Confirm the five rights prior to administration
	Identify patient with 2 identifiers
	Document immediately after administration
	Never borrow meds from another patient
	Educate patient on medications and usage

TABLE 3.9   *(continued)*

	Have knowledge and access to antidotes to high-hazard drugs
	Standardize and limit number of same type of devices (infusion devices)
	Eliminate infusion devices with free flow
	Use flowsheets for selected drugs (e.g., insulin, heparin)
	Use bar coding for medication administration
Monitoring	Have medication reconciliation process
	Use trigger tools to monitor adverse and potential adverse events
	Monitor medication errors for improvement
	Utilize pharmacy and therapeutics committee for reporting
	Have adverse drug reaction (ADR) hotlines
	Specialty clinics for anticoagulation therapy and monitoring
	Conduct self assessment using tools such as ISMP assessment
	Analyze errors for system redesign
	Create nonpunitive culture to encourage error reporting
	Conduct team reviews of errors
	Display error data for feedback and improvement
	Educate staff on problems and solutions
	Benchmark for best medication safety practices

Legend: MAR = medication administration record, PCA = patient-controlled analgesia.
Cohen, 1999; Florida Hospital Association, 2001; Findlay, 2000; JCAHO 1999b; JCAHO, JCAHO, 2001c; JCAHO, 2001d; JCAHO, 2001e; JCAHO, 2002b

are certain characteristics of these organizations that can be used as a model. HROs recognize that health care is a high-risk industry and no longer deny that a safety problem exists. These organizations have applied key lessons from other industries and provide for voluntary reporting and discussion of errors and near misses. Reward, not punishment, for reporting is the cultural norm.

HROs realize that process control will minimize opportunities for errors, and so they have rules, procedures, and training. System and process vulnerabilities are identified and corrected with prompt feedback. Interdisciplinary teams allow all members to participate in patient safety improvement (see chapter 11).

Health care is a complex industry with information overload and expectations for perfect performance 24 hours a day, 7 days a week, 365 days a year. Humans are not perfect so quality management tools are needed to help identify and mitigate errors, control risks, and reduce harm (Turnbull, 2002; White, 2002).

TABLE 3.10 **Surgery Patient Care Practices**

Preoperative	Surgeon to be involved in consent process and marking if possible
	Patient to be involved in marking process
	Clearly mark operative site (Yes/initials not X)
	Ensure all documentation match (chart, images, consent, operating room schedule, etc.)
	Use pre-op checklists; consider body diagram
	Identify patient using two identifiers
	Reduce handoffs when moving patient to operating room and always repeat name, procedure, and site aloud to receiving personnel
	Standardize procedures across settings
Intraoperative	Active oral verification process in operating room
	Verification checklist (written and verbal) that includes all documents
	Have a "stop" or "time out" process if mismatch occurs
Postoperative	Have process for counting sponges and instruments
	Process to monitor adverse events such as reintubation, transfer to critical care, retained foreign body, etc.
	Use triggers for monitoring such as unexpected return to surgery, death in operating room, complications
	Monitor verification procedures for high-risk procedures

Florida Hospital Association, 2001; JCAHO, 1998a; JCAHO, 2001a; JCAHO, 2002b

TABLE 3.11   Falls Prevention Safety Practices

Assessment	Have all information about the patient readily available
	Identify intrinsic factors of patients at risk for falls using established tool, checklist, protocol, etc. Assess patient characteristics and physical functioning; diagnosis and physical changes; medications and drug interactions; mental condition/cognition, and substance use
	Identify extrinsic factors of environment that may predispose patient to fall such as floor surfaces, lighting, bed position, locks on utility rooms, window openings, exits
	Assess policies and procedures on use of restraints and alternatives
	Assess patients in specialty units for additional predisposing factors for falls
	Reassess patients regularly for risk
Implementation	Implement fall prevention program/protocol for those at risk
	Clearly identify patients on fall prevention program (e.g., special arm bands)
	Assess polypharmacy use for patients at risk
	Evaluate toileting routines (especially at night)
	Educate on use of assistive devices
	Maintain bed in low position with locks
	Keep call bell in reach
	Provide access to glasses, hearing aids
	Keep path from bed to bathroom clear
	Keep bathroom light on
	Use raised toilet seat as needed
	Provide aids such as grab bars, railing
	Keep floors dry
	Use bed exit alarms and chair alarms
	Use nonskid footwear
	Use protective hip pads on appropriate patients
	Use stable chairs, and specialty geriatric chairs
	Use floor mats
	Use gait belts for ambulation
	Educate patient and family
Monitoring	Report falls internally (and externally if required) to identify areas for improvement
	Monitor injuries from falls

Florida Hospital Association, 2001; JCAHO, 2000a

TABLE 3.12   Blood Administration Safety Practices

Use two identifiers to identify patient (not room number)
Consider special identification bands
Avoid storing multiple blood products on nursing unit
Avoid taking multiple units for several patients and checking at the same time
Develop policy for double checking products
Assess special identification of patients receiving blood (e.g., colored armbands)
Educate patient about possible adverse reactions and symptoms to report
Limit simultaneous cross matching of multiple patients by the same lab technologist
Use bar coding for administration
Computer verification process
Educate staff and test competency on blood administration (include patients at increased risk for reaction)
Use checklists for blood administration (both assessment and monitoring during and post administration)

JCAHO, 1999a

TABLE 3.13   Restraints Safety Practices

Prevention	Develop policy and procedures on restraint use
	Educate staff on alternatives to restraint use
	Educate staff on aggression control and de-escalation procedures
	Educate staff on appropriate application of restraints using consistent application
	Ensure restraints are in good working condition and can be easily removed as needed (e.g., keys available)
	Provide alternatives to restraints
	Identify patients at greater risk for needing restraints
	Ensure resuscitation equipment is available
Usage	Avoid application with patient in prone position with airway not observable
	Avoid application with patient's face covered and airway at risk
	Have sufficient staff to restrain patient safely and communicate with patient
	Avoid restraining a patient in bed with unprotected split side rails
	Remove all smoking materials
	Ensure protection and monitoring with limb restraints (skin, circulation, nerve)
	Discontinue use of high vest and waist restraints (impairs respiration)
	Assess patient for any deformity or abnormality that may preclude certain types of restraints
	Use only designated devices
	Secure to frame, not to movable bed parts
Monitoring	Conduct continuous observation of patients to monitor safety while restraints in use
	Monitor for hygiene, toileting, nutrition, comfort, as well as clinical assessment of condition, NV checks, and respiratory assessment
	Document and monitor all episodes of restraint use with debriefing and areas for improvement

JCAHO, 1998b

TABLE 3.14   Nosocomial Infections Prevention Practices

Have sufficient hand-washing facilities, including waterless products where needed
Implement CDC hand hygiene guidelines
Develop policies and procedures for instruments used in CJD cases
Process for timely prophylactic antibiotic administration
Administer prophylactic antibiotics as close to incision time as possible
Educate staff on infection control policies and procedures

CMS, 2002; JCAHO, 2003

WEB RESOURCES

Name of Resource/URL	Description
Agency for Healthcare Research and Quality www.ahrq.gov	Making Health Care Safer: A Critical Analysis of Patient Safety Practices
AHRQ book of patient safety indicators www.ahrq.gov	List of patient safety indicators
AHRQ Online journal www.webmm.ahrq.gov	Online journal with sample cases and analyses
AHRQ National Quality Measures Clearinghouse www.qualitymeasures.ahrq.gov	Key quality measures
American Society of Healthsystem Pharmacists www.ashp.org	Numerous resources on medication safety
Anesthesia Patient Safety Foundation www.apsf.org	Anesthesia safety
AORN www.aorn.org/about/positions/correctsite.htm	Position statement on correct-site surgery
AORN www.patientsafetyfirst.org/	Patient safety resource
Association of Professionals in Infection Control and Epidemiology www.apic.org/safety	Infection control practices
Centers for Disease Control and Prevention www.cdc.gov/ncidod/hip/	CDC resources on infection control
Centers for Disease Control and Prevention www.cdc.gov/mmwr/PDF/rr/rr5116.pdf	Handwashing guidelines
Food and Drug Administration www.fda.gov	Rules requiring barcoding on medications
Florida Hospital Association www.fha.org	Practice models for medication safety, surgery safety, and falls safety
Food and Drug Administration www.fda.gov/	FDA checklists for human factors

Institute for Healthcare Improvement www.ihi.org	Sample PDSA model and change concepts
Institute for Safe Medication Practices www.ismp.org	Sample FMEA on infusion devices, medication safety practices
Joint Commission on the Accreditation of Healthcare Organizations www.jcaho.org	Tools on RCA, analysis examples, sentinel event alerts
Joint Commission on the Accreditation of Healthcare Organizations www.jcaho.org	Weaving the Fabric. Strategies for improving our nation's health care report.
Massachusetts Coalition for Prevention of Medical Errors www.macoalition.org/	Medication safety aids
Med Pathways www.hospitalconnect.com/ medpathways/index.jsp	Three tools developed by HRET, ISMP and AHA
National Coalition on Healthcare—Accelerating Change Today www.nchc.org	Reducing Medical Errors and Improving Patient Safety: Success Stories from the Front Lines of Medicine by the National Coalition on Healthcare (NCHC) and the Institute for Healthcare Improvement (IHI)
National Coordinating Center for Medication Error Reporting and Prevention www.nccmerp.org	Medication definitions, classifications
National Patient Safety Center www.patientsafety.gov	Multiple tools on HFMEA
National Patient Safety Center www.patientsafety.gov/ CorrectSurg.html	VA position on marking surgery site
National Patient Safety Center www.patientsafety.gov	Patient Safety Handbook
National Patient Safety Foundation www.npsf.org	Lessons in Patient Safety compendium
Patient Safety Institute www.ptsafety.org	Multiple policies, procedures, and tools developed by the VA
Virginians Improving Patient Care & Safety www.vipcs.org	Multiple resources, links, and statements

VISN 8 Patient Safety Center   Safety practices
www.patientsafetycenter.com
VHA Incorporated   Seven Absolutes on surgery
www.vha.com/releases/020114.asp   marking

REFERENCES

Brassard, M., & Ritter, D. (1994). *The memory jogger*™ II. Methuen, MA: Goal/QPC.

Carey, R. G. (2003). *Improving healthcare with control charts.* Milwaukee, WI: ASQ Quality Press.

Carey, R. G., & Lloyd, R. C. (1995). *Measuring quality improvement in healthcare. A guide to statistical process control applications.* New York: Quality Resources.

Centers for Disease Control (CDC). (n.d.). *National nosocomial infections surveillance system.* Retrieved February 14, 2003, from www.cdc.gov/ncidod/hip/surveill/nnis.htm

Centers for Medicare and Medicaid Services. (CMS). (2003). *Handwashing guidelines.* Retrieved March 3, 2003, from www.cdc.gov/mmwr/PDF/rr/rr5116.pdf

Cohen, M. R. (Ed.). (1999). *Medication errors.* Washington, DC: American Pharmaceutical Association.

Findlay, S. (Ed.) (2000). *Reducing medical errors and improving patient safety: Success stories from the front lines of medicine by the National Coalition on Healthcare (NCHC) and the Institute for Healthcare Improvement (IHI).* Retrieved February 14, 2003, from www.nchc.org/releases/medical_errors.pdf

Institute for Healthcare Improvement. (IHI). (n.d.). *Change concepts: Distinguishing characteristics of a safe medication process.* Retrieved February 14, 2003, from www.ihi.org/resources/patientsafety/concepts/process.asp.

Institute for Healthcare Improvement. (IHI) (n.d). *Change concepts: High hazard drugs to be targeted for specific intervention.* Retrieved February 14, 2003, from www.ihi.org/resources/patientsafety/concepts/high.hazard.asp.

Institute for Healthcare Improvement. (IHI). (n.d). *Change concepts: Key changes for reducing adverse drug events.* Retrieved February 14, 2003, from www.ihi.org/resources/patientsafety/concepts/reduceade.asp.

Institute for Safe Medication Practice. (ISMP). (1998). *Benchmarking—when is it dangerous?* Retrieved February 14, 2003, from www.ismp.org/msaarticles/benchdanger.html

Joint Commission on Accreditation of Healthcare Organizations (JCAHO). (1998a). *Lessons learned: Wrong site surgery.* Retrieved February 12, 2003, from www.jcaho.org/about+us/news+letters/sentinel+event+alert/sea_6.htm

Joint Commission on Accreditation of Healthcare Organizations (JCAHO). (1998b). *Preventing restraint deaths.* Retrieved February 12, 2003, from www.jcaho.org/about+us/news+letters/sentinel+event+alert/sea_8.htm

Joint Commission on Accreditation of Healthcare Organizations (JCAHO). (1999a). *Blood transfusion errors: Preventing future occurrences.* Retrieved February 12, 2003, from www.jcaho.org/about+us/news+letters/sentinel+event+alert/sea_10.htm

Joint Commission on Accreditation of Healthcare Organizations (JCAHO). (1999b). *High-alert medications and patient safety.* Retrieved February 12, 2003, from www.jcaho.org/about+us/news+letters/sentinel+event+alert/sea_11.htm

Joint Commission on Accreditation of Healthcare Organizations (JCAHO). (1999c). *Infant abductions: Preventing future occurrences.* Retrieved February 12, 2003, from www.jcaho.org/about+us/news+letters/sentinel+event+alert/sea_9.htm

Joint Commission on Accreditation of Healthcare Organizations (JCAHO). (2000a). *Fatal falls: Lessons for the future.* Retrieved February 12, 2003, from www.jcaho.org/about+us/news+letters/sentinel+event+alert/sea_14.htm

Joint Commission on Accreditation of Healthcare Organizations (JCAHO). (2000b). *A framework for conducting root cause analysis.* Retrieved January 22, 2003, from www.jcaho.org/sentinel/sentevnt_frm.html

Joint Commission on Accreditation of Healthcare Organizations (JCAHO). (2001a). *A follow-up review of wrong site surgery.* Retrieved February 12, 2003, from www.jcaho.org/about+us/news+letters/sentinel+event+alert/sea_24.htm

Joint Commission on Accreditation of Healthcare Organizations (JCAHO). (2001b). *Exposure to Creutzfeldt-Jakob disease.* Retrieved February 12, 2003, www.jcaho.org/about+us/news+letters/sentinel+event+alert/se a_20.htm

Joint Commission on Accreditation of Healthcare Organizations (JCAHO). (2001c). *Look-alike, sound-alike drug names.* Retrieved February 12, 2003, from www.jcaho.org/about+us/news+letters/sentinel+event+alert/sea_19.htm

Joint Commission on Accreditation of Healthcare Organizations (JCAHO). (2001d). *Medication errors related to potentially dangerous abbreviations.* Retrieved February 12, 2003, from www.jcaho.org/about+us/news+letters/sentinel+event+alert/sea _23.htm

Joint Commission on Accreditation of Healthcare Organizations (JCAHO). (2001e). *Mix-up leads to a medication error.* Retrieved February 12, 2003, from www.jcaho.org/about+us/news+letters/sentinel+event+alert/sea_16.htm

Joint Commission on Accreditation of Healthcare Organizations (JCAHO). (2001f). *Revisions to Joint Commission standards in support of patient safety and medical/ health care efforts.* Retrieved January 22, 2003, from www.jcaho.org/standard/ fr_safety.html

Joint Commission on Accreditation of Healthcare Organizations (JCAHO). (2002a). *2002 Hospital accreditation standards.* Oakbrook Terrace, IL: Joint Commission Resources, Inc.

Joint Commission on Accreditation of Healthcare Organizations (JCAHO). (2002b). *2003 national patient safety goals.* Retrieved January 12, 2003, from www.jcaho.org/ accredited+organizations/patient+safety/npsg/index.htm

Joint Commission on Accreditation of Healthcare Organizations (JCAHO). (2003). *Infection control related sentinel events.* Retrieved February 12, 2003, from www.jcaho.org/about+us/news+letters/sentinel+event+alert/sea_28.htm

Kohn, L. T., Corrigan, J. M., & Donaldson, M. S. (Eds.) (2000). *To err is human: Building a safer health system.* Washington, DC: National Academy Press.

Langley, G. J., Nolan, K. M., Nolan, T. W., Norman, C. L., & Provost, L. P. (1996). *The improvement guide.* San Francisco: Jossey-Bass.

Merry, M. D., & Brown, J. P. (2002). *From a culture of safety to a culture of excellence: The Business of Health Care: A Journal of Innovative Management Collection.* Salem, NH: Goal/QPC.

National Committee on Quality Assurance (NCQA). (2002). *Standards for the accreditation of managed care organizations.* Washington, DC: NCQA.

National Coordinating Council for Medication Error Reporting and Prevention (NCCMERP). (2001). *Types of medication errors.* Retrieved January 14, 2003, from www.nccmerp.org/index.htm?http://www.nccmerp.org/sidebar.htm

National Patient Safety Foundation. (2002). *About NPSF.* Retrieved January 12, 2003 from www.npsf.org/html/pressrel/Krawisz.html

Reason, J. T. (1990). *Human error.* Cambridge: Cambridge University Press.

Shojania, K. G., Duncan, B. W., McDonald, K. M., & Wachter, R. M. (2001). *Making health care safer: A critical analysis of patient safety practices* (Publication 01-E058). Rockville, MD: Agency for Healthcare Research and Quality.

Tague, N. R. (1995). *The quality toolbox.* Milwaukee, WI: ASQC Quality Press.

Turnbull, J. E. (2002). *Process management and systems thinking for patient safety: The Business of Health Care: A Journal of Innovative Management Collection.* Salem, NH: Goal/QPC.

Veterans Affairs National Center for Patient Safety. (n.d.). *Healthcare failure mode and effect analysis course materials (HFMEA™).* Retrieved February 14, 2003, from www.patientsafety.gov/HFMEA.html

White, S. V. (2002). Brief report. Effective practices improve patient safety summit 2001. *Journal for Healthcare Quality, 24*(1), 34–36.

Chapter 4

Evidence-Based Practice to Promote Patient Safety

Jacqueline Fowler Byers

INTRODUCTION

The 2001 Institute of Medicine *Crossing the Quality Chasm* report cites six health care quality aims to address health care quality gaps. These include safe, effective, patient-centered, timely, efficient, and equitable health care (Committee on Quality of Care in America, 2001, pp. 5–6). Of these, safety, effectiveness, and efficiency can be directly addressed by evidence-based practice (EBP). The Committee on Quality of Care in America recommended that health care be based on quality as a system characteristic and the following rules: care based on continuous healing relationships; customization based on patient needs and values; the patient as the source of control; shared knowledge and free flow of information; evidence-based decision-making; safety as a system quality; the need for transparency; anticipation of needs; continuous decrease in waste; and cooperation among clinicians (Committee on Quality of Care in America, 2001, pp. 8–9). Evidence-based practice assists in compliance with several of these rules, including customization based on the individual patient's needs and values, shared knowledge and the free flow of information, evidence-based decision-making, safety as a system property, anticipation of needs, and continuous decrease in waste.

Evidence-Based Practice Defined

Evidence-based practice is not straight empiricism. Sackett and colleagues in the *British Medical Journal* wrote the most widely used definition for evidence-based medicine in 1996. They define EBP as the "conscientious, explicit and judicious use of current best evidence in making decisions about the care of individual patients" (Sackett, Rosenberg, Muir-Gray, Haynes, & Richardson, 1996, p. 71). The term "practice" is substituted for "medicine" in this chapter because not all health care is medical care, and multiple disciplines are involved in health care delivery. This definition clearly indicates that EBP is not cookbook medicine, since the practitioner takes individual situations and preferences into account. Clinicians should base their care not only on the experimental evidence, but consider experiential evidence, physiologic principles, patient and professional values, and system features (Tonelli, 2001). This allows individualized application of aggregate research evidence (Greenhalgh, 1999; Tonelli, 2001). A benefit of EBP is that it requires practitioners to be lifelong learners and to stay current with the research literature and apply it to their practice (Straus & Sackett, 1998). In order to promote safety, one aspect of evidence that should not be applied to individuals is the use of unnecessary or nontherapeutic interventions.

Evidence-based practice promotes patient safety through the provision of effective and efficient health care, resulting in less variation in care and less unnecessary or nontherapeutic interventions (Committee on Quality of Care in America, 2001). EBP as a patient safety strategy is based on well-designed research on clinical practice questions (see chapter 15). Figure 4.1 illustrates this relationship. In order to evaluate the impact of EBP, outcomes evaluation at the individual and aggregate level is an essential step of this process. EBP and outcomes measurement are iterative; one facilitates the other (Deaton, 2001).

Evidence-Based Practice Opportunities

There are challenges related to the implementation of EBP. The first is that evidence does not exist for the majority of clinical situations. The second is that even when guidelines are available, they are not necessarily widely used, despite comprehensive dissemination strategies. This is improving over the past decade (Reikvam, Kvan, & Aursnes, 2002), but significant opportunity still exists. A study of family practice physicians

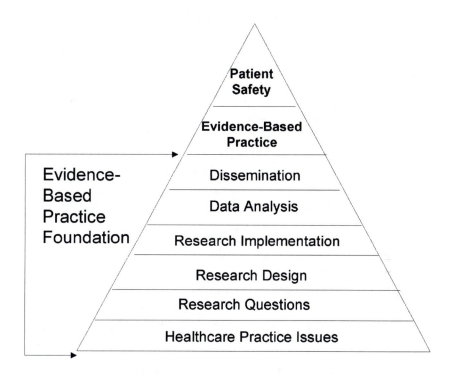

FIGURE 4.1   Foundations for evidence-based practice and patient safety.

from the Netherlands reported high knowledge regarding clinical guide-lines, but only two-thirds of relevant clinical decisions were based on guidelines. The authors cited large individual variation between individual physician practice and guidelines (Grol, 2001).

Well designed evidence-based practice augmented with automated clini-cal information systems provides the greatest opportunity for improvement in the outcomes of chronic diseases in the United States (Committee on Quality of Care in America, 2001). The Committee recommended that the priorities for evidence development should be in the following chronic diseases that have tremendous impact on health expenditures and out-comes: cancer, diabetes, emphysema, high cholesterol, HIV/AIDS, hyper-tension, ischemic heart disease, stroke, arthritis, asthma, gall bladder disease, stomach ulcers, back problems, Alzheimer's disease and other dementias, and depression and anxiety (Committee on Quality of Care in

America, 2001). It is further recommended that the Secretary of Health and Human Services be given responsibility for creating a public-private partnership to ensure ongoing analysis and synthesis of medical evidence, development and dissemination of evidence-based clinical guidelines and best practices, and development of decision support tools to assist clinicians and patients in applying the evidence based on values and preferences (Committee on Quality of Care in America, 2001).

STRATEGIES TO PROMOTE EVIDENCE-BASED PRACTICE

Evidence-Based Practice Steps

EBP is developed, supported, implemented, and evaluated on three distinct levels: the health care provider-patient interaction, the organizational level, and the research team who develops evidence-based knowledge. Although the steps are similar, the specific questions and activities vary. Table 4.1 summarizes the different perspectives at each stage of the EBP process. Since the activities at each step are similar regardless of perspective, they will be discussed together.

Identification of a Clinical Practice Issue/Information
Need and Priority

The need for EBP may come from several sources. At the clinician-patient level, it may come from a rare diagnosis or a request from a patient for a nonstandard treatment. At the organizational level, it may come from introduction of new procedures, risk or quality data, known deviation from benchmarks, or identification of high-volume, high-risk or high-resource diagnoses or procedures. For knowledge development, it may come from a proposed new drug or device, or consideration of a previously approved drug or treatment for a new clinical indication.

Since there are always more questions than there are time and resources to address them, prioritization is key. Factors to consider in prioritization include:

- What is the magnitude of the problem?
- How important is it to safety and outcomes?
- What is the cost of investigation vs. potential cost savings?
- What are the risks if you address it?

TABLE 4.1   Perspectives at Each Phase of the EBP Process

EBP step	Provider–patient (Lipman, 2000)	Organizational	Knowledge development
Identification of a clinical practice issue/information need and its priority	What is the recognized gap in clinical knowledge regarding how to manage a clinical case?	What is my greatest health care quality opportunity?	What clinical practice areas still have no high-level evidence to optimize outcomes? What new potential therapeutic interventions need to be researched?
Converting need into researchable question	What is the context-specific structured answerable question?	What is my specific researchable question?	What are my research questions/ hypotheses?
Efficiently determining best evidence	How to search the evidence? What are the findings?	Perform a literature review; design and implement a research utilization or quality improvement project	Performed well-designed and implemented research study
Critical appraisal of the evidence	How strong are the findings?	What are my findings? Do they justify roll-out to other areas of the organization?	Determine data quality and results
Determining applicability to practice	Are the findings valid and applicable to the current clinical situation? Evidence is used based on shared decision making with the patient.	Determine which organizational areas would benefit from diffusion of the EBP findings.	Discuss based on previous findings and formulate practice implications. What are the study limitations? How generalizable are the findings?
Evaluation of impact of use of the evidence	Evaluation of individual clinical outcomes	What is the EBP compliance? Are the outcome gains sustained? Were similar benefits also found in other areas of the organization?	Do future clinical outcomes and research studies support the prior research findings?

- What are the risks if you don't address it?
- Are there adequate resources available?
- What is the availability of adequate measures to evaluate the problem?
- Are there political/cultural issues?
- What are the organizational priorities, philosophy, mission and vision? (Richmond & Byers, 2000).

These considerations can be quantified on a decision matrix in order to objectively determine the highest priority EBP need (Granger & Chulay, 1999).

Converting Need into a Researchable Question

This is a critical step as it drives the subsequent literature review or clinical research. The question must be defined precisely. Straus and Sackett (1998) describe four necessary components for the researchable question: (1) the patient or problem being addressed, (2) the intervention being considered (a cause, prognostic factor or treatment), (3) another intervention to consider if relevant, and (4) the clinical outcomes of interest. At the clinician-patient level, the question reflects what is the best potential management for a patient based on their presenting symptoms, history, values, and preferences. For the organizational level, it would involve investigating an evidence-based approach to management of a patient population or problem at the group level. For research knowledge development, it requires the development of formal, researchable questions and/or hypotheses.

Efficiently Determining Best Evidence

In the ideal world, there would be systematic reviews of randomized clinical trials (RCTs) for all clinical practice questions, but in reality, most clinical practice is based on tradition and experience, not hard science. Available levels of evidence exist on a continuum based on the quality, quantity, and rigor of the available research.

The goal at this step to promote EBP is to efficiently obtain the highest available level of evidence. Systematic reviews or meta-analyses combine findings across studies and calculate a summary effect size. This allows statistical consolidation of numerous studies to determine the aggregate result (Byers & Stullenbarger, 2003). The steps of systematic reviews include a comprehensive search, critical appraisal, data synthesis, and interpretation (Committee on Quality of Care in America, 2001). Randomized clinical trials are considered the most stringent research design. Therefore systematic reviews of RCTs are the gold standard for the highest level of evidence.

The usefulness of data sources is based on the amount of relevance and validity, divided by the amount of work required to obtain it (Grandage, Slawson, & Shaughnessy, 2002). In order to efficiently obtain the highest level of evidence, searches should initially filter out all studies except for systematic reviews and RCTs (Grandage, Slawson, & Shaughnessy, 2002; Straus & Sackett, 1998). Pertinent evidence-based clinical practice guidelines should also be obtained. A librarian can assist with identifying pertinent key words, search databases, and filter terms to streamline the search. The National Library of Medicine PubMed (MedLine) search engine has an automatic filter available (see Web Resources). In addition to the frequently used MedLine and Cumulative Index of Nursing and Allied Health Literature (CINAHL), some additional helpful search databases are provided in the list of web resources at the end of this chapter. The top databases for systematic reviews are the Cochrane Collaboration, Evidence-Based Medicine, ACP Journal Club, TRIP, and DARE. If systematic reviews or RCTs are not available, the search can be broadened to include less rigorous studies related to the practice question.

Critical Appraisal of the Evidence

Once the highest level of systematic reviews, RCTs, studies, and clinical practice guidelines are obtained, the next step is to critically appraise the evidence. The steps of critical appraisal include systematically reviewing the research evidence and determining the validity and relevance of the findings in order to influence practice (Hill & Spittlehouse, 2001). There are three steps in performing a critical appraisal of an individual study or systematic reviews: review the study/systematic review for an initial overview, complete a critical appraisal checklist, and create a summary table in order to determine scientific merit (Byers & Beaudin, 2001). Tables 4.2 and 4.3 provide critical appraisal checklists for both original research and systematic reviews. Examples of areas to include in research summary tables of original research and systematic reviews are reference, sample and setting, research methods, findings, strengths and weaknesses, and applicability to the practice question (Byers & Beaudin, 2001). Once this process has been completed, a summary level of evidence and grading recommendation can be made based on the highest level reviews and studies.

TABLE 4.2   Critical Appraisal Tool for Original Clinical or Health Services Research Study

---

The purpose of a *critical appraisal* is to critique available research for potential use in the health care quality professional's work setting. This appraisal tool can be used to assist with data gathering at the beginning of a performance improvement initiative or to answer a clinical or nonclinical practice question. Specific questions below are intended to evaluate the quality of the original research and the applicability to your setting. Clarification of questions is in *italics*.

1.   **Merit**

1a.	Was the purpose of the study clear and logical? Is the question of practical significance? *Purposes may relate to patient population, type of intervention, or specific outcomes.*	❐ Yes	❐ No	❐ Unsure
1b.	Did the authors review the literature? *The study report should build on prior research in the area. The report should also compare the current findings to prior research in the field.*	❐ Yes	❐ No	❐ Unsure
1c.	Was an appropriate study design used for the research question? *To definitely answer a research practice question, a randomized clinical trial is needed. To investigate a new (not previously investigated) area, descriptive research is acceptable. The goal is the strongest possible research design possible.*	❐ Yes	❐ No	❐ Unsure

If the above 3 are answered "Yes," you should proceed with the critical appraisal and study summary. In there are any "No" answers in the above, the research is of insufficient merit to proceed further.

2.   **Rigor**

2a.	Was the research design clear? Are there any flaws? *Can you picture the research approach in your mind? Is there a figure to assist in understanding? Is it the best possible design?*	❐ Yes	❐ No	❐ Unsure
2b.	Were all variables clearly identified? *The article should address all types of variables appropriate to the research design. Look for a summary of variables. Examples: descriptive, independent, dependent, confounding, and extraneous variables*	❐ Yes	❐ No	❐ Unsure

---

TABLE 4.2 *(continued)*

2c.	Were all critical variables measured? *For instance, if the study is related to diabetes compliance and HgbA$_1$C is not measured, the study's usefulness is jeopardized.*	❐ Yes	❐ No	❐ Unsure
2d.	Were the research questions/hypotheses appropriate? *Do the questions/hypotheses relate to the study purpose? Do the questions/hypotheses fit with the research design?*	❐ Yes	❐ No	❐ Unsure
2e.	Were subject recruitment and sampling methods acceptable? *Are the recruitment methods and sampling methods clearly described? Does the sample reflect the population of interest? If there is more than one study group, are they comparable?*	❐ Yes	❐ No	❐ Unsure
2f.	Was the sample size adequate to determine a statistical difference if one exists? *Was the rationale for sample size described?* Examples: *Time period, accessibility of subjects, prospective or retrospective power analysis.*	❐ Yes	❐ No	❐ Unsure
2g.	Were the instruments used to measure the variables the strongest possible and practical? Are the reliability and validity of measures discussed? Reliability examples: *test-retest, split-half, or Cronbach's alpha.* Validity examples: *Content, criterion, established in previous studies.*	❐ Yes	❐ No	❐ Unsure
2h.	Were strategies to ensure methodologic and rater consistency described? *Look for data collector training, a clear data collection procedure, and/or assessment of interrater reliability.*	❐ Yes	❐ No	❐ Unsure
2i.	Was protection of human subjects maintained? *Was informed consent obtained? Was there a review or exemption by an Institutional Review Board? An exception would be a public survey or retrospective chart or database review with no subject identifiers recorded.*	❐ Yes	❐ No	❐ Unsure

(continued)

TABLE 4.2 *(continued)*

2j.	Were the authors unbiased in their research study? *Did a manufacturer of the pharmaceutical or device fund the study? Is there any other evidence of conflict of interest?*	❏ Yes	❏ No ❏ Unsure
2k.	Was the study subjected to peer review prior to distribution? *Was the study published in a peer reviewed journal such as* Journal for Healthcare Quality *or published by a government agency such as the Agency for Healthcare Quality and Research which has a peer review process in place?*	❏ Yes	❏ No ❏ Unsure

3. Findings

3a.	Were the overall findings of the study discussed? *What are the "take home" findings of the study? Are all research questions/hypotheses discussed? Are both significant and nonsignificant findings discussed?*	❏ Yes	❏ No ❏ Unsure
3b.	Were the appropriate data analyses/statistics used? *Clearly presented descriptive statistics (frequency, percent) should be used to summarize the setting and sample. Additional statistical analysis will be determined by the research questions/hypotheses.*	❏ Yes	❏ No ❏ Unsure
3c.	Did the discussion of the findings follow from the data? *Discussion and recommendations should not "overreach" beyond concrete findings. Study design or prior research may be used to provide rationale for findings.*	❏ Yes	❏ No ❏ Unsure

4. Subject applicability

4a.	Can the results be applied to a local setting/population? *This is dependent on whether the local setting is similar to the setting/population of the study in terms of structure of health care (setting and provider), and patient population.*	❏ Yes	❏ No ❏ Unsure

TABLE 4.2 *(continued)*

4b.	Were the limitations/weaknesses of the results stated? *Look for any information about small numbers, limited study design, subject withdrawals and loss to follow-up. This limits generalizability of findings to other settings than where the original research was performed.*	☐ Yes ☐ No ☐ Unsure	
4c.	Can you replicate the study in your work setting? *Replication with formal evaluation can determine whether recommendations should be implemented on an ongoing basis.*	☐ Yes ☐ No ☐ Unsure	
4d.	Is there a benefit of implementing the research recommendations in your work setting?	☐ Yes ☐ No ☐ Unsure	
4e.	Is there a cost benefit for implementing the recommendations in your work setting?	☐ Yes ☐ No ☐ Unsure	
4f.	Would only minor to moderate modifications have to be made to implement research recommendations in your work setting?	☐ Yes ☐ No ☐ Unsure	
4g.	Do the benefits of implementing the findings outweigh potential risks or costs? *This is based on your assessment of your practice setting in terms of administrative/ practice priorities, risk, etc. Compare the risks of implementing vs. not implementing.*	☐ Yes ☐ No ☐ Unsure	

5.   Scoring

The strength of the guidelines or review (measured by the total number of questions answered with a "Yes") will determine whether the findings should be used in your setting.

20–24 "Yes's"	Implement recommendations in your work setting
15–19 "Yes's"	Consider implementing recommendations based on priority
≤ 14 "Yes's"	Do not implement recommendations

If there are more than 3 "Unsures," seek assistance from a colleague more familiar with the research process and then rescore.

From "Critical Appraisal Tools Facilitate the Work of the Quality Professional," by J. F. Byers, and C. L. Beaudin, 2001, *Journal for Healthcare Quality, 25*(3), pp. 35–43. Reprinted with permission.

TABLE 4.3   Critical Appraisal Tool for Research Synthesis: Practice Guidelines, Integrated Research Reviews and Meta-Analyses

---

The purpose of a *critical appraisal* is to critique available research for potential use in the health care quality professional's work setting. This appraisal tool can be used to assist with data gathering at the beginning of a performance improvement initiative or to answer a clinical or nonclinical practice question. Specific questions below are intended to evaluate the quality of the research synthesis and the applicability to your setting. Clarification of questions is in *italics*.

1.   **Merit**

1a.   Does the guideline or review article focus on a specific question?   ❒ Yes   ❒ No   ❒ Unsure
Focus areas may include patient population, type of intervention, or specific outcome measures.

1b.   Do the authors review appropriate references?   ❒ Yes   ❒ No   ❒ Unsure
The review should focus on clearly related research based articles that reflect the investigator's research question.

1c.   Are the findings current?   ❒ Yes   ❒ No   ❒ Unsure
In general, reviews more than 5 years old are out of date. The exception would be if no new work has been done in the area.

If the above 3 questions are answered "Yes," you should proceed with the critical appraisal and study summary. In there are "No" answers in the above, the research synthesis is of insufficient merit to proceed further.

2.   **Rigor**

2a.   Are all the important, relevant studies included?   ❒ Yes   ❒ No   ❒ Unsure
Consider whether the appropriate references and/or databases were used (e.g., MedLine, CINAHL, ERIC, PsychInfo, Health Star, Internet search engines). Attempts should be made to find unpublished studies.

2b.   Do the authors evaluate the rigor of the studies?   ❒ Yes   ❒ No   ❒ Unsure
The review should focus on clearly related research based articles. The strongest available research designs should be reviewed. Consensus papers should only be used if no prior research exists.

TABLE 4.3 *(continued)*

2c.	If the results are combined (such as in a meta-analysis), was it justified? *The variables should have been similar across studies. Aggregate and individual results should be noted and the possible rationale for differences discussed.*	❐ Yes	❐ No	❐ Unsure ❐ Not applicable
2d.	Is an appropriate method used to reach recommendations/conclusions? *Were reviewed studies rated by rigor? Was a systematic approach used to formulate recommendations based on reviewed studies?*	❐ Yes	❐ No	❐ Unsure
2e.	Are the authors unbiased in their review of research studies? *Did appropriately qualified people without conflicts of interest do the review? Were the recommendations or findings subjected to peer review prior to distribution?*	❐ Yes	❐ No	❐ Unsure
3.	**Findings**			
3a.	Are the overall findings of the guidelines, review, or meta-analysis clearly described? *Can you understand the "take home" findings of the guidelines, review, or meta-analysis?*	❐ Yes	❐ No	❐ Unsure
3b.	Are the appropriate data analyses/statistics used? *Clearly presented descriptive statistics (frequency, percent) should be used to summarize findings. For meta-analyses, the results should be presented using the Effect Size statistic.*	❐ Yes	❐ No	❐ Unsure
3c.	Do the recommendations logically follow from the findings? *Recommendations should be supported by the statistical analysis or practice results.*	❐ Yes	❐ No	❐ Unsure
4.	**Setting applicability**			
4a.	Can the results be applied to the local setting/population? *This is dependent on whether the local setting is similar to the setting/populations in the guidelines, reviews or meta-analyses in terms of structure of health care (setting and provider), and patient population.*	❐ Yes	❐ No	❐ Unsure

(continued)

TABLE 4.3 *(continued)*

4b.	Are the limitations/weaknesses of the results stated? *Look for any information about small numbers, limited study design, or variable selection. This limits generalizability of findings to other settings than where the original research was performed.*	☐ Yes	☐ No	☐ Unsure
4c.	Are all critical outcomes evaluated? *Ideally, multidimensional outcome measures would be considered based on quality, customer service, and cost.*	☐ Yes	☐ No	☐ Unsure
4d.	Can you pilot the recommendations in your work setting? *Pilot work with formal evaluation can determine whether recommendations should be implemented on an ongoing basis.*	☐ Yes	☐ No	☐ Unsure
4e.	Is there a benefit of implementing the recommendations in your work setting?	☐ Yes	☐ No	☐ Unsure
4f.	Is there a cost benefit for implementing the recommendations in your work setting?	☐ Yes	☐ No	☐ Unsure
4g.	Would only minor to moderate modifications have to be made to implement recommendations in your work setting?	☐ Yes	☐ No	☐ Unsure
4h.	Do the benefits of implementing the findings outweigh potential risks or costs? *This is based on your assessment of your practice setting in terms of the items above as well as administrative/practice priorities, risk, etc. Weigh the risk of implementation vs. the risk of not implementing.*	☐ Yes	☐ No	☐ Unsure

5.   **Scoring**

The strength of the guidelines or review (measured by the total number of questions answered with a "Yes") will determine whether the findings should be used in your setting.

16–19 "Yes's"	Implement recommendations in your work setting
12–15 "Yes's"	Consider implementing recommendations based on priority
≤ 11 "Yes's"	Do not implement recommendations

If there are more than 3 "Unsures," seek assistance from a colleague more familiar with the research process and then rescore.

From "Critical Appraisal Tools Facilitate the Work of the Quality Professional," by J. F. Byers, and C. L. Beaudin, 2001, *Journal for Healthcare Quality*, 25(3), pp. 35–43. Reprinted with permission.

Several ratings and grading systems are in use to determine the level of evidence and the related grading of the recommendation. In general, a level of evidence of "1" or a grading recommendation of "A" is the best, based on either a systematic review of RCTs, or a large randomized clinical trial. A typical level of evidence and grades of recommendation chart is shown in Table 4.4. The level of evidence and grading of recommendation is based on the rigor of the available studies using A–D and 1–5. Less rigorous studies receive lower grades and higher numbers (European Society of Medical Oncology, n.d.; Phillips, et al., 2001). Some term the less rigorous levels of evidence such as consensus as "best practices" or "potentially better practices," since these practices haven't been scientifically validated (Burch, et al., 2003; Driever, 2002).

Determining Applicability to Practice

This step allows interpretation of scientific evidence in combination with additional subjective and objective data. The analysis varies at this phase depending on whether the practice question was framed at the individual, organizational or aggregate level. At this point, the results of the evidence review are combined with clinical expertise and knowledge of unique

TABLE 4.4   Levels of Evidence and Grades of Recommendations*

Grade of recommenda- tion	Level of evidence	Type of data/studies
A	1a	Systematic review of randomized controlled trials
	1b	Randomized controlled trial (adequate power)
B	2a	Systematic review of cohort studies
	2b	Individual cohort study
	3a	Systematic review of case—control studies
	3b	Individual case—control study
C	4	Case series, nonexperimental
D	5	Case reports
		Expert opinion without explicit critical appraisal
		Based on physiologic bench research

*Grading recommendations may vary based on the quantity of studies or the consistency of findings across studies.

European Society of Medical Oncology, n.d.; Phillips, et al., 2001.

features of the target population including values, preferences, specific medical comorbidities, and any other relevant contextual factors (Sackett, Rosenberg, Muir-Gray, Haynes, & Richardson, 1996). Frank discussions and decision analyses can assist with this phase of promoting EBP (Byers & Stullenbarger, 2003). Clinical care is delivered based on the conclusions of this step.

Evidence-Based Practice Evaluation

Like all quality improvement activities, the EBP cycle is not complete until formal evaluation occurs of both processes and outcomes. First, the processes of determining the best evidence are evaluated. Were there ways to be more efficient? Did the process yield a rational, acceptable clinical management strategy (Straus & Sackett, 1998)? An additional area of evaluation is clinical and organizational outcomes. The specific focus of outcomes evaluations depends on whether the EBP question was targeted at the individual, organizational, or knowledge development level. If EBP focused on an individual patient, then that patient's clinical outcomes are evaluated using appropriate, objective clinical measures. If the focus was at the organizational level, clinical outcomes for the target patient population is the level of evaluation. At the knowledge development level, the clinical outcomes of the research subjects are aggregately analyzed. Although not directly related to EBP, the impact of EBP on health care resource use is frequently also assessed.

Key to EBP evaluation is the development of valid, reliable, and easy to measure outcomes indicators. This is the only way to provide meaningful comparisons across patients, organizations, regions, and other aggregate groups for benchmarking and evaluation. The Committee on Quality of Care in America recommends the use of HEDIS, JCAHO ORYX and FAACT measures for this purpose (Committee on Quality of Care in America, 2001).

MAKING EVIDENCE-BASED PRACTICE HAPPEN

Barriers and Facilitators

Even if every clinical practice question had a definitive systematic review or guideline, getting practitioners to use them is a challenge. Singer proposes that EBP only happens when it suits the practitioner based on personal dogma and if implementation of the EBP would be easy (Singer, 2002). The biggest barrier to implementation is resistance to change (Sitzia, 2002). Other cited barriers to EBP in the literature include lack of perceived need, aversion to "cookbook medicine," lack of awareness of EBP guidelines, lack of confidence in the guideline developer, and suspicion that the true goal is cost control (Leape, et al., 2003). Therefore perceived barriers must be reduced, and facilitators provided.

In the study of family practice physicians in the Netherlands, guideline knowledge and use was greater when mailed guidelines were supplemented with two outreach visits to encourage use of the guideline (Grol, 2001). Conversely, an Australian study found that adding local adaptation steps of guideline dissemination did not increase knowledge or use regarding nationally produced clinical practice guidelines (Silagy, et al., 2002).

A survey regarding adherence and barriers to following guidelines to prevent ventilator-associated pneumonia found that the nonadherence rate was 37%. Adherence was better for interventions with a higher level of evidence on nonpharmacologic interventions. Reasons cited for nonadherence included disagreement with the interpretation of the clinical trial findings (35%), unavailability of resources (31.3%) and cost (16.9%) (Rello, et al., 2002). In a study of compliance with specialty society guidelines regarding coronary artery bypass graft and percutaneous transluminal coronary angioplasty, recommendations were more likely to be followed if they were based on randomized clinical trial results (Leape, et al., 2003).

Evidence-Based Practice Culture

The two most important steps in getting EBP to the front line of patient care are to promote a culture of inquiry and EBP accountability (Richmond & Byers, 2000). EBP knowledge must be translated into easy to use information for use by the frontline health care provider and disseminated in such a way that the health care provider sees the value of its use.

According to the research on barriers to EBP, there is no best way to disseminate EBP information to ensure its use by health care providers. The source of information (individual or institutional) is frequently more influential than the information itself (Scullion, 2002). Active engagement of the provider by an opinion leader or consensus development has the best demonstrated success of EBP (Agency for Healthcare Research and Quality, 2001; Eve, Golton, Hodgkin, Munro, & Musson, 1996; Grol & Grimshaw, 1999).

Support by administration and local opinion leaders is critical for EBP success (Agency for Healthcare Research and Quality, 2001; Landry & Sibbald, 2002). Additional allies include early adopters, that is, those health care providers that readily embrace change. A clearly established plan and program in conjunction with clear accountability increases the probability of success. An exemplar of an evidence-based medicine program that won the 2003 Voluntary Hospitals of America Clinical Effectiveness Leadership Award is the Crozer-Keystone Health System in Pennsylvania (Schumacher, Stock, & Richards, 2003).

Several research utilization models have been widely used to promote each step of the EBP process, from practice question determination to evaluation. These models not only provide previously tested structure and process, but also have clinical examples to assist the novice (Grol & Grimshaw, 1999; Rosswurm & Larrabee, 1999; Stetler, 2001; Titler & Everett, 2001; Titler, et al., 1994; Titler, Steelman, Budreau, Buckwalter, & Goode, 2001).

Another strategy to promote the use of EBP recommendations is to automate them in some way, such as standing order sets, practice protocols and computerized prompts. Computer technology can provide automated evidence-based order sets and clinical alerts to prevent errors in planning. A randomized control trial of the use of a Web-based diabetes disease management program found that use of this program significantly increased diabetes appropriate evaluations, and improved hemoglobin A1C levels (Meigs, et al., 2003). Point of care access to Internet-based search engines and systematic reviews also promotes EBP (Schwartz, et al., 2003).

Initial and ongoing education of health care professionals also can positively influence EBP (Paltiel, Brezis, & Lahad, 2002). Implementation of an EBP curriculum in the education of all health care professionals is needed to get all health care providers practicing with an EBP framework. Evidence-based outpatient rounds using previous cases increased the percentage of EBP questions of residents from 13% to 59% over a six-month period (Ozuah, Orbe, & Sharif, 2002). Three-day short courses at McMaster University demonstrated an increase in EBP knowledge (Fritsche, Greenhalgh, Falck-Ytter, Neumayer, & Kunz, 2002).

AREAS FOR FUTURE RESEARCH

Areas for future research regarding promoting evidence-based practice include the following:

- Once technology is more widely available, how will this impact the degree of adherence to EBP?
- What are the definitive dissemination and engagement strategies to promote EBP?
- What is the patient's role in promoting EBP?
- Are there additional strategies that can be successfully employed to promote the conduct and dissemination of systematic reviews?
- What is the direct relationship among EBP, variation in care, and patient outcomes?

CONCLUSION

Evidence-based practice is a critical process to promote patient safety. In order to address gaps in health care quality and safety, EBP must become the standard of care across the United States. Employing the EBP steps at the individual patient, organizational and knowledge development levels ensures the elimination of nontherapeutic interventions, decreases variations in health care, and promotes optimal outcomes.

WEB RESOURCES

Name of Resource/URL	Description
Agency for Healthcare Research and Quality Evidence-Based Practice Centers *http://www.ahrq.gov/clinic/epc/*	Includes history of the centers and their evidence-based practice reports
Centre for Evidence-Based Medicine *http://www.cebm.net/*	Oxford Centre for Evidence-Based Medicine; great educational information and tools
Cochrane Collaboration http://www.cochrane.org	International collaboration dedicated to the creation, review, maintenance, and dissemination of systematic overviews of the effects of health care interventions; systematic review abstracts available for free; full reports require subscription

Critical Appraisal and Using the Literature *http://www.shef.ac.uk/~scharr/ir/ units/critapp/*	Tutorial with working examples
Database of Abstracts of Reviews of Effects (DARE) *http://nhscrd.york.ac.uk/darehp.htm*	From the University of York National Health Service Centre for Reviews and Dissemination
Health Links Evidence-Based Practice and Guidelines http://healthlinks.washington.edu/ clinical/guidelines.html	Numerous helpful links
McMaster University Evidence-Based Practice Internet Resources *http://www-hsl.mcmaster.ca/ebm/*	Another site with numerous helpful links
McMaster University Health Information Resource Unit http://hiru.mcmaster.ca/hiru/ default.htm	Research projects to promote evidence-based practice through the use of information technology
National Guideline Clearinghouse http://guidelines.gov	United States central portal for evidence-based clinical practice guidelines; offers personal digital assistant downloads and weekly updates via e-mail
PubMed Search Queries http://www.ncbi.nlm.nih.gov/ entrez/query/static/clinical.html	Provides automated filters to search MedLine for randomized controlled trials and systematic reviews
Translating Research Into Practice (TRIP) Database *http://www.tripdatabase.com/*	Searches over 75 sites on the Web for evidence-based content, including online journals
What Is Critical Appraisal? http://www.evidence-based-medicine.co.uk/ebmfiles/ WhatisCriticalAppraisal.pdf	Nice review of critical appraisal steps

REFERENCES

Agency for Healthcare Research and Quality (AHRQ). (2001). *Making health care safer: A critical analysis of patient safety practices.* Agency for Healthcare Research and

Quality Evidence Report/Technology Assessment Number 43. Rockville, MD: Author.

Burch, K., Rhine, W., Baker, R., Litman, F., Kaempf, J. W., Schwarz, E., et al. (2003). Implementing potentially better practices to reduce lung injury in neonates. *Pediatrics, 111*(4), Pt 2, e432–436.

Byers, J. F., & Beaudin, C. L. (2001). Critical appraisal tools facilitate the work of the quality professional. *Journal for Healthcare Quality, 23*(5), 35–38, 40–33.

Byers, J. F., & Stullenbarger, E. (2003). Meta-analysis and decision analysis bridge research and practice. *Western Journal of Nursing Research, 25*, 193–204.

Committee on Quality of Care in America (CQCA). (2001). *Crossing the quality chasm: A new health system for the 21st century.* Washington, DC: National Academy Press.

Deaton, C. (2001). Outcomes measurement and evidence-based nursing practice. *Journal of Cardiovascular Nursing, 15*(2), 83–86.

Driever, M. J. (2002). Are evidenced-based practice and best practice the same? *Western Journal of Nursing Research, 24*(5), 591–597.

European Society for Medical Oncology. (n.d.). *Levels of evidence and grades of recommendations.* Retrieved December 7, 2003, from http://www.esmo.org/reference/referenceGuidelines/html/levels%20of%20evidence.htm

Eve, R., Golton, I., Hodgkin, P., Munro, J., & Musson, G. (1996). Beyond guidelines: Promoting clinical change in the real world. *Journal of Management in Medicine, 10*(1), 16–25.

Fritsche, L., Greenhalgh, T., Falck-Ytter, Y., Neumayer, H. H., & Kunz, R. (2002). Do short courses in evidence-based medicine improve knowledge and skills? Validation of Berlin questionnaire and before and after study of courses in evidence-based medicine. *British Medical Journal, 325*(7376), 1338–1341.

Grandage, K. K., Slawson, D. C., & Shaughnessy, A. F. (2002). When less is more: A practical approach to searching for evidence-based answers. *Journal of the Medical Library Association, 90*(3), 298–304.

Granger, B. B., & Chulay, M. (1999). *Research strategies for clinicians.* Stamford: Appleton & Lange.

Greenhalgh, T. (1999). Narrative based medicine in an evidenced based world. *British Medical Journal, 318*, 323–325.

Grol, R. (2001). Successes and failures in the implementation of evidence-based guidelines for clinical practice. *Medical Care, 39*(8, Suppl 2), I146–154.

Grol, R., & Grimshaw, J. (1999). Evidence-based implementation of evidence-based medicine. *Journal on Quality Improvement, 25*(10), 50–513.

Hill, A., & Spittlehouse, C. (2001). *What is critical appraisal?* Retrieved April 14, 2003, from http://www.evidence-based-medicine.co.uk/ebmfiles/WhatisCriticalAppraisal.pdf

Landry, M. D., & Sibbald, W. J. (2002). Changing physician behavior: A review of patient safety in critical care medicine. *Journal of Critical Care, 17*(2), 138–145.

Leape, L. L., Weissman, J. S., Schneider, E. C., Piana, R. N., Gatsonis, C., & Epstein, A. (2003). *Adherence to practice guidelines: The role of specialty society guidelines.* Retrieved March 31, 2003, from http://www.medscape.com/viewarticle/448529_print

Lipman, T. (2000). Power and influence in clinical effectiveness and evidence-based medicine. *Family Practice, 17*(6), 557–563.

Meigs, J. B., Cagliero, E., Dubey, A., Murphy-Sheehy, P., Gildesgame, C., Chueh, H., et al. (2003). A controlled trial of web-based diabetes disease management: The MGH diabetes primary care improvement project. *Diabetes Care, 26*(3), 750–757.

Ozuah, P. O., Orbe, J., & Sharif, I. (2002). Ambulatory rounds: A venue for evidence-based medicine. *Academic Medicine: Journal of the Association of American Medical Colleges, 77*(7), 740–741.

Paltiel, O., Brezis, M., & Lahad, A. (2002). Principles for planning the teaching of evidence-based medicine/clinical epidemiology for MPH and medical students. *Public Health Reviews, 30*(1–4), 261–270.

Phillips, B., Ball, C., Sackett, D., Badenoch, D., Straus, S., Haynes, R. B., et al. (2001). *Oxford Centre for evidence-based medicine levels of evidence.* Retrieved April 14, 2003, from http://www.minervation.com/cebm2/docs/levels.html

Reikvam, A., Kvan, E., & Aursnes, I. (2002). Use of cardiovascular drugs after acute myocardial infarction: A marked shift towards evidence-based drug therapy. *Cardiovascular drugs and therapy/sponsored by the International Society of Cardiovascular Pharmacotherapy, 16*(5), 451–456.

Rello, J., Lorente, C., Bodí, M., Diaz, E., Ricart, M., & Kollef, M. H. (2002). Why do physicians not follow evidence-based guidelines for preventing ventilator-associated pneumonia?: A survey based on the opinions of an international panel of intensivists. *Chest, 122*(2), 656–661.

Richmond, T., & Byers, J. F. (2000). *Inquiring minds want to know: Moving from clinical problems to solutions.* Paper presented at the American Association of Critical Care Nurses National Teaching Institute, Orlando, FL.

Rosswurm, M. A., & Larrabee, J. H. (1999). A model for change to evidence-based practice. *Image: Journal of Nursing Scholarship, 31*(4), 317–322.

Sackett, D., Rosenberg, W. M. C., Muir-Gray, J. A., Haynes, R. B., & Richardson, W. S. (1996). Evidence based medicine: What it is and what it isn't. *British Medical Journal, 312*(13), 71–72.

Schumacher, D. N., Stock, J. R., & Richards, J. K. (2003). Evidence-based medicine: A model structure for multi-hospital systems. *Journal for Healthcare Quality: Official Publication of the National Association for Healthcare Quality, 25*(4), 10–15.

Schwartz, K., Northrup, J., Israel, N., Crowell, K., Lauder, N., & Neale, A. V. (2003). Use of online evidence-based resources at the point of care. *Family Medicine, 35*, 251–256.

Scullion, P. A. (2002). Effective dissemination strategies. *Nurse Researcher, 10*(1), 65–78.

Silagy, C. A., Wellner, D. P., Lapsley, H., Middleton, P., Shelby-James, T., & Fazekas, B. (2002). The effectiveness of local adaptation of nationally produced clinical practice guidelines. *Family Practice, 19*(3), 223–230.

Singer, M. (2002). Evidence-based medicine: CON. *The Journal of the Intensive Care Society, 3*(3), 80–81.

Sitzia, J. (2002). Barriers to research utilisation: The clinical setting and nurses themselves. *Intensive & Critical Care Nursing: The Official Journal of the British Association of Critical Care Nurses, 18*(4), 230–243.

Stetler, C. B. (2001). Updating the Stetler model of research utilization to facilitate evidenced-based practice. *Nursing Outlook, 49*(6), 272–279.

Straus, S. E., & Sackett, D. (1998). Getting research findings into practice: Using research findings in clinical practice. *British Medical Journal, 317,* 339–342.

Titler, M. G., & Everett, L. Q. (2001). Translating research into practice: Considerations for critical care investigators. *Critical Care Nursing Clinics of North America, 13*(4), 587–604.

Titler, M. G., Kleiber, C., Steelman, V., Goode, C., Rakel, B., Barry-Walker, J., et al. (1994). Infusing research into practice to promote quality care. *Nursing Research, 43*(5), 307–313.

Titler, M. G., Steelman, V., Budreau, G., Buckwalter, K., & Goode, C. J. (2001). The Iowa model of evidence-based practice to promote quality care. *Critical Care Nursing Clinics of North America, 13*(4), 497–509.

Tonelli, M. (2001). The limits of evidence-based medicine. *Respiratory Care, 46*(12), 1435–1440.

Chapter 5

Putting Patients in Charge of Their Health Care to Promote Patient Safety

Tania Daniels

INFORMED AND ENGAGED PATIENTS

Doctors, nurses, pharmacists, and other health care professionals continuously strive to keep patient safety a priority. However, when interventions or events do not proceed as planned, medical errors can occur. Errors occur in all health care settings such as clinics, surgery centers, pharmacies, hospitals, and even in the home. Because of the widespread settings in which errors occur, patients play a vital role in partnering with caregivers to make health care as safe as possible.

There is a positive correlation between people who are actively involved in their own health care and better outcomes (Kaplan, Greenfield, Gandek, Rogers, & Ware, 1996). This means not only should patients have more information, but they should be active partners in their health care by making decisions about their care. Patients are more likely to follow the treatment plan when they are involved in the decision making process and understand the plan. In order to be engaged in making decisions, patients and family members are responsible for learning as much as they can about their health prior to their health care visit and to ask questions about proposed treatments and medications.

Preparing Patients for Health Care Visits

Consumers actively seek health care information from a variety of resources including friends and family, health plans, the Internet, magazines and newspapers—even though physicians are still the primary and most trusted source of health care information (Voluntary Hospitals of America [VHA], 2000). To prepare for health care visits, consumers should gather reliable information about their condition and potential treatments or tests from a variety of sources including the library, specialty associations, reliable Web sites, or even support groups. They should write down questions and concerns and bring notes to their health care visit. Patients need to share information they have obtained with their physician or primary caregiver, and also honestly share information about themselves, including sensitive topics such as substance abuse, so the practitioner has all of the needed information for diagnosis and treatment. Without a complete patient history the physician or primary caregiver may not accurately diagnose a condition or may prescribe inappropriate medications thereby contributing to an adverse event. This is more likely to occur when the patient does not report over-the-counter medications, alternative therapies, or medications ordered by other practitioners.

During the health care visit, patients should write down key points to help guide information gathering and improving the ability to recall instructions. Relying solely on memory can lead to errors related to following directions and instructions on medications or other treatments. Visiting a physician's office often contributes to emotional distress and an inability to focus on the information presented. As part of gathering information, consumers should consider seeking more than one opinion, especially for invasive and/or surgical procedures, and in many cases a second opinion is a requirement of some insurers.

Asking Questions

By researching specific health care topics prior to the appointment, patients will be prepared to ask relevant questions, and patients and their family members should be encouraged to raise any concerns. Patients should feel comfortable asking for clarification when answers are not sufficient. Caregiver answers should be delivered in easy to understand terms that the average layperson recognizes.

PATIENT AND PROVIDER COMMUNICATION

A trusting relationship with providers and open, two-way communication is needed for the best care possible. Consumers must be open, honest, and willing to share relevant information by discussing all acute and chronic health conditions, medications, nutritional supplements, and health habits with their health care provider. In return, patients should expect their provider to be open and honest as well. Honest communication with patients, especially in reporting adverse events and errors, has been demonstrated to reduce the risk of lawsuits and increase patients' positive perception of care. "Physicians who attract a disproportionate share of lawsuits tend to have difficulty connecting with patients. In fact, 75% to 85% of awards and settlement costs over a five-year period were made on behalf of just 8% of surgeons, 6% of obstetricians and 1.8% of internists" (Hickson, 2001).

High-quality care depends on shared understanding between physicians and patients regarding the nature of the medical problem and an agreed upon approach to addressing it. One in four patients confessed to not following the doctor's advice on a treatment plan or recommended test because they did not agree with the doctor, or the plan did not consider their personal preferences, beliefs, or other life situations. The end result was these patients did not feel as involved in the decision-making process as they wanted and therefore they did not follow the needed plan (The Commonwealth Fund, 2002). Unfortunately, these patients are often termed "noncompliant" rather than involving the patient in decision making about their care and seeking a mutually agreed on plan.

It is important that the patient understand his/her medical condition, tests, and treatment. Patients should be given information on the expected duration of the condition, resources to obtain more information, and if appropriate, the condition's etiology(ies). Often, the patient can be overwhelmed with the amount of information presented and it is helpful to have written materials to refer to later. Clinical pathways are helpful education tools for patients and can be used to identify treatments with the patient's role and the role of the health care team's daily expectations made clear.

A Case for Disclosure After an Unanticipated Event

Should patients be told when an error occurs? At the Annenberg III Patient Safety Conference in 2001, Hickson reported that 32% of patients' families sue doctors because they were advised to do so by someone influential, such as an attorney; 24% sue because they believe there was a cover-up; and another 20% sue because they feel they need information that the caregivers won't provide. "The single greatest error in health care is failure of communication" (Hickson, 2001).

There is both a business case and an ethical case for being honest with patients and families after an adverse event. The Lexington Veterans Affairs (VA) Medical Center has taken a first step to demonstrate the business case. The center implemented a risk management policy in 1987 requiring full disclosure, which resulted in a decrease in the average malpractice costs. The median medical malpractice settlement in 1999 at Lexington was $98,150; in the private sector it was $497,412, a fourfold increase. In 2000, 28% of Lexington's cases were settled without trial; the remaining 72% were denied (Kraman, Hamm, & Reynolds, 2001).

Health care professionals have a moral responsibility to be honest with their patients that is usually part of a code of ethics. In recent years the ethical responsibility has been strengthened with regulations and accreditation standards. Chapter 9 offers a detailed discussion on reporting errors and adverse events. The following case study from The Lexington VA Medical Center further demonstrates the ethical case of reporting.

Case of Medical Error

A long-term patient with a severe clotting disorder had been on several anticlotting drugs like Warfarin without success. The doctor prescribed injectable Heparin on an outpatient basis. The patient's daughter picked up her father's prescriptions at a VA pharmacy. She had been shown visually how to put enough Heparin in the syringe.

In the beginning, the Heparin was supplied in small vials. Then, one shipment from the pharmacy contained large bottles. In January and February of 1997, things started happening. There was a call from the home health nurse to the primary care clinic. The nurse discovered that the patient had been taking wrong doses of Heparin.

The patient's daughter called a few days later saying her father was in respiratory trouble. He died a few days later; the doctor said it was probably due to a pulmonary embolism. After visiting the patient's home and reviewing the medication vials, it was discovered that some of the bottles said 1,000 units per ml, and others said 10,000 units.

1000 vs. 10,000 Units of Heparin

Checking the prescriptions at the pharmacy revealed that the prescription was written for 10,000 units; but two pharmacists made an identical error on two separate occasions, dispensing 1,000 units instead of 10,000. [The comma in "10,000" had inadvertently been left out on the written prescription.] The difference in dosage was what caused the patient's death.

The Daughter's Perspective

"When Dad was in the ER, I was on a mission," she began. "I was gonna make somebody pay for what they did, because I killed him with those shots."

"Three weeks after Dad died, the VA called and they sent the nurse and Ms. Hamm to see me. Ms. Hamm told me, 'Sandy, you were right. We killed your dad.' I had not shed one tear from the day he died until that day. When she said that, it was like something was taken off of me."

"It makes such a difference when someone says, 'I'm sorry.' I hope just one person understands that it's not about money, it's about being able to heal, to be rid of that anger that eats at you like a cancer" (Kraman, Hamm, & Reynolds, 2001).

PATIENT-CENTERED CARE

The Institute of Medicine (IOM) proposed patient-centered care as one of the six aims for a new health system in the twenty-first century; this concept must first be defined (Committee on Quality of Health Care in America, 2001). Patient-centered care means being respectful and responsive to individual patient preferences, perspectives, values, needs, and beliefs (MAPS, 2002). These aspects should guide clinical decisions, and allow the patient to be involved with their health care decisions as much as they desire, since the level of involvement may vary according to patient preferences and severity of illness. Patient-centeredness also includes customized care with the ability of caregivers to be sensitive to the physical, emotional, and spiritual healing environment provided for patients.

Patients as the Center of the Health Care Team

To succeed at providing patient-centered care, health care organizations must recognize and include patients as members of the team. Patients, family members, and health care professionals need to work together to achieve the best care possible. The Joint Commission on Accreditation of Healthcare Organizations (JCAHO) and the Centers for Medicare and Medicaid Services (CMS) launched a "Speak Up" campaign in April 2002. This educational campaign is intended to reduce errors by increasing patient involvement in care and educating them on key safety issues. More information can be found at www.jcaho.org. In fact, JCAHO Standard PF.3.7 requires patients and their families to play a role in helping health care organizations facilitate the safe delivery of care, and the facility's education efforts should include information on the patient's responsibilities in their own care (JCAHO, 2003). The Agency for Healthcare Research and Quality (AHRQ) also developed *Five Steps to Safer Healthcare* and *Twenty Tips to Help Prevent Medical Errors* among its publications to educate consumers on their role in patient safety (AHRQ, 2003).

Shared Decision Making

Patient-centered care includes six clinical components (Stewart, et al., 1995):

- Exploring both the disease and the illness experience
- Understanding the whole person
- Finding common ground for management of the condition
- Incorporating prevention and health promotion
- Enhancing the doctor-patient relationship
- Being realistic

Shared decision making is a component of patient-centered care that focuses on identifying agreement on the medical management of the disease and illness. Shared decision-making implies participation by both the clinician and patient. The clinician provides information on treatment options, and respects the patient's preference to choose among treatment options (Wensing, Elwyn, Edwards, Vingerhoets, & Grol, 2002). This model of care is participative rather than a traditional paternalistic model. It respects the autonomy of the patient as a partner in care. This role is mediated by the patient's ability to participate and desire to take an active role. Many patients prefer the physician to direct the care and are not comfortable with taking an active role, while other patients assume a stronger role in their care.

Although it is ideal to have patient involvement and better patient adherence as a result, it is a difficult task to achieve. Promoting the patient's understanding is key to achieving informed decision-making. There are seven criteria for ethical, informed decision-making (Braddock III, Edwards, Hasenberg, Laidley, & Levinson, 1999):

- Discussion of the patient's role in decision-making
- Nature of decision
- Alternatives
- Benefits and risks of alternatives
- Uncertainties associated with decision
- Assessment of patient understanding of the decision
- Exploration of patient preferences

Informed decision-making that meets the seven criteria is as low as 9% in many cases (Braddock, Edwards, Hasenberg, Laidley, & Levinson, 1999).

Consent Forms

Informed decision making often requires a consent form. The purpose of obtaining informed consent is to ensure the patient understands the procedure and associated risks and benefits (AHRQ, 2001). This is both ethically and legally required of physicians. The consent process allows patients to decide, along with their care provider, whether to undergo a treatment or procedure. The American Medical Association (AMA) professional guidelines require that patients be informed of the nature of their condition, the proposed procedure, the purpose of the procedure, the risks and benefits associated with the procedure, the alternatives, and the potential risks of not receiving the recommended treatment or procedure. In addition to professional organization standards for informed consent, there may be state regulations or practice acts that address the topic.

Fewer than 40% of consent forms support models of shared decision-making (Bottrell, Alpert, Fischbach, & Emanuel, 2000). Traditional procedures to obtain informed consent do not promote patient-physician interaction and dialogue. In fact, 69% of patients do not even read consent forms before signing (Lavelle-Jones, Byrne, Rice, & Cuschieri, 1993). A more complete description of informed consent is found in the chapter 9 discussion of risk management issues, and informed consent for research subjects is discussed in chapter 15.

Does having detailed information about surgery discourage patients from having needed procedures?

Communication is an essential part of the social contract between physician and patient, as well as risk analysis and risk management (Fischhoff, 2001).

Fifteen percent of patients who are candidates for carotid endarterectomy should decline after learning about the risk of death (Merz, Fischhoff, Mazur, & Fischbeck, 1993).

Effective communication requires a systematic analysis of the patient's information needs. It is important to utilize available research and evaluate each patient's situation (Fischhoff, 2001).

SOCIODEMOGRAPHIC FACTORS

Many factors impact the patient's involvement in their care. One in four patients did not follow their doctor's advice because they disagreed with their doctor, the procedure was too costly, or the advice conflicted with their personal beliefs (Davis, et al., 2002). Sociodemographic factors that influence health care outcomes include age, education, gender, and culture.

Age

Older Adults

Significantly more consumers age 55 and older depend on their doctors rather than seek information from other sources, as compared with consumers age 25–34. Only 1 in 63 consumers age 25–34 relied solely on their doctor for health care information (VHA, 2000). Nearly 66% of United States (U.S.) adults over age 60 have inadequate or marginal literacy skills, compared with 50% of the general U.S. population. Up to 25% of older adults report having difficulty reading written information provided by their doctor (Center for Health Care Strategies, Inc. [CHCS], 1997a).

Certain medicines are considered high-risk for the elderly and are listed in the *Merck Manual of Geriatrics* (Merck & Co. Inc., 2000). As patients age, their metabolism slows and kidney and liver function may be impaired so that patients require lower doses of medicine to achieve therapeutic benefits. When multiple medications are prescribed, it is therefore recommended that the physician or pharmacist review medications every six months. One in five Americans over 65 takes at least one inappropriate prescription drug (American Association of Retired Persons [AARP], 2003). See chapter 13 for more discussion on this population.

Not only are the elderly vulnerable to incorrect dosages of medications, they also face challenges in taking medications as prescribed. According to the American Pharmacy Association, patients should be encouraged to take medicine in well-lit areas so they can clearly read the label. Other aids can be used to take medicines safely such as containers marked with days of the week with daily doses prepared for each day. Calendars, timers, and other tools can also be used. All patients can encounter difficulties with taking medications correctly, but the elderly may be more susceptible to mistakes because of problems with eyesight, memory, and manual dexterity.

Children

Each type of patient population is at risk for errors or adverse events due to unique characteristics. Rates of medication errors and adverse drug events for hospitalized children are comparable to rates for hospitalized adults. However, the rate for potential adverse drug events has been reported as three times higher in children and substantially higher still for babies in neonatal intensive care units (Kaushal, et al., 2001). This research indicates the importance of a parent's role in being engaged and vigilant and to be the watchful eyes for their child's safety. Refer to chapter 10 for further discussion of pediatric patient safety.

Education

Most health care information is printed at a twelfth-grade reading level or higher, even though the average U.S. adult reads at an eighth-grade level.

Patients prefer simple and easy to understand health care information. Content should be limited to those aspects that patients need to know to safely follow instructions. Adult education theory proposes that adults prefer information that helps solve their problems, rather than background information (Ad Hoc Committee on Health Literacy for the Council on Scientific Affairs of the American Medical Association, 1999).

Consumers rarely rely on their physician as their sole source of information and actively seek other resources to help them become more involved in their care. However, this varies by education level. Significantly more consumers with a high-school education or less depend on their doctors rather than seeking information from other sources (VHA, 2000). Patients with higher education levels seek out information from other sources such as the Internet.

Gender

Gender differences are also a consideration for patient safety. For example, gender differences should be considered when prescribing drugs. Women have a different metabolism than men and are often smaller in size. This may be one reason that women are often more sensitive to the same dose of the same medication than men. For example, the 1997 withdrawal of the antihistamine Seldane® occurred because of heart problems that occurred primarily in women (American Association of Retired Persons [AARP], 2003). Providers should be sure to explain to patients if there are expected gender differences when prescribing and administering medication. Another condition that impacts women is heart disease. Patient education for women with heart disease may vary from what is taught to men due to the different presentation of symptoms of the same condition.

Ethnicity

The majority of drug trials are performed on Caucasians. But differences in genes can affect the body's reaction to a drug. For example, studies show that four times the amount of Prilosec® accumulates in the blood stream and lasts 50% longer in Asian Americans as it does in Caucasians. Providers should be sure to consider pharmaceutical dose adjustments in various patient populations to ensure safety (AARP, 2003).

HEALTH ILLITERACY

Illiteracy in the U.S. is more prevalent than most health care providers recognize. Forty-two percent of patients in one study were unable to comprehend directions for not taking medication on an empty stomach, 26% could not understand appointment information, and 60% could not understand a consent form (Ad Hoc Committee on Health Literacy for the Council on Scientific Affairs of the American Medical Association, 1999). Low literacy is associated with poorer self-reported health, less knowledge of self-care, increased doctor visits, and greater hospitalization rates.

Health literacy includes the ability to perform basic reading and numerical tasks required to function in the health care environment. Patients with adequate health literacy can read, understand, and act appropriately on health care information. Patients with inadequate health literacy are five times more likely to misinterpret their medication prescriptions. Studies show a strong positive correlation between health literacy and knowledge of illness. In fact, literacy is a stronger correlate of health status than education, age, or race (Ad Hoc Committee on Health Literacy for the Council on Scientific Affairs of the American Medical Association, 1999).

According to the AMA, nearly 50% of adult Americans have inadequate literacy skills. These 90 million adults have difficulty with or are unable to read and understand health consent forms, patient rights statements, appointment forms, and medication labels. In addition, less than half of the adult U.S. population understands many commonly used medical words. Despite these facts, only 2% of physicians assess their patient's understanding of instructions (Braddock, Fihn, Levinson, Jonsen, & Pearlman, 1997). One strategy to overcome this barrier is to assess literacy levels. There are screening tools, such as the Rapid Estimate of Adult Literacy in Medicine (REALM), Test of Functional Health Literacy in Adults (TOFHLA) and the shortened version of the TOFHLA (S–TOFHLA). The REALM tool can provide an approximate grade level of reading in three minutes (Ad Hoc Committee on Health Literacy for the Council on Scientific Affairs of the American Medical Association, 1999).

Patients typically are ashamed to admit to illiteracy, supported by the fact that 67% have never even told their spouse. Providers can make a difference in reducing the stigma associated with illiteracy when they ensure the patient understands medication labels, consent forms, follow-up instructions, and other health care forms by reviewing instructions, having the patient verbalize or demonstrate instructions, or conducting a follow-up call to check understanding and compliance. There is limited

TABLE 5.1   Improving Health Care Communication

Improve Verbal Communication	Modify Written Language
Speak slowly	Material should be no higher than a 4th
Provide only 2–3 concepts at a time	to 5th grade level
Use layperson terms	Use pictures or diagrams
Have patient repeat instructions	Use common words rather than medical
	terms
	Focus on two to three key concepts
	Emphasize desired behavior/outcome
	rather than specific medical information

AMA Discussion Guide, 1999.

research addressing effective solutions to improve health literacy, however communication and health educators recommend some of the strategies in Table 5.1, Improving Health Care Communication.

Thirty-four percent of English speaking, 50% of Hispanics, 40% of African Americans, and 33% of Asian Americans have literacy problems (AMA Health Literacy Introductory Kit, 1999). Simply translating written materials into multiple languages will not reach the diverse populations in the U.S. Much of the population within each culture is not functionally literate. More effective strategies may include use of multiple media such as video, audio, or cable television.

'NOTHING ABOUT ME WITHOUT ME'

The Institute for Healthcare Improvement (IHI) instituted the "Nothing About Me Without Me" program in 1999. Recommendations for policies and practices include the involvement of patient and family in every decision. Patients should be encouraged and educated to participate in the care and decision-making process to the extent they are willing and able. Patients, families, and staff who perceive a risk to safety should have the right to stop the process at any time and ask questions (Berwick, 1999). This program has been expanded by the National Patient Safety Foundation in 2003 as a national agenda of the organization.

Patients and family members should pay attention to the health care they receive. They need to agree on exactly what the care will be; know who will be taking care of them; how long the treatment or test will last;

and how they should expect to feel. Patients should receive health care knowing they will be encouraged to be involved in every step.

PATIENT'S ROLES AND RESPONSIBILITIES

How can we close the gap between patients who do not actively participate with health care decisions and those patients who are actively engaged with all aspects of their health care? There are specific ways that patients can be involved in their care to help reduce the risk of a medical error. First and foremost, patient and family partnerships are essential in all aspects of health care. Patients should appoint a spokesperson, advocate, or legally designated surrogate in the event that they are unable to be active decision makers. Patients should ask questions about their care and look for practitioners and settings that will best meet their needs and preferences. Selections for a health care facility and provider should be based on criteria such as ample experience and successful outcomes with the recommended treatment, procedure, or test. Patients should ask the provider the number of procedures performed, the percentage of positive outcomes, as well as the number of complications, expected or unexpected. Patients tend to have better results when they are treated in hospitals that have a great deal of experience with their condition (McGrath, et al., 2000).

When being discharged from a health care facility or leaving a health care appointment, patients should be sure they understand orders, medications and schedule, activity level, treatment plan, follow-up appointment, and expected outcomes. This impacts the patient's ability to properly follow their treatment.

If any concerns arise, patients should be encouraged to seek a second opinion to instill confidence that the recommended treatment is right for them. Open communication is essential. Patients should tell their health care professional if something does not seem right. If it does not feel right, then something may be amiss, and additional discussion should ensue. Patients have a right to ask questions of anyone involved in their care. This is especially important when multiple health professionals are involved. The patient's personal physician is the leader of the health care team and is responsible for coordinating the overall care process and communication. It is the patient's responsibility to learn about the care and treatment prescribed.

Appoint a Patient Advocate

Being active and engaged during times of medical illness or hospitalization can be difficult, stressful, and tiring. For this reason it is recommended that patients have an advocate—someone who can help by taking notes, asking questions, making sure the right things are done at the right time, speaking up if the patient cannot, and assisting with continuity of information and care. Overall, the patient advocate assumes the role of acting in the patient's best interest and helping to ensure the patient receives the best care possible (Minnesota Alliance for Patient Safety [MAPS], 2002).

Health care facilities often have a patient representative that serves as a professional advocate. Patients may want to ask a family member or friend to act on their behalf, to ensure their wishes are carried out, and be the family spokesperson during health care visits and hospitalizations. The patient advocate's name and contact information should be documented and communicated to the health care team and other family members to prevent any miscommunication about wishes.

The JCAHO Speak Up! Campaign recommends that an advocate stay overnight in the hospital, since family members and friends can also offer comfort and support during stressful times. Advocates should also be allowed to accompany the patient to tests, appointments, and procedures, if the patient requests.

Medication Safety

Only 50% of all patients take medications as directed, so medication safety is definitely an important health concern (CHCS, 1997b). Medication tips to educate patients include: timing, form, dose, pharmacies, costs, food cautions, sharing medical history, and checking medications.

Timing

The hour of day to take a drug can greatly alter its effectiveness based on circadian rhythms, hormonal cycles, and release of chemicals in the body during a 24-hour cycle. Studies indicate there is a 40% higher risk of heart attack and 49% higher risk of stroke in the morning, so it is essential to educate patients when to take their medicine so it is working at its peak effectiveness when needed most (AARP, 2003). Timing of medications is also critical for specific conditions such as diabetes. Timing is important not only for effectiveness but also because it can contribute to adverse events when prescribed medications are given along with over-the-counter medications, thus enhancing or limiting the therapeutic benefit. Timing may also precipitate problems based on sleep habits. For example diuretics and laxatives taken in the evening may create urgency at night and cause slips and falls to the bathroom in the middle of the night.

Form

Medication should be taken as prescribed. According to the American Pharmacy Association, if pills are crushed and put into liquid, some drugs become less effective. Other drugs have slow release actions and if these medications are crushed, chewed, or capsules opened, the body absorbs the medicine too quickly. There are a few drugs that should never be crushed including all extended release drugs such as Procardia XL®, aspirin, and nitroglycerin (AARP, 2003). The form of the medication can precipitate errors if instructions are not clear. For example, liquid medications can be given via several routes such as oral, in the ears, in the eyes, or applied topically, and the form of the medication is not self-evident. So the form of the medication and the manner of modifying the form and administration must all be communicated precisely.

Dose

The American Pharmacy Association also describes cautions for the right way to measure doses of medications. For liquid medications, many patients use household teaspoons, which often do not hold a true teaspoon of liquid. Special devices, such as marked syringes, help measure the correct dose. Being instructed on the use of the devices improves the patient's ability to measure medicine accurately. Be sure to explain the dose clearly. For example, does "four doses daily" mean the patient should take a dose every six hours around the clock or just during regular waking hours? If the prescription requires splitting the medicine, be sure the patient uses a pill splitter and does not split the drug in advance, as it may affect the medication (AARP, 2003). Because medication costs have increased, some groups have advocated splitting pills to save money. Not all pills can be safely split, so the health care provider should review the manner in which the patient is to take their medicine and discuss which pills have been approved to be safe for splitting.

Pharmacies

The patient should obtain all prescription medications at one pharmacy. This allows the pharmacist to be a knowledgeable partner in preventing medication errors. By developing a relationship with the patient, pharmacists can document the patient's history and medication record, and can monitor therapy and provide education.

Costs

According to the Food and Drug Administration (FDA) (2002), there are no differences in the active ingredients of generic medicines compared with brand medicines. Generic brands often cost significantly less than brand-name drugs. Drugs that have been on the market for a period of time are less expensive. Also, drug prices vary from pharmacy to pharmacy, so patients should shop around before choosing one pharmacy. As of June 2002, there is a prescription savings service available through a Medicare program called "Together Rx" at www.together-rx.com or (800) 865-7211. The program offers discounts on products from major drug companies. Many other organizations also offer services with discounted drugs (www.aarppharmacy.com). Additional Medicare drug benefits will be implemented between now and 2006.

Food Cautions

Potential food and drug interactions may occur with many medications. For example, asparagus, broccoli, and spinach are high in Vitamin K, which promotes blood clotting. This can neutralize the effect of anticoagulants (AARP, 2003). Patients should be informed which medicines should be taken with food as this varies the absorption rate. For example, if the osteoporosis drug Fosamax® is taken with food, it will reduce the absorption rate by half (AARP, 2003).

Sharing Medication History

It is imperative that patients write down and communicate their medication information to all caregivers, since some drugs can complicate certain conditions. For example, many bronchodilators can be dangerous when taken by patients with heart disease, high blood pressure, or diabetes (FDA, 2003). Patients should share information on all prescriptive medicines, over-the-counter medicines, and alternative medicines or herbals with all of their health care providers. Many of these drugs will interact with medicines and other treatments. There is less research on alternative medications and herbals and unfortunately several complications have been identified after a thorough review of the interactions of all medications consumed by the patient.

Checking Medicines

Patient identification, medication type and dose, and patient allergies should be double-checked. The patient should bring medicines or a list to appointments, including over-the-counter, herbal, or dietary drugs to have them reviewed for safety. When filling a prescription from the pharmacy, patients should examine their purchase to make sure it is the right medicine.

Prior to leaving an appointment, patients should know what the prescribed medication looks like; why they are taking it; what to expect from taking the drug; how much to take; when and how to take it; when to discontinue it; what to do if they miss a dose; if they should discontinue any current medications; and how they should store it.

Health care providers should provide written information about the side effects the medicine could cause. Patients, who are instructed about expected drug actions, will be better prepared for normal responses and side effects. If something unexpected happens patients can report the problem right away and get help before the drug side effect gets worse.

Prevent Infections

Hand washing is the most important way to prevent the spread of infections (Boyce & Pittet, 2002), yet, it is not done regularly or thoroughly enough. Studies find that the health care worker compliance rate with good hygiene practice is at 25–50% (JCAHO, 2001). Refer to chapter 11 for further discussion of this topic.

Safe Surgery

The more patients know before surgery, the more they can prepare and be involved, which will lead to a better experience. Being informed and getting ready for surgery makes for a faster recovery (National Institute on Aging [NIA], 2002). Patients should ask their surgeon questions such as how many of these operations have been done successfully; what is the success rate of the operation; how many of these surgeries has this surgeon performed; what kinds of problems or pain can be expected; will they be staying in the hospital over night; how long is the expected recovery; will they be receiving rehabilitation; and is there a process in place for the surgical team to conduct a final verification for safety prior to the start of the surgery (NIA, 2002)?

Strategies to reduce the risk of wrong-site surgery include involving the patient with marking the surgical site. There must be a process to monitor compliance with policies and procedures set to eliminate wrong surgeries (JCAHO, 2003). Chapter 11 discusses this in more detail.

DO CONSUMERS USE INFORMATION TO MAKE INFORMED DECISIONS?

Physicians are typically the central source of reliable information, along with personal recommendations from friends and family. A national survey performed by the Kaiser Family Foundation and the AHRQ (Kaiser Family Foundation, 1996) indicated that seven out of ten people regard their family and friends as good sources of health care information. When making health care decisions, personal recommendations from family, friends, or physician are the most likely information used. When it comes to making health care choices, personal recommendations weigh heavier than comparative quality information. Seventy-six percent of consumers would see a surgeon they know over one they do not know, even if the latter had reports of much higher quality ratings. Seventy-two percent of consumers would go to a hospital they are familiar with over a hospital that has ranked much higher in quality. In fact, when there is information indicating poor or below average quality, 39% of consumers would not choose a different hospital if they had a previous positive experience with that hospital (Kaiser Family Foundation, 1996).

However, consumers are beginning to consider objective information such as the use of evidence-based treatment plans and whether or not expected outcomes are achieved (VHA, 2000). Refer to chapter 4 for more information on evidence-based practices.

Nearly 50% of consumers are turning to printed materials while 26% are obtaining information on the Internet (Davis, et al., 2002). However, most data available to date have a purpose for internal quality improvement, not providing comparative information to the public. Quality health care information is very complex and difficult for consumers to translate into meaningful information. It is essential that information made public have an explanation of the purpose, value, and how to appropriately use the information.

Report Cards

Public and private groups are working on ways to measure and report the quality of health care. This will equip health care consumers with comparative information to allow them to make informed decisions. Some organizations are providing hospital specific quality information, such as Health Care Choices, a New York not-for-profit corporation dedicated to educating the public about the nation's health care system. The Health Care Choice Web site (see web resources) provides hospital-specific volume data on breast cancer, cardiac, colon cancer, esophageal cancer, lung cancer, pancreatic cancer, and stomach cancer surgeries for California, Florida, Iowa, Illinois, Maryland, New Jersey, and New York. The site also provides information on research. For example, the site provides breast cancer surgical volume data and links to resources that cite a correlation between higher hospital volumes and better patient outcomes for breast cancer surgery (Health Care Choices, 2003).

Despite the publication of hospital specific quality data, consumer research indicates that patient satisfaction surveys are more influential than objective quality information. Forty-five percent of Americans indicate that after personal recommendations from physicians, friends, and family members, the information on patient experiences and attitudes from consumer surveys are the most influential resource. Only 39% of Americans reported seeing quality comparative information in the last year. Of those persons, 83% say the information would be useful, although only 30% have actually used it (Kaiser Family Foundation, 1996).

Patient Satisfaction Surveys

Almost every health care organization surveys patients to assess their experience during their health care visit. In fact, CMS is in the process of developing a nationally standardized patient satisfaction tool for hospitals called the Hospital Consumer Assessment of Health Plans Survey (HCAHPS, 2002) to give consumers the ability to compare hospital specific patient satisfaction data. This information has typically been used for internal quality improvement processes. However, more recently organizations have begun to publish this data to provide consumers comparative information.

The Massachusetts Health Quality Partnership (MHQP) utilizes patient satisfaction data to measure quality performance. The MHQP, established in 1995 to develop health care performance measurements for public accountability, surveyed 600 hospitalized patients in 1998. The hospital-specific results are posted on their Web site at www.mhqp.org. Other states have publicly reported data for consumers, such as California, Pennsylvania, and Florida, but there is no standard format, system, or conditions reported which makes it difficult for patients to interpret these data.

Medical Records

Personal medical records are another way to provide patients information. By allowing patients access to their own health records containing information about their medical condition and treatment options, they are more likely to be active partners in their care, understand their condition, and comply with a recommended treatment plan. However, some debate exists that allowing patients access to their medical records might cause health care professionals to alter the information. In addition, it might be difficult for a patient to appropriately understand and interpret what they read. Some states require patient access, while other states leave it to the professional to deem appropriateness and level of access. In Britain, providers are mandated to allow patients full access to their medical records (AHRQ, 2001).

Direct-to-Consumer Marketing

Since the Food and Drug Administration (FDA) relaxed restrictions on pharmaceutical companies direct-to-consumer (DTC) marketing in 1997, there has been a significant increase in the number of advertisements for medications in magazines and on radio and television. There are both pros and cons to DTC marketing. It provides more information to consumers on treatment alternatives; however it can also interfere with the patient/physician relationship. As a result of DTC marketing, if physicians do not recommend the patient's desired medication, 46% of patients will try to persuade their physician to prescribe, and another 24% will attempt to obtain, requested drugs from another physician (AHRQ, 2001). DTC marketing also encourages the prescription of new, latest generation medications. This is not necessarily advantageous for positive patient outcomes. Newer medications have a less well-known side effect profile, cost more, and may be no more effective than older medications. In the case of antibiotics, they may promote development of medication resistant bacteria.

PATIENT EDUCATION

There are a number of resources and practices available to engage the patient as an active participant with their health care decisions. The purpose is not to shift the burden to patients, but to encourage a shared responsibility for their safety (AHRQ, 2001).

Tools for Patients

Medical Information Cards

Many organizations have made available medication or medical information cards. Cards are a good resource for patients to track key medical information such as medication lists, emergency contact information, allergies, medication "do not take" lists, immunization records, and important medical history. This serves as a communication tool to share health care information. Organizations such as the National Council on Patient Information and Education (NCPIE) also make medical information cards available in large print, English, Spanish, and other languages by calling (301) 656-8565.

Personal Health Guides

There are pocket-sized consumer booklets for adults and children that help track key health care information such as immunizations, blood pressure, growth/weight, and cholesterol. Tools such as AHRQ's "Put Prevention Into Practice" provide additional preventive information on topics such as diabetes, nutrition, and activity. Consumers can receive a free copy by calling (800) 358-9295.

Decision Support Tools

Decision support tools can help consumers identify their interests, needs, and values relative to their decision. These tools help consumers focus on what is important for their decision. Support can be described as directive support or non-directive support. Directive support explicitly points consumers to choices that seem best for them. This may be in the form of a worksheet or a computer-aided application that ranks the best choices based on the consumer's response to a set of questions. This type of decision aid can be very sophisticated incorporating the patient's responses to formulate a decision, or they can be basic. For example, a computer application tool called "The Decision Helper" provides information on types of health plans, benefits, costs, and providers. It is also designed to help people navigate through Consumer Assessment of Health Plans Survey (CAHPS) results. These tools can add value, but they can be time consuming for the patient to use, which may limit their application (Talking Quality, 2003).

A less time consuming tool is non-directive support. This tool helps consumers identify the issues they need to consider, rather than asking questions that lead to a decision. This type of tool is often a list of questions or a checklist that identifies issues patients need to consider during the decision-making process such as "Your Guide to Choosing Quality Health Care" (AHRQ, 2002). This process does not guide consumers to reach a decision and it is unclear whether this type of tool helps consumers make better choices.

Health Care Information on the Internet

Consumers are turning to the Internet for medical information about health issues and medical problems. In fact, six million people log on to the Internet everyday in search of health information (Lewis, 2003). There are many Web sites available for health care information, some more reliable than others. Government sites such as the AHRQ and Healthfinder are considered reliable and provide health care information based on evidence. Refer to the Web Resources section at the end of this chapter for reliable Web-based consumer resources.

The following tips can be used to verify that information from non-government Web sites is reliable:

- Check the author's credentials and find out if he/she is affiliated with any major institutions

- Look for a site that is reviewed by a medical advisory group
- Review the organization's purpose and goal
- Make sure the information is current
- Check for resources of cited medical data and be wary of information that is provided for marketing purposes.

Dot.com Pharmacies

With more Americans turning to the Internet for health care information, some consumers are even buying prescription medicines online. The challenge is to make sure that the Internet site is reliable. CybeRx Smart Safety Coalition involves the National Council on Patient Information and Education, the FDA, consumers, and dot.com pharmacies as joint forces to educate Internet users on buying prescription medicines from reputable sites. The risks of online ordering include fake, unapproved, outdated, or substandard products; little or no quality control over packaging; purity of ingredients or storage; possibility of obtaining an inappropriate medicine; breach of patient confidentiality; and insecure transactions. Some sites even diagnose and prescribe online, which leads to a high chance of incorrect diagnosis or incorrect medicine prescription (NCPIE, 2002).

There are strategies to reduce these risks including meeting with your personal physician to obtain any new prescription. It is also key to verify that the online pharmacy is licensed through the National Association of Boards of Pharmacy (refer to the Web Resources section at the end of this chapter for more information). Internet consumers should be sure to report any problems to the FDA.

Specific precautions include instructions to **not**:

- (a) Buy online from sites that do not require an examination by a doctor
- (b) Buy online from sites that do not require a prescription
- (c) Provide any personal identifiable information
- (d) Buy from sites that do not provide citations with case histories (NCPIE, 2002)

Consumer Based Clinical Guidelines

Health care quality and helping people stay healthy and recover during illness varies across the country. The Institute of Medicine *Crossing the Quality Chasm* (2001) reports that even after 17 years when evidence-based practice has been scientifically proven, only 25% of clinicians use the practice. Clinical practice guidelines are a road map for evidence-based practice. The Web Resources section at the end of this chapter provide suggested Web sites for consumer based clinical practice guidelines. Refer to chapter 4 for more information on evidence-based practices.

ENGAGING CONSUMERS IS EVERYBODY'S ROLE

The IOM recommends that there be efforts put in place to increase public awareness of patient safety issues. The government, health plans, purchasers, and even employers are taking an active role.

Government's Role

The federal government is the primary agent that has put mechanisms in place to assure a safe health care system. There are many government initiatives underway, such as the establishment of the National Patient Safety Center and the creation of the National Quality Forum. The National Patient Safety Center coordinates and oversees safety activities across the U.S., particularly in the Veterans Affairs medical system. The National Quality Forum was created to develop consensus on standardized quality and patient safety measures. Information about these federal initiatives was discussed in chapter 2.

Government should also balance the role of public accountability with the role of creating an environment to support learning and prevent future medical accidents. The typical "blame" culture is misguided and counterproductive, and state and federal governments should develop regulations and guidelines that facilitate a blameless or nonpunitive reporting system to allow information on medical accidents to be shared so learning can occur from these situations and prevent future harm. The clinician's fear of discovery and punishment of accidents drives reporting underground and decreases organizational learning.

Health Plan's Role

The National Committee for Quality Assurance (NCQA, 1990) is a not-for-profit organization dedicated to measure and publicly report the quality of America's health care based on health plans. Through the Health Plan Employer Data Information Set (HEDIS), NCQA evaluates over 60 standards and performance measures. The measures provide information to consumers on member satisfaction, effectiveness of care, finances, and health plan activities to provide patients with information to compare health plans based on performance. NCQA posts HEDIS data results on a report card on their Web site at www.healthchoices.org.

Individual health plans such as HealthPartners of Minneapolis are also taking the lead on providing facility-specific safety and quality information to patients. HealthPartners assesses and makes public the quality of care provided by medical groups and hospitals, as rated by patient satisfaction and evidence-based clinical quality measures. Topics include heart disease, diabetes, preventive care, healthy lifestyle counseling, and smoking cessation education. Information is released publicly on their Web site at www.consumerchoices.com to give consumers information to make more informed health care choices. This is one example in which health plans are taking a proactive role to engage patients by providing comparative information to the public. There are many plans across the country that are also tackling this issue.

Purchaser's Role

The Leapfrog Group

Representing approximately 33 million health care consumers and composed of more than 130 public and private organizations, the Leapfrog Group aims to provide consumers information on three specific patient safety standards. The Leapfrog Group posts on their Web site whether or not hospitals meet the three following standards:

- *Computer Physician Order Entry (CPOE)*: Some studies show that a computerized prescription system can reduce serious medication mistakes by up to 88% (Bates, et al., 1999).
- *Evidence-Based Referrals*: Studies suggest that 4,500 lives could be saved each year if evidence-based hospital referrals were successfully implemented for the procedures and conditions selected by Leapfrog (Birkmeyer, Birkmeyer, Wennberg, & Young, 2000).
- *Intensivists*: Some studies have associated intensivist model intensive care units with lower mortality rates (Pronovost, Young, Dorman, Robinson, & Angus, 1999). (see also chapter 11).

By posting the results on their Web site, they are encouraging the employees of the organizations within Leapfrog Group organizations to choose hospitals that have implemented the three standards. Unfortunately, these standards are not widely agreed upon, and the information provided to consumers is limited in scope. The information is process-oriented rather than focused on outcomes, and does not provide patients with practical information to become engaged with their health care, nor does it provide a full picture of a hospital's safety.

The Pacific Business Group on Health (PBGH)

The PBGH is a nonprofit coalition of major California employers that focuses on quality, availability, and cost of health care. The coalition provides to patients hospitals, physicians, and health plans specific, comparative information. For example, hospitals are ranked based on a combination of hospital-specific data on surgery and treatment outcomes, patient satisfaction ratings on ability to meet patient needs, and the steps California hospitals have taken to reduce errors. To assess the ability of providers and hospitals to meet patient needs, patients are surveyed on their hospital experience. The survey addresses patient's perception on the hospital's ability to meet their personal preferences, coordinate care, provide physical and emotional comfort, involve family and friends, and ease the transition to home (Pacific Business Group on Health [PBGH], 2003).

Employer's Role

Employers can engage employees to become active in health care decisions by taking steps such as offering incentive programs for participating in wellness programs, providing more transparency with actual health plan prices, and offering innovative health packages.

Wellness Programs

Incentive-based wellness programs allow employees to earn points for smoking cessation, weight loss programs, and physical exercise programs that can accrue to buy benefits such as higher interest levels on their personal medical funds, waivers of plan premiums, frequent-flyer programs, fitness club benefits and even hotel vacation packages.

Health Care Premiums

It is likely that employees would be more engaged in the process of choosing health plans if health care premiums paralleled actual health care prices. Health insurance is very price sensitive. In fact, researchers of consumer-driven health care indicate that when all health plans are subsidized equally, consumers switch to lower-cost plans (Herzlinger, 2002).

Innovative Health Packages

Employers can offer health packages that allow their employees more flexibility with health care dollars through programs such as company-paid personal care accounts. For example, in 2001 Medtronic, a $5.5 billion medical device company headquartered in Minneapolis, offered personal care accounts (PCAs) to its employees. Medtronic contributed $2,000 to the employee's PCA and also paid 100% of preventive services. If employees chose a health package with a $3,000 deductible they would first use the $2,000 contributed to the PCA from Medtronic, then the employee would be responsible for the next $1,000 of expenses. Insurance would then cover any additional in-network health care costs. The PCA could also be used for any out-of-pocket expenses that typically are not covered by traditional health plans, such as prescriptions, weight loss plans, and eyeglasses. Unspent balances are rolled into the next year (Herzlinger, 2002).

AREAS FOR FUTURE RESEARCH

Other than physician and family/friend referrals, there is little evidence of the type of objective information consumers use to make health care decisions. As more safety and quality data become available, will patients use this information to choose providers with a better safety and quality record?

There is a gap between patients engaging in their health care choices and providers encouraging patients to be engaged. So which tools and resources would be most effective to support both providers and patients with the shared decision making approach to patient-centered care?

And what is the full impact of health illiteracy on safety? Understanding the impact of illiteracy on safety is crucial to fully understanding patient's needs and supporting their engagement in their own health care. With 60% of patients unable to understand a consent form, 42% unable to comprehend directions for not taking medication on an empty stomach, and 26% unable to understand appointment information, how can patients be active participants in their health care within the current system?

CONCLUSION

There are many efforts underway to support patients being in charge of their health care. As consumers take part in health care decisions, better outcomes will result so that utmost safety can be achieved. Whether resources are for educating providers or patients on why and how to be engaged, quality and safety will be best achieved with patients being active members of the health care team.

WEB RESOURCES

Name of Resource/URL	Description
Agency for Healthcare Research and Quality consumer site www.ahrq.gov/consumer	The AHRQ has developed materials that help patients be informed about health care. The consumer Web site provides materials on specific consumer tips to help prevent medical errors. This agency also has an extensive list of quality health care guides that provide useful information to assist consumers when choosing health plans, hospitals, doctors and nursing homes.
Agency for Healthcare Research and Quality, Your Medicine: Play It Safe www.ahrq.gov/consumer/safemeds/safemeds.htm or www.talkaboutrx.org.	A consumer guide to help consumers use prescription medicines safely. Available from AHRQ and NCPIE
American Medical Association Physician Select http://www.ama-assn.org/aps/amahg.htm	The AMA has developed a Web-based tool, AMA Physician Select, to assist consumers searching for a physician. The Web site provides

reliable information on more than 690,000 medical doctors and doctors of osteopathic medicine. Information includes credential data, practice philosophy, physician achievements, and other helpful information for consumers.

American Association of Retired Persons
www.aarp.org/wiseuse

AARP provides educational resources to prepare consumers to 'Take Charge' of their health care. Resources include 'How to be Drug Smart', a guide to prescription drugs, helpful Web links, and AARP bulletins.

American Association of Retired Persons pharmacy site
www.aarppharmacy.com

This AARP Web site provides pharmacy services to AARP members with a goal to ensure access to competitively priced, quality pharmaceutical products. Purchase prescription medications, vitamins, home aids, or access AARP's resources on 'wise use of medications', a drug digest, or FAQs.

Five Steps to Safer Health Care
http://www.ahrq.gov/consumer/
5steps.htm (English)
or http://www.ahrq.gov/consumer/
cincorec.htm (Spanish)

Patient fact sheet developed by the Agency for Healthcare Research and Quality, Centers for Medicare and Medicaid Services, and the Office of Personnel Management, the Department of Labor, the American Hospital Association, and the American Medical Association.

Food and Drug Administration
www.fda.gov/opacom/
morecons.html

This Web site provides links to FDA information written especially for consumers. Education topics include clinical conditions, medications, administering medications to children, and how to contact the FDA to report adverse reactions.

Health Care Choices for Patients
www.healthcarechoices.org

Health Care Choices is a New York not-for-profit corporation

	dedicated to educating the public about the nation's health care system. The Web site provides hospital specific quality information, such as volume data on breast cancer, cardiac, colon cancer, esophageal cancer, lung cancer, pancreatic cancer, and stomach cancer surgeries for California, Florida, Iowa, Illinois, Maryland, New Jersey, and New York. The site also provides research and resources on volume data and patient outcomes.
Healthfinder www.healthfinder.gov	The U.S. Department of Health and Human Services developed the Healthfinder Web site to provide reliable consumer health information and resources such as frequently asked questions (FAQs), brochures on specific clinical topics and links to hundreds of consumer health Web sites. Healthfinder also has a library for specific health topics such as asthma and diabetes.
Institute for Safe Medication Practices www.ismp.org/Pages/ Consumer.html	ISMP Web site lists safety alerts specific to consumers on topics such as safe medication use and safety with cancer treatment, and lists actual cases that highlight safety issues. They also publish 'Safe Medicine' which focuses on the prevention of medication errors by teaching consumers how to become active partners with their health care practitioners and take a leading role in preventing medication errors.
Joint Commission on Accreditation of Healthcare Organizations—Speak Up!	The Joint Commission, together with the Centers for Medicare and Medicaid Services (CMS),

www.jcaho.org/ accredited+organization/speak+up/ speak+up+index.htm	launched a national program to urge patients to take a role in preventing health care errors by becoming active, involved, and informed participants on the health care team. Program brochures, posters, and buttons are available for purchase online or through Joint Commission Resources at (877) 223-6866.
MedlinePlus www.medlineplus.gov	To provide health information specifically for consumers, the National Library of Medicine (NLM) along with the National Institutes of Health (NIH) created MEDLINEplus. MEDLINEplus provides consumer specific information on conditions, diseases, and wellness for over 590 topics.
National Association of Boards of Pharmacy www.napb.org	This Web site provides information on licensed online pharmacies. The site lists whether the online pharmacy meets state and federal requirements for licensure and if they have a Verified Internet Pharmacy Practice Sites seal through the National Association of Boards of Pharmacy.
National Council on Patient Information and Education www.talkaboutrx.org	The National Council on Patient Information and Education (NCPIE) is dedicated to improving communication about the safe, appropriate use of medicines. Their Web site is designed to help consumers make sound decisions about the use of medicines. The Web site provides direct links to timely, authoritative guidelines, tips, and resources to help patients use medicines safely and appropriately.

National Library of Medicine
www.nlm.nih.gov/pubs/cbm/
hliteracy.html

The National Library of Medicine
(NLM) is the world's largest medical library. The Web-based library
lists consumer versions of clinical
practice guidelines such as cardiac
rehabilitation and prevention of
pressure sores. Through MED-
LINE, created by NLM, there are
references to more than 11 million
abstracts and articles published in
4,300 biomedical journals written
for health care professionals.

National Patient Safety Foundation
www.npsf.org/html/psaw/patient
advocate_factsheet.pdf
www.npsf.org/download/
agendaFamilies.pdf
http://www.npsf.org/html/
online_resources.html
http://www.npsf.org/download/
AgendaFamilies.pdf

NPSF is dedicated to improving
the safety of patients through education, research, and providing resources. These Web sites contain
general and topic specific patient
safety resources for patients and
families, quality and patient safety
specialists, administrators, and
health care providers.

Pharmacy and You
www.pharmacyandyou.org

The "Pharmacy and You" Web site
is sponsored by the American Pharmaceutical Association and the National Professional Society of
Pharmacists. This Web site has the
latest information about how patients can work with their pharmacist to help make the most of
medicines. Sections include health
news, pharmacists' education and
licensure requirements, and facts
about patients.

Talking Quality
www.talkingquality.gov

Talking Quality is a Web site that
supports efforts to educate and inform consumers about health care
quality. It is designed for people
and organizations trying to educate consumers about health care
quality. In particular, it is intended to help those who are pro-

viding consumers with information on the performance of health plans and providers. Talking Quality offers the latest research findings, real-world examples, and innovative ideas on ways to communicate complex information on health care quality to consumers.

Together Rx
www.together-rx.com

Together Rx is a prescription savings program with free membership that provides savings to eligible Medicare enrollees on more than 150 widely prescribed medicines—right at the pharmacy counter. Multiple pharmaceutical companies participate in Together Rx including Abbott Laboratories, AstraZeneca, Aventis Pharmaceuticals, Inc., Bristol-Myers Squibb Company, GlaxoSmithKline, Janssen Pharmaceutical Products, L.P., Novartis, and Ortho-McNeil Pharmaceutical, Inc. Each company has its individual savings program.

WebMD
www.webmd.com

WebMD provides practical, relevant, and credible health and medical information on a variety of topics. The site posts an A–Z health guide and offer answers to consumer questions by medical professionals. It also provides education services through their WebMD University.

REFERENCES

Ad Hoc Committee on Health Literacy for the Council on Scientific Affairs of the American Medical Association. (1999). Health literacy: Report of the Council on Scientific Affairs. *Journal of the American Medical Association, 281*(6), 552–557.

Agency for Healthcare Research and Quality (AHRQ). (2001). *Making health care safer: A critical analysis of patient safety practices.* Evidence Report/Technology Assessment Number 43, Part III, Section H: Role of the patient, pp. 551–559, 575–576.

Agency for Healthcare Research and Quality (AHRQ). (2001a). *Your guide to choosing quality health care* (Publication number 99–0012). Retrieved May 23, 2003, from www.ahrq.gov or (800) 358-9295.

Agency for Healthcare Research and Quality (AHRQ). (2003). *Patient fact sheet. Five steps to safer health care.* Retrieved August 24, 2003, from www.ahrq.gov/consumer/5steps.htm

American Medical Association Health Literacy Introductory Kit. (1999). *Low health literacy: You can't tell by looking. Discussion guide.* Health literacy kit. Available through the American Medical Association at (312) 464-5355.

American Association of Retired Persons (AARP). (2003). *How to be drug smart. 35 easy-to-take tips.* Retrieved May 23, 2003, from www.aarpmagazine.org/health/articles/a2003-01-16-drugsmart

Bates, D. W., Teich, J. M., Lee, J., Seger, D., Kuperman, G. J., Ma'Luf, N., et al. (1999). The impact of computerized physician order entry on medication error prevention. *Journal of the American Medical Informatics Association, 6,* 313–321.

Berwick, D. (1999). *Institute for healthcare improvement national quality forum escape fire plenary presentation.* Retrieved May 28, 2003, from www.ihi.org

Birkmeyer, J. D., Birkmeyer, C. M., Wennberg, D. E., & Young M. P. (2002). *Leapfrog safety standards: Potential benefits of universal adoption.* Washington, DC: The Leapfrog Group.

Bottrell, M., Alpert, H., Fischbach, R. L., & Emanuel, L. (2000). Hospital informed consent for procedure forms: Facilitating quality patient-physician interaction. *Archives of Surgery, 135,* 26–33.

Boyce, J. M., & Pittet, D. (2002). *Guideline for hand hygiene in health-care settings.* Recommendations of the Healthcare Infection Control Practices Advisory Committee and the Hand Hygiene Task Force (HICPA, SHEA, APIC, and IDSA) at the Centers for Disease Control and Prevention, Atlanta, GA. Retrieved May 28, 2003, from www.cdc.gov/mmwr

Braddock, C. H., Fihn, S. D., Levinson, W., Jonsen, A. R., & Pearlman, R. A. (1997). How doctors and patients discuss routine clinical decisions: Informed decision in the outpatient setting. *Journal of General Internal Medicine, 12,* 339–345.

Braddock, C. H. III, Edwards, K. A., Hasenberg, N., Laidley, T. L., & Levinson, W. (1999). Informed decision-making in outpatient practice: Time to get back to basics. *Journal of the American Medical Association, 282*(24), 2313–2320.

Center for Health Care Strategies, Inc. (CHCS). (1997a). Who suffers from poor health literacy? Fact sheet. Available in the American Medical Association Health Literacy Introductory Kit, Low Health Literacy: You Can't Tell by Looking. Available at (312) 464-5355.

Center for Health Care Strategies, Inc. (CHCS) (1997b). Health literacy and understanding medical information fact sheet. Available in the American Medical Association Health Literacy Introductory Kit, Low Health Literacy: You Can't Tell By Looking. Available at (312) 464-5355.

Committee on Quality of Health Care in America (2001). *Crossing the quality chasm: A new health system for the 21st century.* Washington, DC: National Academy Press.

The Commonwealth Fund. (2002). *Room for improvement: Patients report on the quality of their healthcare.* Retrieved December 7, 2003, from http://www.cmwf.org/programs/quality/davis_improvement_534.pdf

Davis, K., Schoenbaum, S. C., Collins, K. S., Tenney, K., Hughes, D. L., & Audet, A. J. (2002, April). *Room for improvement: Patients report on the quality of their health care.* The Commonwealth Fund Program on Quality Improvement. Retrieved May 29, 2003, from www.cmwf.org

Fischhoff, B. (2001, May). *The power of words: Communicating.* Presentation from Annenberg III Patient Safety Conference in St. Paul, Minnesota. Retrieved December 19, 2002, from www.mederrors.org

Food and Drug Administration (FDA). (2002). *Generic drugs: Questions and answers.* Retrieved March 10, 2003, from www.fda.gov/cder/consumerinfo/generics_q&a.htm

Food and Drug Administration (FDA). (2003). *Drug interactions—What you should know.* Retrieved March 10, 2003, from www.fda.gov/cder/consumerinfo/generics_q&a.htm

Health Care Choices. (2003). Retrieved January 25, 2003, from www.healthcarechoices.org

Herzlinger, R. E. (2002, July). Let's put consumers in charge of health care. *Harvard Business Review, 80,* 44–55.

Hickson, G. (2001, May). *Communication: It's more than just talking.* Presentation at the Annenberg III Patient Safety Conference in St. Paul, Minnesota. Retrieved March 10, 2003, from www.mederrors.org

Hospital Consumer Assessment of Health Provider Survey (HCAHPS). (2002). Retrieved March 24, 2003, from www.cahps-sun.org/products/HCAHPS.asp

Joint Commission Benchmark. (2001). Getting the real skinny on hand hygiene. *Joint Commission Benchmark, 3*(9), 3.

Joint Commission on the Accreditation of Healthcare Organizations (JCAHO). (2003). *Comprehensive accreditation manual for hospitals: The official handbook.* Oakbrook Terrace, IL: Joint Commission Resources, Inc.

Joint Commission on the Accreditation of Healthcare Organizations (JCAHO). (2003). *Universal protocol for preventing wrong site, wrong procedure, wrong person surgery*™. Retrieved December 7, 2003, from http://www.jcaho.com/accredited+organizations/patient+safety/universal+protocol/universal+protocol.pdf

Joint Commission on Accreditation of Healthcare Organizations (JCAHO). (2003) *Speak up! Campaign brochure.* Retrieved May 28, 2003, from www.jcaho.org

Kaiser Family Foundation. (1996, September). *Americans as health care consumers: The role of quality information.* Retrieved May 29, 2003, from www.ahrq.gov/quality/kffhigh.htm

Kaplan, S. H., Greenfield, S., Gandek, B., Rogers, W. H., & Ware, J. E. (1996). Characteristics of physicians with participatory decision-making styles. *Annals of Internal Medicine, 124,* 497–504.

Kaushal, R., Bates, D. W., Landrigan, C., McKenna, K. J., Clapp, M. D., Federico, F., et al. (2001). Medication errors and adverse events in pediatric inpatients. *Journal of the American Medical Association, 285*(16), 2114–2120.

Kraman, S., Hamm, G. M., & Reynolds, S. (2001). *We made a mistake: A case of medical error.* Presentation from the Annenberg III Patient Safety Conference, St. Paul, Minnesota, May 2001. Retrieved May 30, 2003, from www.mederrors.org

Lavelle-Jones, C., Byrne, D. J., Rice, P., & Cuschieri, A. (1993). Factors affecting quality of informed consent. *British Medical Journal, 306,* 885–890.

Lewis, R. (2003). Quotation from Regina Lewis, America OnLine Internet Advisor during interview on CBS Saturday Morning Show, January 2003.

Minnesota Alliance for Patient Safety (MAPS). (2002). *Patient safety: Your role.* Retrieved May 30, 2003, from www.mnpatientsafety.org

Merck & Co., Inc. (2000). *The Merck manual of geriatrics.* Retrieved March 10, 2003, from www.merck.com/pubs/mm_geriatrics/

Merz, J., Fischhoff, B., Mazur, D. J., & Fischbeck, P. S. (1993). Decision-analytical approach to developing standards of disclosure for medical informed consent. *Journal of Toxics and Liability, 15,* 191–215.

McGrath, P., Wennberg, D., Dickens, J., Siewers, A., Lucas, L., Malenka, D., et al. (2000). Relation between operator and hospital volume and outcomes following percutaneous coronary interventions in the era of the coronary stent. *Journal of the American Medical Association, 284*(24), 3139–3144.

National Committee on Quality Assurance (NCQA). (1990). *HEDIS data on health plans.* Retrieved December 7, 2003, from www.healthchoices.org

National Council on Patient Information and Education (NCPIE). (2002). *Buying prescription medicines online: Be cyberRx smart!* Retrieved December 19, 2002, from www.talkaboutrx.org/cyberx.html

National Institute on Aging. (2002). *Talking with your doctor: A guide for older people* (Publication Number 02-3452). Retrieved May 29, 2003, from www.nia.nih.gov

National Patient Safety Foundation. (2003). *National agenda for action: Patient and families in patient safety nothing about me without me.* Retrieved December 7, 2003, from http://www.npsf.org/download/AgendaFamilies.pdf

Pacific Business Group on Health (PBGH). (2003). *About PBGH.* Retrieved December 7, 2003, from www.pbgh.org/about_pbgh/default.asp

Pronovost, P. J., Young, T., Dorman, T., Robinson, K., & Angus, D. C. (1999). Association between ICU physician staffing and outcomes: A systematic review. *Critical Care Medicine, 27,* A43.

Stewart, M., Brown, J., Weston, W., McWhinney, L., McWilliam, C., & Freeman, T. (1995). *Patient-centered medicine: Transforming the clinical method.* London: Sage.

Talking Quality. (2003). *Talking to consumers about health care quality.* Retrieved January 6, 2003, from www.talkingquality.gov

Voluntary Hospitals of America. (2000). Consumer demand for clinical quality: The giant awakens. *VHA 2000 Research Series,* Volume 3. Retrieved May 30,2003, from https://www.vha.com/pagebuilder.asp?url=/public/research_consumerissues.asp

Wensing, M., Elwyn, G., Edwards, A., Vingerhoets, E., & Grol, R. (2002, January). Deconstructing patient centered communication and uncovering shared decision making: An observational study. *BMC Medical Informatics and Decision Making, 2,* 2. Retrieved December 19, 2002, from http://www.biomedcentral.com/1472-6497/2/2

Chapter 6

Impact of Nurse Staffing on Patient Safety

Lynn Unruh

INTRODUCTION AND CASE STUDY

Becky Ellis, RN is in the second hour of her eight-hour 3:00–11:00 p.m. shift at St. Francis Regional Medical Center. She has yet to start passing her 4:00 p.m. medications. She is late because shift report on the medical-surgical unit's 25 patients took one-half hour. Then, when she emerged from report, she discovered several new sets of orders for her eight patients, including new and changed medications that required checking prior to administration.

She also had to check on a patient of the licensed practical nurse (LPN) assigned to her. She ended up having to call the physician about the patient's blood sugar level of 49, and then administer intravenous (IV) glucose. She made a quick assessment on five out of her own eight patients—the three that needed accuchecks before their dinner trays came at 5:00 p.m., the one that had a new subclavian central venous catheter placed at 2:00 p.m., and the one that had just returned from the recovery room. Her assessment of the other three patients consisted of a glance through the doorway—breathing, alert, good color. Her nursing assistant would provide her with patient vital signs, including the every 15-minute vital signs of the postoperative patient. That would be all she could do until she had caught up on passing medications.

Now, at 5:00 p.m, she was just beginning her 4:00 p.m. medications. She prioritized the medications so that those with the most serious consequences would be given first. While passing the medications she was interrupted several times to answer the unit phone (which was unattended), and to patients' bedsides (intravenous fluid pumps alarming, patients needing the bedpan but no assistants available, a patient's dressing was saturated). She finished distributing medications an hour later with an antibiotic to be administered to a newly admitted dialysis patient. This medication was one the patient had been on at home, and had been transcribed and signed off by the first shift. The medication sheet indicated that it was to be given at 4:00 p.m. She hurriedly gave the medication, and then raced to finish her initial patient assessments and otherwise get caught up.

It wasn't until 10:00 p.m that night that she discovered, as she was finishing up transcribing and checking new medication orders, that the antibiotic she had given earlier in the shift actually had the following time written in the medication Kardex: "4 p.m. q 72 hours." In other words, the medication was to be given once every 72 hours, at 4:00 p.m. Becky had not noticed the "q 72 hours," and the exact days the medication was to be given had not yet been blocked out on the Kardex. With a sinking feeling, she rushed into the patient's room and inquired as to the patient's home schedule. She was dismayed to hear that the patient had just taken the medication yesterday. She called the physician about the error and filled out an incident report. The medication was put on hold and the patient suffered no ill effects. Becky was shaken, however. She thought about how, going by the book, she actually made a medication error for every medication she gave that night, since she gave all of them late, and how several of her patients could have developed complications while she was too busy to assess them or check on them.

A few years ago we would have said that Becky made a mistake by not properly checking the medication administration record. She violated one of the "rights" of medication administration—the right time and therefore needs to be more careful. We would then have closed the book on the investigation into the error. But our current systems approach to medical errors attempts to look deeper into the source of errors. Was there anything in Becky's environment that contributed to the active medication error? What failures in the hospital's system of nursing care allowed Becky to make this error? What latent errors were waiting to happen in the system in which Becky worked?

Clearly, we can see several problems with change of shift routines and medication transcription. Perhaps the unit could be better organized. We see that the multiple tasks she was performing and her constant interruptions may have caused her to make this slip. She got behind in her work, so she hurried and did not take appropriate precautions. But what else is at play in this scenario?

Aside from the organizational and psychological factors (see chapter 1), one underlying theme runs through this scenario: Becky did not have enough human resources to do her job properly. She did not have enough support personnel, such as nursing assistants and unit secretaries, and more important, she did not have enough registered nurses (RNs). A patient load of eight patients, along with supervision of LPNs and nursing assistants, appears to have been too high a workload in this situation. Therefore, one of the contributing causes of her error was too great a workload, resulting from the latent error of understaffing.

By understaffing, we are referring to a situation of inadequate human resource allocation in which the workload or the nature of the work exceeds the number and/or abilities of the available staff. This definition refines the one by Yoe (1988) in which understaffing ("undermanning") is defined as too few staff for the adequate maintenance of the unit. It is both quantitative and qualitative; quantitative in the sense that there may not be enough personnel to do the job; qualitative in that the personnel may not have the necessary education or skills. It also encompasses all types of health care workers involved in patient care. Staffing considerations, therefore, must take into account both the quantity and type of staff. To be adequately staffed requires the right amount and the right type of staff.

Nurse understaffing has received significant press lately due to the 1990s downsizing and the current nursing shortage. Surveys of nurses report that workloads are unmanageable, and that patient care quality is suffering (Shindul-Rothschild, Berry, & Long-Middleton, 1996; Aiken, et al., 2001). Several new studies point to an inverse relationship between staffing levels or mix on the one hand, and patient outcomes on the other (Aiken, Clarke, Sloane, Sochalski, & Silber, 2002; Kovner & Gergen, 1998; Kovner, Jones, Zhan, Gergen, & Basu, 2002; Needleman, Buerhaus, Mattke, Stewart, & Zelevinsky, 2002; Unruh, 2003). Yet until recently, understaffing has not been addressed as a safety issue. For example, in the two initial Institute of Medicine (IOM) reports on patient safety that came out in 2000 and 2001, many systems changes were suggested to improve safety; but ensuring adequate staffing was not one of them (Kohn, Corrigan, & Donaldson, 2000; Committee on Quality of Health Care in America (CQHCA), 2001).

The first definitive statement regarding understaffing and safety came from the Joint Commission on Accreditation of Health Care Organizations

(JCAHO) in its 2002 report on the nursing shortage: Health Care at the Crossroads. In this document, JCAHO reveals that staffing was analyzed to be a factor in 24% of the 1,609 sentinel events reported to them as of March 2002. JCAHO wrote that, "When there are too few nurses, patient safety is threatened and health care quality is diminished" (JCAHO, 2002, p. 5). JCAHO recommended that institutions set staffing levels based on nurse competency, skill mix, patient mix, and patient acuity. In November of 2003, the IOM issued their report on *Keeping Patients Safe: Transforming the Work Environment of Nurses* (Page, 2003). This report calls for a supportive leadership structure, work design, safety culture, and adequate staffing of licensed and unlicensed nursing personnel to promote patient safety.

This chapter examines understaffing as a significant source of medical error. It develops a framework for the role of understaffing in medical error, drawing upon human factors and systems analyses. Understaffing is identified as a latent cause of medical error. Understaffing causes work overload, which creates conditions for slips, mistakes, and rule violations. The chapter discusses how understaffing impacts patient safety through a structure-process-outcomes framework. It also considers that institutional staffing decisions are not the most distal latent error in the system. Reimbursement mechanisms that place financial pressures on institutions, and the lack of supply of appropriate nursing staff, may lead to poor staffing decisions.

In this chapter, research that supports the understaffing-medical error connection is reviewed. Studies find that lower RN/patient ratios, licensed nurse levels, and RN/nurse or licensed nurse/nurse ratios are associated with higher institutional rates of complications, falls, failure to rescue, medication errors, mortality, nosocomial infections, patient/family complaints, and skin breakdown (Flood & Diers, 1988; Kovner & Gergen, 1998; Needleman, Buerhaus, Mattke, Stewart, & Zelevinsky, 2002; Blegan, Goode, & Reed, 1998; Tarnow-Mordi, Hau, Warden, & Shearer, 2000; Aiken, Clarke, Sloane, Sochalski, & Silber, 2002; Fridkin, Pear, Williamson, Galgiani, & Jarvis, 1996; Unruh, 2003). Studies of nursing care in nursing homes also show that lower nurse staffing is related to poorer resident outcomes (Cohen & Spector, 1996; Anderson, Hsieh, & Su, 1998; Johnson-Pawlson, & Infield, 1996).

The chapter concludes with policy and research suggestions. It calls for a reexamination of public and private payment systems that may not adequately reimburse organizations for their costs of hiring the proper numbers of appropriately skilled nurses. It discusses the current nursing shortage and measures to overcome it. Finally, it suggests various ways to improve staffing at the institutional level.

UNDERSTAFFING AS A SOURCE OF MEDICAL ERROR

Our current approach to medical error has turned from blaming the individual to assessing and changing the system (Dekker, 2002; Leape, 1994; Leape, et al., 1995; Reason, 2000; Vincent, Taylor-Adams, & Stanhope, 1998). We now know that focusing on active failure, sometimes called the "sharp end" of the error cascade, does little to reduce or minimize future error. It does not support a proactive process of anticipating errors and assessing the multiple sources of, or inadequate barriers to, those errors (Croteau & Schyve, 2000; Dekker, 2002; McClanahan, Goodwin, & Houser, 2000; Reason, 2000).

What patient safety experts now look at in detecting the source of errors, or possible future errors, are the paths backward from the active error. The focus is on the ways in which the underlying system contributed to the error. In so doing, latent failures, root causes, or the "blunt end" of the error cascade are determined and then corrected or minimized. Latent failures or conditions can also be identified and remedied prior to an active error (Leape, 1994; Reason, 2000; Ternov, 2000). Chapter 1 covers the human factors and systems approach to patient safety in detail.

Understaffing and Latent Failures

System components that have been identified as latent failures in health care include problems with the following: technological design and maintenance, procedures, supervision and training of staff, communication between staff, workplace design and environment, and the working environment (Reason, 1997; Ternov, 2000). Understaffing is a *part* of the working environment component: It is the "too few nurses" that a staff nurse grapples with as she performs her job. Understaffing is also a *result* of problems in several of the other components, for example supervision, communication, and workplace design, which can lead to staff recruitment and retention problems and result in understaffing in the working environment (Aiken, et al., 2001; Aiken, Clarke, Sloane, Sochalski, & Silber, 2002; Tai, Bame, & Robinson, 1998; Unruh & Fottler, 2002). Understaffing itself can lead to recruitment and retention problems, further promoting understaffing (Tai, Bame, & Robinson, 1998; Unruh & Fottler, 2002). Therefore, understaffing is not only a latent failure, it can also be the result of other latent failures, including that of understaffing itself.

These latent failures are the result of administrative and managerial decisions, which may or may not be mistakes (Reason, 1997, 2000). For example, a decision may be made to downsize staff when other cost-cutting options are available. This would constitute a mistake. In a contrasting case, an administrator responding to nursing personnel supply constraints may make a decision to place fewer staff on night shift in order to adequately staff the busier shifts. In this case, the decision may be the best option open to the unit or institution, and although it threatens patient safety, it would not necessarily constitute a mistake.

The second decision-making case draws out an additional point about latent failure: system components of medical error also extend beyond institutional boundaries (Reason, 1997; Croteau & Schyve, 2000). Institutional decisions and actions concerning levels of nursing staff are not necessarily the most distal latent failure in the system. Financial pressures on hospitals and nursing homes, and the lack of skilled nursing staff, may prompt the poor staffing decisions at the institutional level. It is important to consider the impact of prospective payment systems, such as DRG-based payments and managed-care contracts, on the ability of hospitals to hire qualified nursing personnel (Grazier, 1999; Levey, 1999). Furthermore, the impact of payer cost cutting on institutional resource allocation has been deepening. For example, the Balanced Budget Act of 1997 sharply reduced in- and outpatient and long-term care payments from Medicare (Stahl, 2000; Turnbull, 2000). Institutions already feeling the pinch of the various prospective payment systems have had to tighten their belts even further.

It is also important to consider personnel supply issues, such as the current nursing (more specifically, an RN or skilled nursing) shortage. This shortage, which became noticeable around 1999 (AHA, 1999), is thought to be a very serious problem now and for the future (Bednash, 2001; Kimball & O'Neil, 2001; White, 2001). Current hospital RN staffing problems are largely attributed to this shortage (Crawshaw, 2001). Obviously, if the numbers of needed and demanded RNs or LPNs are not engaging in hospital employment, and work redesign cannot streamline or rationalize the nursing process any further, understaffing of skilled nursing personnel is unavoidable. In this case, the latent failures needing attention are not ones of fixing staffing decision-making, but of *recruitment to* and *retention in* the institution and profession.

These financial and supply constraints are no less latent failures than understaffing. They are just temporally and spatially farther away from the active errors due to understaffing. In a systems analysis, therefore, medical errors can be traced all the way back to public and private payment systems and actions, and personnel supply factors. These, in turn, can be traced back even farther into analyses of societal values and culture, in an infinite progression of more removed, yet still pertinent, latent failure. For the most part, however, analyses tend to focus on what institutions can do to control internal latent failures and protect against external failures.

Understaffing and Barriers to Error

A final consideration in the current approach to medical error is the existence or absence of barriers to the error. Institutions cannot remove or control all possible latent failures at all times. In the case of understaffing, institutions may have periods of time or areas of work in which staffing is a problem. Understaffing will more likely lead to active failure if there are not enough safe practices in place to safeguard patient care. In this chapter's case study, Becky might not have made the medication error had a supervisor noted the chaotic atmosphere at shift change and made arrangements to help the understaffed unit until it quieted down. Likewise, different medication transcription procedures or the adoption of a new technology might have been a barrier to her error. As is noted in Reason's (1997) "Swiss Cheese" model of defenses (see chapter 1), because barriers themselves have a tendency to break down, the more defenses a system has against error, the more likely a latent failure will not poke through all the defenses to cause an active failure.

In summation, latent failures create conditions of work that contribute to active failures, especially if there are inadequate barriers to error (Meurier, 2000; Reason, 1990, 1997, 2000; Ternov, 2000). In the case of understaffing, latent failures are the financing and/or supply constraints, and the administrative and/or managerial decisions that result in understaffing. Understaffing produces conditions of work that open the door to active errors. If barriers to the active failure are weak or nonexistent, sooner or later errors will occur.

In the next section, we look more closely at the mechanisms of the relationship of understaffing to medical error. What conditions does understaffing create that lead to medical error? In particular, we use a structure-process-outcomes model to hypothesize how understaffing leads to slips, mistakes, and rule-based errors, and the types of active errors characterized in human factors analysis.

HOW UNDERSTAFFING COMPROMISES PATIENT SAFETY

If we are only beginning to recognize the role of understaffing in medical error, we are even less aware of the mechanisms involved in this relationship. No framework exists, and little information is available to help explain why understaffing compromises patient safety. In what follows, a framework is built based on the Donabedian structure-process-outcomes model of health care quality as it applies to human factors analysis of errors. Based on the framework, we hypothesize the ways in which understaffing could impact nursing performance and cause medical error.

A Structure-Process-Outcomes/Human Factors Framework

Donabedian's structure-process-outcomes (SPO) framework has been used to assess quality in health care institutions and to model relationships between structure, process and outcomes (Donabedian, 1966, 1969, 1988). In this framework, health care quality is composed of components that relate to the organizational characteristics of health care providers (structure), the clinical and nonclinical processes involved in care delivery (process), and the effect of care on the health status of patients and populations (outcomes). These components also relate to each other. Institutional structure, such as financial status, the physical facilities, equipment, and other physical resources, and the human resources such as physicians, nurses, and other personnel, impact the processes involved in delivering patient care, which in turn affect patient outcomes.

Utilizing this framework, staffing is a structural component, a part of the quantity and quality of the human resources of the institution. It may be linked to other structural components such as the financial status of the institution and the organization of the physical and human resources. Staffing can either be adequate (or more than adequate), or inadequate (in which case we characterize the situation as "understaffed").

The provision of patient care is part of process. It is the activities carried out by the health care staff, including their communications and interactions with each other and the patients, and the things they do to, or for, patients that contribute to the patients' health and well-being. For nursing care in particular, it includes the assessment, planning, delivery, and evaluation of nursing care. As with structure, patient care processes can either be performed well, for example, according to professional standards and guidelines, and in a timely manner, or they can be performed poorly, such as outside standards and guidelines, and performed late or not at all.

Poor performance may or may not constitute medical error. To be considered a medical error, the practitioner would have to make a slip, mistake, or rule violation (Feldman & Roblin, 1997, 2000). Slips are unintended deviations from an intended plan. In the chapter case study, Becky's wrong-time medication error was a slip. Mistakes are poor judgments and faulty reasoning. Becky's decision to answer phones and patient call lights while administering her medications may have been a mistake. Rule violations are conscious violations of established practices or procedures. When Becky waited until later in the shift to assess her patients, she was committing a rule-based error, since standard nursing practice is to complete an initial assessment early in the shift. Also, when Becky was unable to administer her medications within the hour of their ordered time, she was committing a rule violation.

Performance, or provision of patient care, results in patient outcomes that can be measured through patient satisfaction, functional status, recovery from illness, mental and social health, management of pain and chronic illness, and other factors. The outcomes can be either positive states such as improved health status and freedom from illness, or negative states such as acquired infections, injuries, or even death.

Poor performance to the point of medical error may or may not cause demonstrably poor patient outcomes. In the case study, Becky administered the medication on the wrong day, a potentially serious error, yet the patient was not demonstrably harmed. Becky was not able to adequately assess all of her patients at the beginning of the shift. However, she was "lucky" in that "nothing happened to them" as a result of this failure. Her "luck" was due to situational factors such as the stability of her patients, the expertise and attentiveness of other staff, and other factors. Also, per policy, all of her late medications were medication errors, and some of them may have to some degree harmed the patient by not being on time. The potential harm was not considered because delays are common occurrences in short-staffed situations and no investigation was conducted.

Figure 6.1 presents highlights of the algorithm just discussed. The diagram shows that inadequate staffing can result in processes and outcomes that follow several different paths. Only the path following the shaded boxes results in medical error.

The Relationship Between Understaffing and Medical Error

The above model provides a framework for understanding the relationship between understaffing and medical error. With this framework we can begin to fill in the details of the path from understaffing to medical error. When staffing is not adequate, i.e., when understaffing occurs, it creates

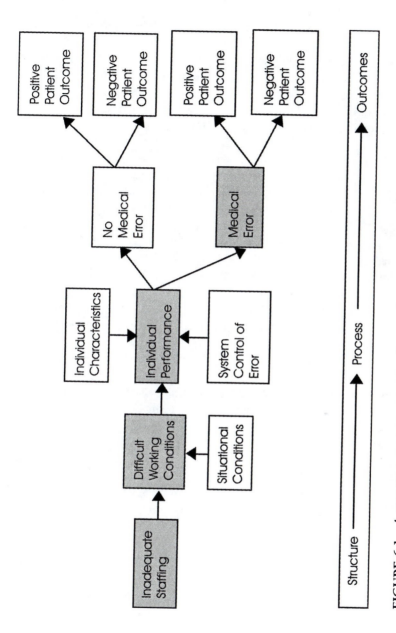

FIGURE 6.1 A structure-process-outcomes/human factors framework for understaffing and medical error.
Adapted from the Donabedian structure-process-outcomes framework (1996, 1969, 1988).

adverse working conditions that affect individual performance. Difficult working conditions that might occur with understaffing include heavy workloads, inadequate knowledge or experience, inadequate supervision, inadequate communication, and stressful environment (Leape, et al., 1995; Vincent, Taylor-Adams, & Stanhope, 1998). Understaffing causes tight time constraints, or coupling, which has been identified as increasing the risk of a process failure (McClanahan, Goodwin, & Houser, 2000).

The adverse working conditions listed above pave the way for performance problems. Studies have demonstrated that work overload and time pressures lower the quality of care provided and create stress in the workforce (Bridger, 1997; Bryant, Fairbrother, & Fenton, 2000; Fox, Dwyer, & Ganster, 1993; Motowidlo, Packard, & Manning, 1986; Taylor, White, & Muncer, 1999; Williams, 1998). Stress in the workforce has been associated with reduced competence and lower quality of care (Arnetz, 1999; Firth-Cozens & Greenhalgh, 1997; Leveck & Jones, 1996; Williams, 1998).

Although our knowledge of specifics is extremely limited, we do have research on the impact of nurse staffing on adverse events among hospital patients. Studies of this nature connect the structural, staffing component with the patient outcomes component, skipping over an analysis of the processes involved. They rarely look at medical error *per se*, but at a broader category called adverse events, defined below. Despite these limitations, they can tell us whether we are on the right track in assuming a relationship between understaffing and medical error. Likewise, studies of nursing home quality have linked nurse staffing to certain processes and resident outcomes. These, too, can show the connection between staffing and unsafe care in nursing homes.

The next section reviews results from empirical studies on the relationship between nurse staffing and adverse events in hospitalized patients. Following that, the chapter examines research on staffing and nursing home resident outcomes.

STUDIES ON NURSE STAFFING AND ADVERSE EVENTS

Researchers have explored the relationship between adverse events and the characteristics and processes of health care organizations for several decades. Nurse staffing is a more recent focus of the research; several studies have been published since the early 1980s.

In these studies, adverse events are defined as injuries caused by medical management rather than by the underlying disease or condition of the patient (Brennan, et al., 1991; Leape, et al., 1991; Thomas, et al., 2000; Unruh, 2002). Since adverse events are due to medical management, they may occur due to medical error, but they may also happen even when the correct treatment has been given. Therefore, not all adverse events are the result of medical error. Likewise, not all medical errors become adverse events. Recall that a medical error may have been committed, yet no harm occurs to the patient, and therefore no adverse event is recorded.

Adverse events, therefore, will capture more than medical error, yet at the same time will not capture all medical error. Nevertheless, medical error does cause a certain proportion of adverse events, and that proportion has been explored. One study estimates that 69% of adverse medical injuries are due, in part, to error (Bates, et al., 1995). Another finds 58% to be due to error (Leape, et al., 1991). Figure 6.2 demonstrates the relationships just described.

In the studies that examine the impact of nurse staffing on adverse events, the staffing variables have included raw numbers of nurses, ratios of nurses to patients, nurses to patient days of care, nurses to hours of care, and types of skill mix. Categories of nurses include RNs, LPNs, licensed nurses (both RNs and LPNs) and a usually undefined category of "nurses." Sources of data differ from nationwide to statewide databases, and from governmental to private. This variety of staffing categories, mea-

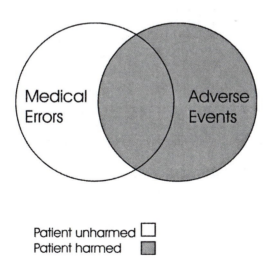

FIGURE 6.2   Relationship between medical errors and adverse events.

sures, and sources has on the one hand encouraged a large number of independent studies, but on the other hand has made it difficult to compare results across studies.

In addition to the nurse staffing variables, the studies usually control for other variables that could contribute to adverse events. Control variables also differ from study to study, but frequently include other hospital characteristics such as size, teaching status, ownership, and patient characteristics such as acuity.

The adverse events that have been studied in relation to nurse staffing are: complications; falls; failure to rescue; medication errors; mortality; nosocomial infections such as blood stream infections, pneumonia, and urinary tract infections; and skin breakdown. Studies may examine more than one type of adverse event. Table 6.1 lists the types of adverse events and the studies that found significant inverse relationships between the events and various types of nurse staffing.

Complications

Complications and nurse staffing have been examined in nine studies since 1988. Complications were greater in a short-staffed unit than in an adequately staffed unit in a 1988 study (Flood & Diers). In a 1993 study, Giraud and colleagues discovered that a high or excessive nursing workload was associated with a higher incidence of iatrogenic complications in two intensive care units in France. Kovner and Gergen (1998) found that a lower RN/adjusted inpatient day is related to greater incidences of thrombosis after surgery. Amaravadi and colleagues (2000) found increased pulmonary and infectious complications among patients undergoing esophageal resection when ICU nurses cared for more than two patients. Dimick and colleagues (2001) discovered that patients with fewer ICU nurses had increased risks for pulmonary failure, and reintubation.

In a study by Needleman and colleagues (2002), more patients experienced upper gastrointestinal bleeding in hospitals with lower proportions of hours of RN care and lower absolute hours of RN care. Unruh (2003) found that after controlling for hospital characteristics and the number and acuity of patients, hospitals with more complications in general, and atelectasis in particular, were the ones with fewer licensed nurses.

Related to complications is failure to rescue, which is defined as death within 30 days of admission among patients who experienced complications (Needleman, et al., 2002). Only two nurse staffing studies have looked

TABLE 6.1 Research Literature Showing a Significant Inverse Relationship Between Nurse Staffing and Adverse Events in Hospitals

	Complications	Falls	Failure to Rescue	Medication Errors	Mortality	Nosocomial Infections	Skin Breakdown
RN staffing	Kovner & Gergen, 1998 Needleman, et al., 2002	NA	Aiken, et al., 2002 Needleman, et al., 2002	Bond, et al., 2001	Aiken, et al., 2002	Kovner & Gergen, 1998 Kovner, et al., 2002 Needleman, et al., 2002	NA
Licensed nurse staffing	Unruh, 2003	Unruh, 2003	NA	NA	NA	Unruh, 2003	Unruh, 2003
Nurse staffing	Flood & Diers, 1988* Giraud, et al., 1993 Amaravadi., et al., 2000 Dimick, et al., 2001 Giraud, et al., 2001	NA	NA	NA	Provonost, et al., 1999 Tarnow-Mordi, et al., 2000	Haley & Bregman, 1982 Haley, et al., 1995 Fridkin, et al., 1996 Archibald, et al., 1997 Harbarth, et al., 1999 Vicca, 1999 Stegenga, et al., 2002	NA

(continued)

TABLE 6.1 (*continued*)

	Complications	Falls	Failure to Rescue	Medication Errors	Mortality	Nosocomial Infections	Skin Breakdown
RN skill mix	Needleman, et al., 2002	Blegan & Vaughn, 1998	Needleman, et al., 2002	Blegen, Goode, & Reed, 1998 Blegan & Vaughn, 1998	NA	Needleman, et al., 2002	Blegen, Goode, & Reed, 1998
Licensed nurse skill mix	NA	NA	NA	NA	NA	Unruh, 2003	Unruh, 2003

The literature cited above showed a statistically significant inverse relationship between the nurse staffing variable and the negative patient outcome, except for Flood and Diers, 1988.

RN staffing = any of the following: RN/patient; RN/APD; RN hrs/patient; RN/occupied bed.

Licensed nurse staffing = licensed nurses (RNs + LPNs), controlling for the number of patients.

Nurse staffing = an undefined term that could mean all nursing staff, including RNs, LPNs, and nursing assistants, or any one of these types.

RN skill mix = RNs/total nursing staff; or the proportion of RN hours of care.

Licensed nurse skill mix = (RNs + LPNs)/total nursing staff.

*Statistical significance was not reported.

NA = none available.

at this adverse event. Needleman and colleagues (2002) found greater failure to rescue in hospitals with lower hours of RN care and proportions of RN hours of care. Aiken and colleagues (2002) found greater failure to rescue with each additional patient per RN.

Falls and Medication Errors

Regarding falls, Blegan and Vaughn (1998) and Unruh (2003) found that the proportion of RN hours of care and the number of licensed nurses, respectively, were inversely related to the number of falls in hospitals. Medication errors have been examined in three studies. Increased medication errors have been associated with fewer numbers of RNs/occupied beds (Bond, Raehl, & Franke, 2001), proportion of hours of RN care (Blegen, Goode, & Reed, 1998), and low and high proportions of RN hours of care (Blegan & Vaughn, 1998).

Mortality

Studies of patient mortality in hospitals have a long history. Most were interested in looking at hospital structural characteristics, some included nurse staffing. Of these early studies relating hospital characteristics to mortality, a few found an inverse relationship between nurse staffing and mortality (Hartz, et al., 1989; Krakauer, Bailey, & Skellan, 1992; Manheim, Feinglass, & Shortell, 1992). Two more recent studies are listed in the table. Using several measures of nurse workload, Tarnow-Mordi, Hau, Warden, and Shearer (2000) found that the odds of mortality were two times higher in patients exposed to higher ICU workload. Aiken and colleagues (2002) found a 7% greater likelihood of dying within 30 days of admission with each additional patient per nurse.

Nosocomial Infection

The category of adverse event most studied in relationship to nurse staffing is that of nosocomial infections. There have been twelve studies since 1996, and one was conducted as far back as 1982. Several types of nosocomial infections have been examined, including staphylococcal and enterobacter bacteremia, pneumonia, viral gastrointestinal infections, and urinary tract infections.

The 1982 study by Haley and Bregman found staphylococcal infection rates to be 16 times higher after periods when the infant to nurse ratio was greater than seven. In 1995, Haley and colleagues also found lower staffing to inhibit eradication of Methicillin-Resistant *Stapholococcus Aureus* (MRSA) in a neonatal unit. Similarly, in a study by Vicca (1999), MRSA outbreaks were related to high nursing staff workload and reduced nurse/patient ratios. In another study, the patient-to-nurse ratio was significantly related to central venous catheter-associated bloodstream infections (Fridkin, Pear, Williamson, Galgiani, & Jarvis, 1996).

Nosocomial infection risk was assessed by Archibald, Manning, Bell, Banerje, and Jarvis (1997), and found to be associated with nursing hours/patient day. Kovner and Gergen (1998) found higher rates of urinary tract infections and pneumonia after surgery in hospitals with lower RN/adjusted inpatient days. A few years later, Kovner and colleagues (2002) found that pneumonia and RN hours/adjusted inpatient days were inversely related. Harbarth and colleagues (1999) found an increased risk of infant Enterobacter clocae infection rates with understaffing. The monthly viral gastrointestinal infection rate correlated significantly with the patient-to-night nurse ratio in Stengenga, Bell, and Matlow (2002). Significant findings in the (2002) study by Needleman and colleagues were associations between the absolute number of hours and proportion of hours of RN care on the one hand and urinary tract infections on the other hand, and between the proportions of hours of care and pneumonia. Pneumonia was also significantly inversely related to licensed nurse/nurse skill mix in a study by Unruh (2003), while urinary tract infections were significantly negatively related to the numbers of licensed nurses (controlling for the number and acuity of patients).

Skin Breakdown

Skin breakdown is the final category of adverse events under investigation. Its relationship to nurse staffing has been examined in two studies. The already mentioned studies by Blegan, Good, and Reed (1998) and Unruh (2003) examined the incidence of decubitus ulcers and found significantly inverse relationships between this complication and the proportion of nursing hours of care and the number and proportion of licensed nurses respectively.

STUDIES ON NURSE STAFFING AND LONG-TERM CARE RESIDENT OUTCOMES

Other empirical evidence that inadequate nurse staffing compromises patient safety comes from the long-term care setting. Due to long-standing problems with staffing and quality in nursing homes, abundant data and research exist on the subject. Table 6.2 lists some of the more important studies that have been conducted, categorized by the type of problem found in nursing homes. In these studies, the resident problems range from behavioral, emotional, and basic physical problems, to complications involving skin breakdown and mortality. The staffing variables include RN/resident, LPN/resident, and LPN/nursing assistants, among others. Nursing turnover and nursing pool labor are two additional variables.

Lower total nursing staff/resident and the use of nursing pool labor were found to contribute to poorer mental status of residents (Porell, Caro, Silva, & Monane, 1998). Elimination and continence problems, including urinary tract infections and increased use of urinary catheters, were found in facilities with lower RN hours per day per resident (Cherry, 1991). Cohen and Spector (1996) found that the number of LPNs per resident was important in preventing poor physical functioning, while Spector and Takada (1991) found total nursing staff/resident ratios to be important.

Restraint use has been an issue in nursing homes. Studies have indicated that facilities with a greater use of restraints tend to have fewer RNs per resident (Castle & Fogel, 1998) and LPNs per resident (Graber & Sloan, 1995), and lower nursing staff skill mix (Castle & Fogel, 1998).

As in hospitals, understaffing in nursing homes is implicated in pressure ulcers and other skin care problems. This has been found to be an issue when the RN/resident ratio is low (Cohen & Spector, 1996; Cherry, 1991), or when the total nursing staff/resident ratio is low (Aaronson, Zinn, & Rosko, 1994).

Another major issue in nursing homes is inappropriate medication use. Cherry (1991) found that low RN/resident ratios contributed to overuse of antibiotics. Schmidt and colleagues (1998) found a greater deviation from psychotropic drug use criteria among nursing homes with low nurse/resident ratios.

Greater than expected mortality has been attributed to lower RN/resident ratios (Cohen & Spector, 1996), licensed nurse/resident ratios (Bliesmer, Smayling, Kane, & Shannon, 1998), and nursing staff skill mix (Porell, et al., 1998). Undetermined deficiencies and poor patient outcomes have

TABLE 6.2 Research Literature Showing a Significant Inverse Relationship Between Nurse Staffing and Negative Resident Outcomes

	Behavioral/ Cognitive emotional problems	Elimination and continence problems/ Prevalence of catheters	Poor physical functioning	Prevalence of daily physical restraints	Prevalence of Pressure ulcers/Other skin care problems	Mortality	Deficiencies/ Poor outcomes	Inappropriate Medication Use
RN/resident	NA	Cherry, 1991	NA	Castle & Fogel, 1998	Cherry, 1991 Cohen & Spector, 1996	Cohen & Spector, 1996	Anderson, Hsieh, & Su, 1998 Harrington, Zimmerman, et al., 2000	Cherry, 1991
LPN/resident	NA	NA	Cohen & Spector, 1996	NA	NA	NA	NA	NA
LPN/nursing assistants	NA	NA	NA	Graber & Sloan, 1995	NA	NA	NA	NA
Licensed nurse/resident	NA	NA	NA	NA	NA	Bliesmer, et al., 1998	NA	NA
Nurse/ resident	NA	NA	NA	NA	NA	NA	NA	Schmidt, et al., 1998
Total nursing staff/resident	Porell, et al., 1998	NA	Spector & Takada, 1991	NA	Aaronson, Zinn, & Rosko, 1994	NA	Johnson-Pawlson & Infield, 1996	NA

212

TABLE 6.2 (continued)

	Behavioral/ Cognitive emotional problems	Elimination and continence problems/ Prevalence of catheters	Poor physical functioning	Prevalence of daily physical restraints	Prevalence of Pressure ulcers/Other skin care problems	Mortality	Deficiencies/ Poor outcomes	Inappropriate Medication Use
Nursing staff skill mix	NA	NA	NA	Castle & Fogel, 1998	NA	Porell, et al., 1998	Anderson, Hsieh, & Su, 1998 Munroe, 1990	NA
Nursing pool labor	Porell, et al., 1998	NA	NA	NA	NA	NA	NA	NA
Nursing turnover	NA	NA	NA	NA	NA	NA	Munroe, 1990	NA

The literature cited above showed a statistically significant inverse relationship between the nurse staffing variable and the negative patient outcome.
NA = none available.
RN/resident = RNs/nursing home residents.
LPN/resident = LPNs/nursing home residents.
LPN/nursing assistants = LPNs/nursing assistants.
Licensed nurse/resident = RNs + LPNs/nursing home residents.
Nurse/resident = all nursing personnel/nursing home residents.
Total nursing staff/resident = all nursing personnel/nursing home residents.
Nursing staff skill mix = any of the following: RNs/total nursing staff; LPN expenses/total nursing staff expenses; RN hours/LPN hours.
Nursing pool labor = total nursing expense for nonstaff nursing services as a percent of total annual nursing personnel expenses.
Nursing turnover = annual percent turnover for all facility personnel.

213

been reported with low RN/resident ratios (Anderson, Hsieh, & Su, 1998; Harrington, Zimmerman, Karon, Robinson, & Beutel, 2000), low total nursing staff/resident ratios (Johnson-Pawlson & Infeld, 1996), low nursing staff skill mix (Anderson, Hsieh, & Su, 1998), and high nursing turnover (Munroe, 1990).

These studies indicate that understaffing negatively impacts nursing care and resident outcomes in nursing homes. Some of these results indicate that understaffing is directly related to adverse events and patient safety in nursing homes. Pressure ulcers, mortality, and certain deficiencies are included in this category. Some of these negative outcomes may *develop into* adverse events, and therefore *contribute to* patient safety problems. For example, patients with poorer mental status are more likely to fall. Patients who are restrained or who are in poor physical condition are also more likely to fall, acquire pneumonia, or experience other adverse events.

ADDRESSING THE UNDERSTAFFING—PATIENT SAFETY ISSUE

There appears to be a substantial relationship between adequate nurse staffing and safety. First, human factors theory indicates that understaffing and its antecedents in supply and resource allocation issues are latent system failures that, sooner or later, surface as active failures, i.e., medical errors. Second, SPO, psychological, and managerial theories suggest that understaffing produces working conditions that set the stage for individual reactions and behaviors that lead to errors (see Figure 6.1). Third, empirical evidence suggests that inadequate nurse staffing in hospitals contributes to adverse events, about one-half of which could be the result of medical error. Understaffing also has been implicated in poorer outcomes for nursing home residents. These negative outcomes in nursing homes either are themselves adverse events, or could contribute to adverse events, and therefore could be considered patient safety problems.

So what can be done about this situation? In order to address the problem of understaffing and its contribution to unsafe conditions and medical error, let us return to the earlier discussion about latent failures. This discussion revealed several areas from which to approach improvements, including external latent failures such as reimbursement systems and workforce supply issues, internal latent failures of understaffing decisions and recruitment/retention problems, and inadequate barriers such as safe practices and lack of redundancy. In what follows, policies and strategies that address each of these areas are discussed. In addition, the chapter suggests future research directions.

Policies and Strategies Addressing External Latent Failures

Starting with the external latent failures, a society that is genuinely interested in improving patient safety will ensure that health care providers and institutions are reimbursed at rates that support the maintenance of adequate numbers of qualified staff. Without adequate payment, health care institutions have a choice of falling behind in technology and physical growth, or trying to care for patients with inadequate staff, or some combination of both.

According to the American Hospital Association (AHA), payment rates need to be adequate for hospital care, and for improvements in information technology that could streamline work (AHA, 2002). In addition, regulatory reform is necessary to reduce administrative burdens (AHA, 2002). Payment systems should encourage efficiency, but not at the expense of quality. Of course, payers cannot guarantee that institutions will make good use of the payments. Administrators of health care institutions have a responsibility to balance quality with efficiency, while payers and regulators have a responsibility to monitor quality and efficiency.

What is important for health care providers and administrators to consider is the need to publicize current institutional financial shortfalls, and how they affect adequate staffing and patient outcomes. The AHA recommends "building societal support for the public policies and resources needed to help hospitals hire and retain a qualified workforce" (AHA, 2002, p. 5). In order to move public opinion in favor of greater spending for hospital or nursing home care, or in favor of a national health program that could lower administrative costs, people need to be more aware of the problems that ensue when funding is inadequate. Once aware of the problems, consumers and political leaders must consider health care policy alternatives to adequately fund health care institutions and ensure that the increased funds go toward staffing needs.

The other major external latent failure is the issue of the supply of nurses. Currently, the supply of skilled nurses falls short of the demand for them. This nursing shortage is a major stumbling block to patient safety. Until the crisis is relieved, there will be a continuing, and perhaps deepening, undersupply-understaffing-undersupply cycle, and patient safety will be severely threatened. Many reports and articles have been written on the shortage, with many good solutions proposed. Some of the main suggestions (American Organization of Nurse Executives, 2000; Nevidjon & Erickson, 2001; Purnell, Horner, Gonzalez, & Westman, 2001) are to:

- Improve the image of nursing
- Develop successful recruitment strategies
- Develop successful retention strategies
- Fund and support nursing education
- Create federal and state agencies and funding for research and projects on improving the supply of nurses
- Develop ongoing partnerships between educators, employers and regulatory bodies

Much can be said for each of these suggestions. According to the American Association of Colleges of Nursing (AACN), programs addressing these strategies are underway or being proposed in legislatures, schools of nursing, and workplaces at national, state, and local levels. One significant federal legislative development has been the Nurse Reinvestment Act of August 2002. This act amends the prior Public Health Service Act (42 U.S.C. 296) that funded nursing education and promotion. It directs the development of public service announcements that "advertise and promote the nursing profession, highlight the advantages and rewards of nursing, and encourage individuals to enter the nursing profession." It adds scholarships to the loan repayment program. Grants are to be awarded to eligible institutions to initiate nurse retention programs. Also, student loan funds may be set up to educate students for faculty status. Congress appropriated funding for this law in February 2003 (AACN, 2003).

Of the items in the list above, recruitment and retention strategies are of particular interest. Recruitment and retention refers to activities at both the professional and institutional level. Therefore, recruitment and retention have both an external and internal focus. External professional recruitment and retention interplays with other solutions already listed, such as improving the image of nursing, funding research and projects, and developing partnerships. Internal recruitment and retention interplays with policies addressing internal latent failures, and will be addressed directly.

Policies and Strategies Addressing Internal Latent Failures

Internal latent failures include staffing decisions and other resource and managerial decisions that impact staffing and workload. Among these considerations, the most important is to plan for and implement safe levels of nursing staff. From the institutional strategic planning level down to the daily management of units, the need to ensure adequate numbers of qualified nurses cannot be understated. If units are chronically and grossly understaffed, no amount of positive management and communication will be enough to compensate for the inadequacies. Every effort needs to be made to attract and retain the necessary numbers and skill mix of nurses. At a time of shortage, this may require that extra financial resources go into staffing. Administrators must be careful, however, that methods used to attract staff are truly effective and long-lasting (White, 2001). An example of a mistaken strategy, the sign-on bonus, has not brought more nurses back into hospitals, but merely resulted in nurse "swapping" (Groeller, 2001).

Out of frustration with hospital staffing problems over the past few years, government-mandated minimum staffing ratios are being implemented in California, and have been or are being considered in other states such as Florida, Massachusetts, New Jersey, New York, Pennsylvania, and West Virginia (Spetz, 2001; Safe Staffing, 2003). The 1999 California Assembly Bill 394 required the California Department of Health Services to issue minimum staffing ratios for licensed nurses in hospitals. After 3 years of study, the DHS issued ratios specific to various types of nursing units on January 22, 2003. The ratios are not tied to any patient acuity or case-mix system (*USA Today,* 2002).

While the verdict is still out on how well mandated ratios work, the California experience is instructive of the difficulty in establishing mandatory ratios that will ensure adequate staffing in all hospitals. While mandated minimum staffing ratios look good to nurses working in understaffed conditions, hospital administrators decry them because of the added financial burden imposed on those hospitals previously staffed under the minimum. Health care policy analysts worry about increases in overall health care costs and lack of nursing supply (*USA Today,* 2002). However, the most important issue is whether staffing systems can be properly designed and used to improve staffing and the quality of care.

It would seem that in order to work, a mandated approach to staffing requires that 1) the supply of nurses be available to meet increased demand mandated by the ratios, *or* the supply could fairly rapidly become available given improvements in salaries and working conditions; 2) hospitals can afford the wage and benefit enticements necessary to pull more nurses back into the supply and into employment in their institution; 3) workload for a given patient load on a given patient care unit be uniform enough (or can be averaged) across hospitals, across patient case mix/severity, and over time to establish one minimum ratio for each type of patient care unit; and 4) the ratios established by the governmental agency adequately reflect this fairly uniform workload. Further, given the fact that workload/patient assignment varies from hospital to hospital, and over time within each hospital, the efficacy of mandated ratios requires that hospitals not use the ratios as inflexible maximum indicators, but as minimum requirements that are upwardly flexible, i.e., when their staffing needs are greater than those mandated by the ratios, they staff above the ratios.

Whether these requirements will come to pass in the states that have mandated or will mandate minimum staffing requirements remains to be seen. If it is discovered that there are problems in these areas, one solution is to devise a mandated *system* of staffing that requires hospitals to calculate workload based on certain resource factors, such as support personnel, and patient case mix/severity, and to staff according to the workload calculation. Such a system of staffing would be a refinement of mandated staffing by raw numbers of patients.

Mandated ratios or not, internal strategies for ensuring adequate staffing should include a focus on recruitment and retention, and one of the best ways to attract and retain nurses is to improve working conditions. In numerous surveys, nurses state that a major factor driving them out of nursing or out of a particular institution is the extremely stressful and physically demanding nature of their job (Federation of Nurses and Health Professionals, 2001; McNeese-Smith, 2001; North Carolina Center for Nursing, 2002). In turn, the need to improve working conditions brings the problem of understaffing to the fore. The difficulty of the situation is that staffing needs to be improved in order to improve recruitment and retention, which needs to be improved in order to make staffing better.

The situation is not hopeless, however. There are two ways to look at understaffing—one is through patient load, and the other is through workload. In the first case, staffing adequacy is assessed only through the number of patients that a nurse has. In the second case, it is not just the number of patients, but also the *work* associated with caring for those patients that determines the staffing adequacy (Smith, 1980). Factors such as the nursing model, management styles, staff communication, and physical workplace affect both work culture (see chapter 7) and workload, and therefore can moderate or accentuate staffing problems by reducing or increasing workload for any given number of patients. For example, a study of nursing shortages indicated that hospitals using a primary nursing model were less likely to report a shortage than those using a team model (Seago, Ash, Spetz, Coffman, & Grumbach, 2001). If there are ways to lighten the workload despite the patient load, these methods should be sought out and implemented. Some examples of ways to lighten workload include computerized physician order entry systems that are integrated with computerized ordering and charting, or redesign of nursing care model and roles with appropriate use of nursing assistants and support personnel.

In order to implement workplace redesign that decreases workload, a unit-by-unit assessment of staffing needs and ways to reduce workload is required. Staffing changes and work redesign can be planned based on this assessment. Staffing plans should take into account the patient's needs and nurses' skills and competencies (JCAHO Call for Action, 2002), and other factors affecting workload. Work redesign to decrease workload should not be confused with the redesign that occurred in the 1990s that resulted in staff downsizing (Aiken, Clarke, & Sloane, 2000; Barry-Walker, 2000; Ingersoll, Fisher, Ross, & Kidd, 2001; Shindul-Rothschild, 1994; Urden & Walston, 2001). The point of the redesign spoken of here is to reorganize the physical, technological, and human resources on the unit so as to allow the *same number of staff (or more)* to have a lower workload.

One suggestion for improving staffing and reducing workload is to make proper use of nursing assistants and other unlicensed personnel by using them as complements to, not substitutes for, RNs. If available, LPNs could be hired to supplement the RN staff. Existing levels of unlicensed personnel would be maintained or increased and used in non-nursing and custodial nursing roles, while the numbers of licensed personnel (RNs and LPNs) would be increased. In this case, overall staffing increases and skill mix may remain neutral or increase. Advantages of this redesign are that the patient load for each licensed nurse will decrease, and they will also have greater support from assistants. Each skill level of nurse will be performing the nursing care they are educated for, communication will improve, work-load will decrease, and patients will have skilled nurses at the bedside. While this model results in higher labor costs, savings may come from fewer patient complications and shorter lengths of stay (Flood & Diers, 1988; Pittet, Tarara, & Wenzel, 1994; Cody, Friss, & Hawkinson, 1995; Bates, et al., 1997). This model also works to improve nurse satisfaction and retention.

The staffing suggestion above has an added advantage: it is possible to do this even with the current nursing shortage. First, there is no shortage of nursing assistants and other support personnel, and they are relatively inexpensive to employ, so they can be hired in whatever quantity is needed to give RNs the support they need. Second, while attempting to attract RNs, LPNs can also be employed and used to supplement the RN staff.

In addition to these points, the AHA has five recommendations for building "a thriving workforce" (2002, p. 5):

- Foster meaningful work by designing the work around the patients and the staff that takes care of them
- Improve the workplace by building a culture that values, listens to, and rewards staff
- Broaden the base of staff by promoting diversity
- Collaborate (hospitals, associations, educational institutions, corporations, philanthropic organizations and government) to attract new entrants to the health professions
- Build societal support for public policies and resources that support a qualified workforce

Barriers to Errors Related to Understaffing

A final way to lessen medical error due to understaffing is to establish barriers to these errors. Human-factor approaches to error have suggested many ways to establish barriers to error. Two important techniques are safe practices and redundant systems (see chapter 1).

Safe practices are policies and procedures that enable staff to perform in a safe manner (Agency for Healthcare Research and Quality (AHRQ), 2001). Examples of safe practices include hand washing, guidelines for handling of needles, standardized shift routines, and written procedures for nursing care. Important points about safe practices are that they be realistic for the staffing levels, that staff review them and demonstrate competency on a periodic basis, and that staff be monitored for compliance.

The policies and procedures that form safe practices should be evidence based (see chapter 4). However, they should also be realistic so that they do not overburden an already taxed workforce. It might be a good idea to review and revise existing policies and procedures to shorten and simplify them so that overworked staff are more likely to follow them. Or a review of policies and procedures may reveal that they can be followed in a more efficient manner if changes are made to the environment. Once evidence-based, realistic, and efficient policies and procedures are established, staff must be knowledgeable about them and demonstrate competency. In addition to periodic assessment of knowledge and competency, staff should be actively monitored regarding compliance. The institution's quality improvement and/or risk management personnel will want to take an active role in ensuring that these steps are carried out.

An example of safe practices can be found in one of the most important practices related to understaffing and medical error: hand washing. Because of understaffing (as many of the studies on staffing and nosocomial infections bring out), one of the first safe practices to be abandoned is hand washing. Therefore, realistic and efficient hand washing policies must be established, including providing staff with quick and easy access to sinks in all patient rooms and work areas. Second, staff must be educated and monitored to adhere to proper hand washing technique. Staff members need to know that it is not all right to skip this step because they are in a hurry. Then, because overwork will provide an impetus to neglecting this practice, personnel need to be reminded to continue the practice. Impediments to hand washing should be eliminated through mechanisms such as providing waterless alcohol scrubs at each bedside. (See chapter 11 for further discussion of this topic).

Redundancies are systems of repeated checks, such as several people checking narcotic or insulin medication doses, or blood transfusion matches (Leape, 1994). These systems are crucial to preventing medical error. They also take time, so even if the systems are in place, procedures may be skipped when nurses are under time pressures. Therefore, compliance with these systems should be monitored. In our case study, the medical transcription/verification process seemed to lack redundancies. Having two different nurses verify the correctness/clarity of the medication order transcription might have prevented Becky's medication error.

AREAS FOR FURTHER RESEARCH

This chapter has explored a relatively new issue in patient safety investigation and promotion—that of the connection between nurse staffing and patient safety, or rephrased, between understaffing and medical error. The framework developed here, and the studies supporting that framework, are only preliminary work on the subject. Much more needs to be learned about each of the relationships demonstrated in Figure 6.1. We need to better understand the complexities of the structure-process-outcomes triad, including the relationships between structure and process, between process and outcomes, and between components within each category. For example, researchers need to explore the relationships between:

- Inadequate staffing and difficult working conditions (structure to structure)

- Difficult working conditions and individual performance (structure to process)
- Individual performance and medical error (process to outcomes)

We also need more information about how situational conditions affect working conditions, how individual characteristics of nurses affect their performance given the staffing and working conditions, and what system barriers to error help reduce staffing-related errors.

The subject is complex, and research can be approached through studies that examine various pieces of the total picture in detail, or through more complex studies that attempt to study several of the relationships simultaneously. Qualitative studies, using grounded theory, case study, or ethnographic methods, may be used to explore the details and complexities of the relationships. Systems equation modeling may be used to obtain a quantitative analysis of the relationships. Currently, several studies funded by the Agency for Healthcare Research and Quality (AHRQ) are investigating the impact of nurses' workload and working conditions on patient safety (AHRQ, 2002). In addition to these studies, the framework itself could be further developed. Are there other factors that enter the structure-process-outcomes diagram in Figure 6.1? How do the external latent failures referred to in this chapter relate to the internal SPO components in Figure 6.1? What are the psychological and behavioral responses to the difficult working conditions that lead to medical error? Guidance for expanding the framework in these directions could come from empirical research on these questions.

Other useful studies are ones that assess the issue of adequate nurse staffing. We need to explore methods of measuring staffing and workload. How appropriate are currently used methods of assessing the adequacy of staffing in hospitals? Should a standardized method be explored? What should be taken into account in order to estimate workload and assign adequate staffing? Evaluation of nursing process and patient outcome factors in states with mandated staffing ratios will also be important in assessing the positive and negative effects of mandated ratios. Finally, as we become clearer in defining adequate staffing levels for varying workplaces, we can begin to study the relationship of staffing and patient safety from the positive, instead of negative, side. In other words, we can research the impact of adequate staffing on positive patient outcomes in a manner similar to magnet hospital research (Scott, Sochalski, & Aiken, 1999).

In sum, the research needs in the area of nurse staffing and patient safety are many. Some research in the area is already funded and underway.

Much more awaits implementation. These studies will be very helpful in improving nurse staffing and related patient safety issues.

CONCLUSION

This chapter explored the contribution of understaffing to medical error from the theoretical standpoint and from empirical research. Understaffing creates the conditions for medical error, and understaffed hospitals and nursing homes have been shown to have more negative patient outcomes. The evidence is strong that adequate staffing is necessary for patient safety. The chapter discussed policies, strategies, and research for improving staffing and reducing medical error associated with inadequate staffing. As we become more aware of the impact of understaffing on working conditions and on staff performance, we will be able to design safer systems of patient care.

WEB RESOURCES

Name of Resource/URL	Description
Advocacy for Nurses in the Workplace http://nursingworld.org/wpa/	ANA website for workplace advocacy
Health Care at the Crossroads Executive Summary http://www.jcaho.org/news+room/press+kits/executive+summary.htm	JCAHO report on patient safety, speaking to the impact of understaffing on patient safety 2002)
Impact of Working Conditions on Patient Safety http://www.ahrq.gov/news/workfact.htm	Agency for Healthcare Research and Quality fact sheet on research projects currently funded; AHRQ Publication No. 03-P003 (October 2002)
In Our Hands: How Hospital Leaders Can Build a Thriving Workforce http://www.hospitalconnect.com/aha/key_issues/workforce/commission/InOurHands.html	American Hospital Association report on strategies to overcome the nursing shortage (2002)

Keeping Patients Safe: Transforming the Work Environments of Nurses
http://books.nap.edu/books/0309090679/html/index.html

Institute of Medicine Report—readable online.

National Industry—Specific Occupational Employment and Wage Estimates
http://www.bls.gov/oes/2001/oesi2_80.htm

Bureau of Labor Statistics (BLS) industry-specific employment and wages in Health Services

Nurse Reinvestment Act at a Glance
http://www.aacn.nche.edu/media/nraataglance.htm.

American Association of Colleges of Nursing (AACN) report on the act and copy of the act (2002)

Nursing Shortage Poses Serious Health Care Risk: Joint Commission Expert Panel Offers Solutions to National Health Care Crisis
http://www.jcaho.org/news+room/news+release+archives/nursing+shortage.htm

JCAHO statement that the nursing shortage is putting patient lives in danger and issues a call for action on the nursing shortage (August 7, 2002)

Occupational Outlook Handbook, 2002–2003 Edition
http://www.bls.gov/oco/home.htm

Bureau of Labor Statistics manual on the nature of work, employment, training, earning, and employment projections of occupations

Perspectives on the Nursing Shortage: A Blueprint for Action
http://www.ahaonlinestore.com.

Report by AONE (American Organization of Nurse Executives), (2000)

Projected Supply, Demand, and Shortages of Registered Nurses: 2000–2020
http://bhpr.hrsa.gov/healthworkforce/reports/rnproject/default.htm

U.S. Department of Health and Human Services (HRSA) analysis of findings from the 2000 national sample survey of RNs (2002, July)

Staff Nurse Satisfaction, Patient Loads, and Short Staffing Effects in North Carolina
http://www.nursenc.org/research/staff_sat.pdf

Findings from the 2001 Survey of Staff Nurses in North Carolina; In which nurses mention that understaffing is a major source of dissatisfaction and poor quality

The Nursing Shortage: Solutions for the Short and Long Term

Article from the American Nurses Association's (ANA) *Online Journal*

http://www.nursingworld.org/ojin/
topic14/tpc14_4.htm
The Registered Nurse Population:
Findings from the National Sample Survey of Registered Nurses
http://bhpr.hrsa.gov/healthworkforce/
reports/rnsurvey/defa ult.htm

of Issues in Nursing with solutions
for the nursing shortage
U.S. Department of Health and Human Services (HRSA) report on
the nursing supply (2000, March)

REFERENCES

Aaronson, W., Zinn, J., & Rosko, M. (1994). Do for-profit and not-for-profit nursing homes behave differently? *The Gerontologist, 34*(6), 775–786.

Agency for Healthcare Research and Quality (AHRQ). (2002). *Impact of working conditions on patient safety* (Publication No. 03–P003, October 2002). Retrieved May 6, 2003, from http://www.ahrq.gov/news/workfact.htm

Agency for Healthcare Research and Quality (AHRQ). (2001). *Making health care safer: A critical analysis of patient safety practices.* Retrieved May 6, 2003, from http://www.ahrq.gov/clinic/ptsafety/summrpt.htm

Aiken, L., Clarke, S., & Sloane, D. (2000). Hospital restructuring: Does it adversely affect care and outcomes? *Journal of Nursing Administration, 30*(10), 457–465.

Aiken, L., Clarke, S., Sloane, D., Sochalski, J., Busse, R., Clarke, H., et al. (2001). Nurses' report on hospital care in five countries. *Health Affairs, 20*(3), 43–53.

Aiken, L., Clarke, S., Sloane, D., Sochalski, J., & Silber, J. (2002). Hospital nurse staffing and patient mortality, nurse burnout, and job dissatisfaction. *Journal of the American Medical Association, 288*(16), 1987–1993.

Amaravadi, R., Dimick, J., Pronovost, P., & Lipsett, P. (2000). ICU nurse-to-patient ratio is associated with complications and resource use after esophagectomy. *Intensive Care Medicine, 269*(12), 1857–1862.

American Association of Colleges of Nursing (AACN). (2002). *Nurse Reinvestment Act at a glance.* Retrieved April 24, 2003, from http://www.aacn.nche.edu/media/nraataglance.htm

American Hospital Association (AHA). (2002). *In our hands: How hospital leaders can build a thriving workforce.* Retrieved May 6, 2003, from http://www.hospital connect.com/aha/key_issues/workforce/commission/InOurHands.htm

American Hospital Association (AHA). (1999, March). *Trend watch report.* Washington, DC: Author.

American Organization of Nurse Executives (AONE). (2000). *Perspectives on the nursing shortage: A blueprint for action.* Retrieved May 6, 2003, from http://www.ahaonlinestore.com

Anderson, R., Hsieh, P., & Su, H. (1998). Resource allocation and resident outcomes in nursing homes: Comparisons between the best and worst. *Research in Nursing & Health, 21*(4), 297–313.

Archibald, L., Manning, M., Bell, L., Banerjee, S., & Jarvis, W. (1997). Patient density, nurse-to-patient ratio and nosocomial infection risk in a pediatric cardiac intensive care unit. *The Pediatric Infectious Disease Journal, 16,* 1045–1048.

Arnetz, B. B. (1999). Staff perception of the impact of health care transformation on quality of care. *International Journal for Quality in Health Care, 11*(4), 345–351.

Barry-Walker, J. (2000). The impact of systems redesign on staff, patient, and financial outcomes. *Journal of Nursing Administration, 30*(2), 77–89.

Bates, D., Spell, N., Cullen, D., Burdic, E., Laird, N., Peterson, L. A., et al. (1997). The costs of averse drug events in hospitalized patients. *The Journal of the American Medical Association, 277*(4), 307–311.

Bates, D., Cullen, D., Laird, N., Petersen, L., Small, S., Servi, D., et al. (1995). Incidence of adverse drug events and potential adverse drug events. *The Journal of the American Medical Association, 274*(1), 29–34.

Bednash, G. (2001). A nursing leader speaks out on the nursing shortage: Creating a career destination of choice. *Policy, Politics, & Nursing Practice, 2*(3), 191–195.

Blegen, M., Goode, C., & Reed, L. (1998). Nurse staffing and patient outcomes. *Nursing Research, 47*(1), 43–50.

Blegan, M., & Vaughn, T. (1998). A multisite study of nurse staffing and patient occurrences. *Nursing Economics, 16*(4), 196–203.

Bliesmer, M., Smayling, M., Kane, R., & Shannon, I. (1998). The relationships between nursing staffing levels and nursing home outcomes. *Journal of Aging and Health, 10*(3), 351–371.

Bond, C., Raehl, C., & Franke, T. (2001). Medication errors in United States hospitals. *Pharmacotherapy, 21*(9), 1023–1036.

Brennan, T., Leape, L., Laird, N., Hebert, L., Localio, A., Lawthers, A., et al. (1991). Incidence of adverse events and negligence in hospitalized patients: Results of the Harvard Medical Practice Study I. *The New England Journal of Medicine, 324*(6), 370–376.

Bridger, J. C. (1997). A study of nurses' views about the prevention of nosocomial urinary tract infections. *Journal of Clinical Nursing, 6,* 379–387.

Bryant, C., Fairbrother, G., & Fenton, P. (2000). The relative influence of personal and workplace descriptors on stress. *British Journal of Nursing, 9*(13), 876–880.

Castle, N., & Fogel, B. (1998). Characteristics of nursing homes that are restraint free. *The Gerontologist, 38*(2), 181–188.

Cherry, R. (1991). Agents of nursing home quality of care: Ombudsmen and staff ratios revisited. *The Gerontologist, 31*(3), 302–308.

Cody, M., Friss, L., & Hawkinson, Z. (1995). Predicting hospital profitability in short-term general community hospitals. *Health Care Management Review, 20*(3), 77–87.

Cohen, J., & Spector, W. (1996). The effect of Medicaid reimbursement on quality of care in nursing homes. *Journal of Health Economics, 15,* 23–48.

Committee on Quality of Health Care in America, IOM. (2001). *Crossing the quality chasm: A new health system for the 21st century.* Washington, DC: National Academy Press.

Crawshaw, J. (2001). New staffing report claims nursing shortages worse. *Critical Care Alert, 9*(4), 48.

Croteau, R., & Schyve, P. (2000). Proactively error-proofing health care processes. In P. Spath (Ed.), *Error reduction in health care: A systems approach to improving patient safety*. San Francisco: Jossey-Bass.

Dekker, S. (2002). *The field guide to human error investigations*. Burlington, VT: Ashgate.

Dimick, J. B., Swoboda, S. M., Pronovost, P. J., & Lipsett, P. A. (2001). Effect of nurse-to-patient ratio in the intensive care unit on pulmonary complications and resource use after hepatectomy. *American Journal of Critical Care, 10*, 376–382.

Donabedian, A. (1966). Evaluating the quality of medical care. *Milbank Memorial Fund Quarterly, 44*(1), 166–203.

Donabedian, A. (1969). Some issues in evaluating the quality of nursing care. *American Journal of Public Health, 59*(10), 1833–1836.

Donabedian, A. (1988). The quality of care: How can it be assessed? *Journal of the American Medical Association, 260*(12), 1743–1748.

Federation of Nurses and Health Professionals (FNHP). (April 2001). *The nurse shortage: Perspectives from current direct care nurses and former direct care nurses*. Retrieved December 12, 2003, from http://www.aft.org/healthcare/downloadfiles/Hart_Report.pdf

Feldman, S., & Roblin, D. (1997). Medical accidents in hospital care: Applications of failure analysis to hospital quality appraisal. *The Joint Commission: Journal on Quality Improvement, 23*(11), 567–580.

Feldman, S., & Roblin, D. (2000). Accident investigation and anticipatory failure analysis in hospitals. In P. Spath (Ed.), *Error reduction in health care: A systems approach to improving patient safety*. San Francisco: Jossey-Bass.

Firthe-Cozens, J., & Greenhalgh, J. (1997). Doctors' perceptions of the links between stress and lowered clinical care. *Social Science Medicine, 44*(7), 1014–1022.

Flood, S. D., & Diers, D. (1988). Nurse staffing, patient outcome and cost. *Nursing Management, 19*, 34–43.

Fox, M. L., Dwyer, D., & Ganster, D. C. (1993). Effects of stressful job demands and control on physiological and attitudinal outcomes in a hospital setting. *Academy of Management Journal, 36*(2), 289–318.

Fridkin, S., Pear, S., Williamson, T., Galgiani, J., & Jarvis, W. (1996). The role of understaffing in central venous catheter-associated bloodstream infections. *Infection Control and Hospital Epidemiology, 17*, 150–158.

Giraud, T., Dhainaut, J. F., Vaxelaire, J. F., Joseph, T., Journois, D., Bleichner, G., et al. (1993). Iatrogenic complications in adult intensive care units: A prospective two-center study. *Critical Care Medicine, 21*(1), 40–51.

Graber, D. R., & Sloane, P. D. (1995). Nursing home survey deficiencies for physical restraint use. *Medical Care, 33*(10), 1051–1063.

Grazier, K. (1999). Managed care and hospitals. *Journal of Healthcare Management, 44*(5), 335–337.

Groeller, G. (2001, July 4). Result of $15,000 signing bonuses: 'Nurse swapping' among hospitals. *Orlando Sentinel*.

Haley, R., Cushion, N., Tenover, F., Bannerman, T., Dryer, D., Ross, J., et al. (1995). Eradication of endemic Methicillin-resistant Staphylococcus aureus infections from a neonatal intensive care unit. *Journal of Infectious Diseases, 171*, 614–624.

Haley, R., & Bregman, D. (1982). The role of understaffing and overcrowding in recurrent outbreaks of Stephylococcal infection in a neonatal special-care unit. *The Journal of Infectious Diseases, 145*(6), 875–885.

Harbarth, S., Sudre, P., Dharan, S., Cadenas, M., & Pittet, D. (1999). Outbreak of *Enterobacter cloacae* related to understaffing, overcrowding, and poor hygiene practices. *Infection Control and Hospital Epidemiology, 20*(9), 598–603.

Harrington, C., Zimmerman, D., Karon, S., Robinson, J., & Beutel, P. (2000). Nursing home staffing and its relationship to deficiencies. *Journal of Gerontology, 55B*(5), S278–S287.

Hartz, A. J., Krakauer, H., Kuhn, E. M., Young, M., Jacobsen, S. J., Gay, G., et al. (1989). Hospital characteristics and mortality rates. *New England Journal of Medicine, 321*, 1720–1725.

Ingersoll, G., Fisher, M., Ross, B., Soja, M., & Kidd, N. (2001). Employee response to major organizational redesign. *Applied Nursing Research, 14*(1), 18–28.

Johnson-Pawlson, J., & Infeld, D. (1996). Nurse staffing and quality of care in nursing facilities. *Journal of Gerontological Nursing, 22*(8), 36–45.

Joint Commission for Accreditation of Healthcare Organizations (JCAHO). (2002). *Health care at the crossroads.* Retrieved May 6, 2003, from http://www.jcaho.org/news+room/news+release+archives/health+care+at+the+crossroads.pdf

Joint Commission for Accreditation of Healthcare Organizations (JCAHO). (2002, August). *Nursing shortage poses serious health care risk: Joint Commission expert panel offers solutions to national health care crisis.* JCAHO Call for Action. Retrieved May 6, 2003, from http://www.jcaho.org/news+room/news+release+archives/nursing+shortage.htm

Kimball, B., & O'Neil, E. (2001). The evolution of a crisis: Nursing in America. *Policy, Politics, & Nursing Practice, 2*(3), 180–186.

Kohn, L. T., Corrigan, J. M., & Donaldson, M. S. (Eds.). (2000). *To err is human: Building a safer health system.* Washington, DC: National Academy Press.

Kovner, C., Jones, C., Zhan, C., Gergen, P., & Basu, J. (2002). Nurse staffing and post surgical adverse events: An analysis of administrative data from a sample of U.S. hospitals, 1990–1996. *Health Services Research, 37*(3), 611–629.

Kovner, C., & Gergen, P. (1998). Nurse staffing levels and adverse events following surgery in U.S. hospitals. *Image: Journal of Nursing Scholarship, 30*(4), 315–321.

Krakauer, H., Bailey, R. C., & Skellan, K. J. (1992). Evaluation of the HCFA model for the analysis of mortality following hospitalization. *Health Services Research, 27*, 317–335.

Leape, L. (1994). Error in medicine. *Journal of American Medical Association, 272*(23), 1851–1857.

Leape, L., Bates, D., Cullen, D., Cooper, J., Demonaco, H., Gallivan, T., et al. (1995). Systems analysis of adverse drug events. *Journal of American Medical Association, 274*(1), 35–43.

Leape, L., Brennan, T., Laird, N., Lawthers, A., Localio, A., Barnes, B., et al. (1991). The nature of adverse events in hospitalized patients: Results of the Harvard Medical Practice Study II. *New England Journal of Medicine, 324*(6), 377–384.

Leveck, M., & Jones, C. (1996). The nursing practice environment, staff retention, and quality of care. *Research in Nursing & Health, 19*, 331–343.

Levey, S. (1999). Painful medicine: Managed care and the fate of America's major teaching hospitals. *Journal of Healthcare Management, 44*(4), 231–251.

Manheim, L. M., Feinglass, J., Shortell, S. M., & Hughes. (1992). Regional variation in Medicare hospital mortality. *Inquiry, 29,* 55–66.

McClanahan, S., Goodwin, S., & Houser, F. (2000). A formula for errors: Good people + bad systems. In P. Spath (Ed.), *Error reduction in health care: A systems approach to improving patient safety.* San Francisco: Jossey-Bass.

McNeese-Smith, D. (2001). A nursing shortage: Building organizational commitment among nurses. *Journal of Healthcare Management, 46*(3), 173–187.

Meurier, C. (2000). Understanding the nature of errors in nursing: Using a model to analyze critical incident reports of errors which had resulted in an adverse or potentially adverse event. *Journal of Advanced Nursing, 31*(1), 202–207.

Motowidlo, S. J., Manning, M. R., & Packard, J. S. (1986). Occupational stress: Its causes and consequences for job performance. *Journal of Applied Psychology, 71*(4), 618–629.

Munroe, D. (1990). The influence of registered nurse staffing on the quality of nursing home care. *Research in Nursing and Health, 13,* 263–270.

Needleman, J., Buerhaus, P., Mattke, S., Stewart, M., & Zelevinsky, K. (2002). Nurse-staffing levels and the quality of care in hospitals. *New England Journal of Medicine, 346*(22), 1715–1722.

Nevidjon, B., & Erickson, J. (2001). The nursing shortage: Solutions for the short and long term. *Online Journal of Issues in Nursing, 6*(1), Manuscript 4. Retrieved May 6, 2003, from http://www.nursingworld.org/ojin/topic14_4.htm

North Carolina Center for Nursing. (2002, July). *Staff nurse satisfaction, patient loads, and short staffing effects in North Carolina.* Findings from the 2001 Survey of Staff Nurses in North Carolina. Retrieved May 6, 2003, from http://www.nursenc.org/research/staff_sat.pdf

Page, A. (Ed.). (2003). *Keeping patients safe: Transforming the work environments of nurses.* Washington, DC: National Academies Press.

Pittet, D., Tarara, D., & Wenzel, R. P. (1994). Nosocomial bloodstream infection in critically ill patients: Excess length of stay, extra costs, and attributable mortality. *Journal of the American Medical Association, 271*(20), 1599–1601.

Porell, F., Caro, F., Silva, A., & Monane, M. (1998). A longitudinal analysis of nursing home outcomes. *Health Services Research, 33*(4), 835–865.

Purnell, M., Horner, D., Gonzalez, J., & Westman, N. (2001). The nursing shortage: Revisioning the future. *Journal of Nursing Administration, 31*(4), 179–186.

Reason, J. (2000). Human error: Models and management. *British Medical Journal, 320,* 768–770.

Reason, J. (1997). *Managing the risks of organizational accidents.* Brookfield, VT: Ashgate.

Reason, J. (1990). *Human error.* Cambridge, MA: Cambridge University Press.

Service Employees International Union. (2003). *Safe staffing news from states.* Retrieved April 24, 2003, from http://www.seiu.org/health/nurses/safe_staffing/states.cfm

Schmidt, I., Claesson, C., Westerholm, B., & Svarstad, B. (1998). Residents characteristics and organizational factors influencing the quality of drug use in Swedish nursing homes. *Social Science and Medicine, 47*(7), 961–971.

Scott, J. G., Sochalski, J., & Aiken, L. (1999). Review of magnet hospital research: Findings and implications for professional nursing practice. *Journal of Nursing Administration, 29*(1), 9–19.

Seago, J., Ash, M., Spetz, J., Coffman, J., & Grumbach, K. (2001). Hospital registered nurse shortages: Environmental, patient, and institutional predictors. *Health Services Research, 36*(5), 831–852.

Shindul-Rothschild, J. (1994). Restructuring, redesign, rationing, and nurses' morale: A qualitative study on the impact of competitive financing. *Journal of Emergency Nursing, 20*(6), 497–504.

Shindul-Rothschild, J., Berry, D., & Long-Middleton, E. (1996). Where have all the nurses gone?: Final results of our patient care survey. *American Journal of Nursing, 96*(11), 25–39.

Smith, C. (1980). Adequate staffing: It's more than a game of numbers. In B. Brown (Ed.), *Nurse staffing: A practical guide*. Germantown, MD: Aspen Systems Corporation.

Spector, W., & Takada, H. (1991). Characteristics of nursing homes that affect resident outcomes. *Journal of Aging and Health, 3*(4), 427–454.

Spetz, J. (2001). What should we expect from California's minimum nurse staffing legislation? *Journal of Nursing Administration, 31*(3), 132–140.

Stahl, D. (2000). Implications of the Balanced Budget Act of 1997. *Clinics in Geriatric Medicine, 16*(4), 757–774.

Stegenga, J., Bell, E., & Matlow, A. (2002). The role of nurse understaffing in nosocomial viral gastrointestinal infections on a general pediatrics ward. *Infection Control and Hospital Epidemiology, 23*(3), 133–140.

Tai, T. W., Bame, S. I., & Robinson, C. D. (1998). Review of nursing turnover research, 1977–1996. *Social Science and Medicine, 47*(12), 1905–1924.

Tarnow-Mordi, W., Hau, C., Warden, C., & Shearer, A. (2000). Hospital mortality in relation to staff workload: A 4-year study in an adult intensive-care unit. *The Lancet, 356*, 185–189.

Taylor, S., White, B., & Muncer, S. (1999). Nurses' cognitive structural models of work-based stress. *Journal of Advanced Nursing, 29*(4), 974–983.

Ternov, S. (2000). The human side of medical mistakes. In P. Spath (Ed.), *Error reduction in health care: A systems approach to improving patient safety*. San Francisco: Jossey-Bass.

Thomas, E., Studdert, D., Burstin, H., Orav, E., Zeena, T., Elliot, J., Williams, J., Howard, K., Weiler, P., & Brennan, T. (2000). Incidence and types of adverse events and negligent care in Utah and Colorado. *Medical Care, 38*(3), 261–271.

Turnbull, G. (2000). Thriving and surviving in home care and skilled nursing facilities under the Balanced Budget Act of 1997. *Journal of Wound, Ostomy, and Continence Nursing, 27*(2), 79–82.

Unruh, L., & Fottler, M. (2002). Nurse staffing and nursing performance: A review and synthesis of the relevant literature. *Advances in Healthcare Management, 3*, 11–44.

Unruh, L. (2002). Trends in adverse events in hospitalized patients. *Journal for Healthcare Quality, 24*(5), 4–10.

Unruh, L. (2003). Licensed nurse staffing and adverse events in hospitals, *Medical Care, 41*(1), 142–152.

Urden, L., & Walston, S. (2001). Outcomes of hospital restructuring and reengineering: How is success or failure being measured? *Journal of Nursing Administration, 31*(4), 203–209.

USA Today. (2002). California proposes nurse staffing limits. January 23, 2002.

Vicca, A. F. (1999). Nursing staff workload as a determinant of Methicillin-resistant Staphyloccus aureus spread in an adult intensive therapy unit. *Journal of Hospital Infections, 43,* 78–80.

Vincent, C., Taylor-Adams, S., & Stanhope, N. (1998). Framework for analyzing risk and safety in clinical medicine. *British Medical Journal, 316*(11), 1154–1157.

White, K. (2001). A new and very real nursing shortage. *Policy, Politics, & Nursing Practice, 2*(3), 200–205.

Williams, A. M. (1998). The delivery of quality nursing care: A grounded theory study of the nurse's perspective. *Journal of Advanced Nursing, 27,* 808–816.

Yoe, J. (1988). The effects of workload and understaffing on staff in an educational service setting. *Journal of Environmental Psychology, 8,* 107–121.

Chapter 7

Improving the Nursing Work Culture

Jo Ann Miller and Mary Lou Brunell

INTRODUCTION

Work culture plays a significant role in the success or failure of a health care organization and in patient safety. Simply defined, work culture is the way people do things in the workplace. Schein (1992) defines work culture as the behavioral regularities of how people react in a working group—their values, philosophy, and rules for getting along. For the purpose of this chapter, work culture is defined as including the culture of the organization, the nurse work culture, and the work environment. The significance of work culture to patient safety is in its influence on retention of nurses, patient and nurse satisfaction, patient outcomes, and organizational success or failure.

Systems theory provides a framework for conceptualizing and defining the issues and problems related to work culture in health care organizations. This chapter describes strategies to promote a positive nursing work culture, including those acknowledged by the Magnet Recognition Program and the Clinical Governance Model. The Magnet Recognition Program identifies excellence in nursing and is an exemplar culture of care for both nurses and patients. The Clinical Governance Model provides a framework to improve patient safety and the nurse work culture.

ORGANIZATIONAL WORK CULTURE

Organizational culture provides a pervasive framework for everything done and thought in an organization (McLean & Marshall, 1983). For health care, the culture of the organization could not be more critical to the achievement of positive outcomes and patient safety. An organization is designed to incorporate the efforts of individuals and groups to accomplish the work that needs to be done. Organizational culture consists of the fundamental assumptions and beliefs that are shared by members of the organization (Schein, 1992). The shared beliefs, values, and feelings that exist within the organization influence the perception of and the approach to work that is to be completed, and affect how it is done (Sovie, 1993). Within the organization there may also be subcultures shaping the perceptions, attitudes, and beliefs of individuals in specific departments and/or professional disciplines.

One of the most crucial elements affecting the organizational culture is leadership. The first-line manager plays a significant role in fostering a positive organizational and work culture. Organizational culture helps determine the success of the organization. Therefore, in order for organizational leadership to successfully implement change, it must actively manage both the culture and subcultures within the organization (Jones, DeBaca, & Yarbrough, 1997).

Nurse Work Culture

The global shortage of nurses is putting patient lives in danger. Inadequate staffing is frequently cited as the cause of decline in the quality of patient care (see chapter 6). Although nurse staffing is extremely important, it is the nurse work culture that detracts from, or enhances the effect of, nurse staffing on patient and nurse outcomes. Decades of research indicate that high-quality nursing care reduces the rate of complications and the length of stay in hospitals (Nursing's Agenda for the Future Steering Committee, 2002). Research also provides substantial evidence that organizational attributes that support professional nurses in hospitals reduce mortality rates and increase nurse and patient satisfaction (Havens & Aiken, 1999). Safety can be thought of as the minimum standard of adequate patient care. Failure to address the nurse work culture is likely to increase medical errors, adverse events, deaths, complications, and other undesirable patient outcomes.

Nurses are the human interface between the health care organization and the patient. While a physician's time with patients is measured in minutes, nurses spend hours with patients (Greenberg, 2002). The fundamental role of the nurse is to provide quality patient care and support for those suffering from health problems, yet these functions have often been disregarded by health care organizations. Nurses have not been treated as professional caregivers even though their presence at the bedside can literally mean life or death for their patients. With the changes in the health care environment (restructuring, downsizing, managed care), nurses have been forced to perform an array of non-nursing responsibilities, which take them away from the bedside and the provision of professional nursing care (Greenberg, 2002). Typically, paperwork consumes an additional half-hour for every hour of patient care. In settings such as emergency departments, paperwork can consume up to an hour for every hour of patient care [American Hospital Association (AHA), 2001].

A nurse is a physician's primary source of information regarding changes in a patient's condition. They detect impending complications and then act upon them in a timely manner. While nurses observe the patient more than any other professional, their observations do not drive the health care system. The public image of nursing as a technical versus professional field has handicapped nurses from gaining the respect their profession deserves. An additional problem is the failure of organizations to recognize the value of nurses and to invest in them as vital, irreplaceable resources. Until there is recognition and investment in changing this image of nursing, short-term solutions will continue to generate, mediocre short-term results, thus limiting the opportunity to facilitate a positive work culture (Taft, 2001).

Nursing care involves performance of critical assessments, technical tasks, and patient education, although the essence of a nurse's professional obligation is patient advocacy (Hall, 2001). In a more efficient system, the data revealed by nurses' notes, including the use of supplies and services, would be integral to individual patient and organizational health care planning, implementation, and evaluation, and would thus promote patient safety and positive outcomes. The activities of nurses are not a by-product of the treatment process but are, or should be, the central focus of the routine management of the patient during the course of hospitalization.

Nurses have been described as the "glue" that keeps the highly specialized, often fragmented system of hospital care together (Thomas, 1983). Nurses, as direct care providers, are often "in between" patients and their physicians, patients and institutional expectations, and their immediate manager and higher-level administration (Hamric, 2001). With the changes that have occurred in the health care environment, this puts the nurse in a difficult position and often poses significant ethical challenges (Hamric, 2001).

Two ethical issues that nurses face in their clinical practice and work environment are related to the principles of autonomy and beneficence, characterized by lack of control over practice, and the potential for harm to patients and themselves. Strategies to increase control over their practice and decrease the risk of harm to patients include shared decision making with administrators, participating in a process for quality improvement, and creating a more positive image of nursing (Erlen, 2001).

At the same time that nurses are struggling to satisfy patients and employers, the majority of nurses are forgoing breaks, working overtime, and feeling less and less appreciated. In a work environment fueled by severe cost-cutting, nurses have lost trust in a system that instead of supporting them has betrayed them. Effective communication and visibility are crucial components to rebuilding trust in an organization. Trust could be restored by a caring administrator who cultivates relationships and is a competent role model politically, economically, and ethically (Ray, Turkel, & Marino, 2002).

Assuring an adequate nurse work force has been referred to by Disch (2001) as a three-legged stool, and increasing the supply of nurses is just one leg. The second leg involves decreasing the demands made on nurses. Given that nurses are a valued resource, nursing care delivery models need to allow nurses to practice nursing, rather than requiring them to perform other tasks unrelated to patient care. When nurses spend time on the phone ordering supplies, transporting noncritical patients, passing food trays, running to the pharmacy for medications, and making empty beds they waste precious time that could be best utilized in direct care delivery. The third leg of the stool is improving the environment of care. This includes the ergonomics of the work setting and the work culture. When a healthy nurse work culture is present, anything is possible. (Disch, 2001). Improving the environment of care as a critical aspect of patient safety is further supported by the November 2003 report from the Institute of Medicine (IOM) titled: *Keeping Patients Safe: Transforming the Work Environment of Nurses* (Page, 2003). This report calls for a change in both the work culture and environment to promote patient safety.

SYSTEMS THEORY

Health care is a complex organizational system combining technology, treatment, processes, and human interactions. With this complexity is the risk that something will go wrong, and when things go wrong, patient safety is at risk and the consequences can be devastating (O'Neil, 2001). Many of the problems and issues in the nurse work culture can be identified using systems theory. A system is a complex of elements in interaction, which on first appearance may not seem interconnected or related. A systems perspective gives the greatest depth and understanding between multiple variables (Gillies, 1994) that influence work culture, the work environment, and ultimately patient safety and outcomes.

The four classic elements of systems theory are input, throughput, output, and feedback. Input is the operating substance and energizer of a system. Input consists of information, materials, or forces that enter a system (Gillies, 1994). Throughput is the process by which a system converts input into output (Rowland & Rowland, 1997). Output is the end result of system throughput. Feedback loops are an essential mechanism used to monitor and evaluate performance of a system. Examples of input, throughput, output, and feedback in the nurse work setting are found in Figure 7.1.

Nursing is enmeshed in many systems. More than 65% of the work performed by nurses is influenced in some way by others, including physicians, regulatory agencies, or professionals from other disciplines (Murphy, Ruch, Pepicello, & Murphy, 1997). Yet nurses are ultimately responsible for quality patient care. A study of more than 170,000 health care workers, including 47,692 registered nurses (RNs), supports the theory that complexity in health care systems has led to complicated work lives for nurses, accompanied by poor morale, increased levels of stress, and fragmented care delivery systems (Murphy, Ruch, Pepicello, & Murphy, 1997).

A systems approach is particularly useful for the planning and control functions of management. A nurse manager must be the link between a variety of systems. A systems approach investigates the whole situation, rather than considering one or two of the more troublesome aspects (Narrow & Buschler, 1982). Systems awareness is essential in planning a positive approach to improving the quality of health care and providing a safe culture for both nurses and their patients. Systems thinking goes beyond "fault finding" and blaming individuals; instead it examines structures, processes, and relationships. It provides a method of understanding what works well, what is dysfunctional, and what needs to be improved (O'Neill, 2001). Systems thinking encourages a broader view of how the organization actually functions and its interactions instead of viewing individual parts of the system as "good" or "bad," "right" or "wrong" (O'Neil, 2001).

Poor system designs are a threat to patient safety. A means of accountability focused on blame offers little hope of significant improvements. This

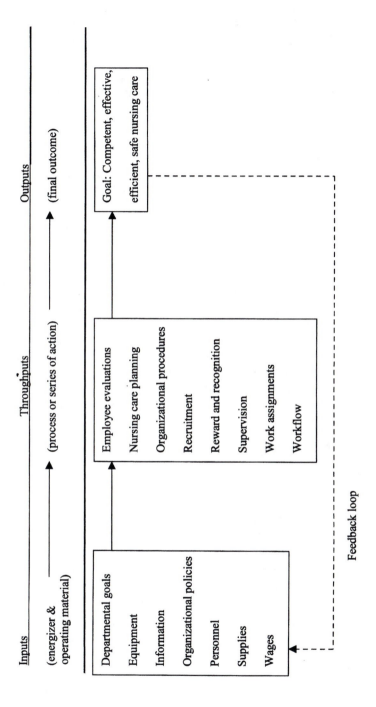

FIGURE 7.1   Systems theory in the nurse work setting.

is because a culture that seeks to blame leads to secrecy, mistrust, and a failure to report mistakes (McSherry & Pearce, 2002), thus disabling the necessary feedback loop for a well-functioning system. As discussed in chapter 1, a major challenge to providing a safer health care system is changing the culture from one of blaming individuals for errors, to one in which errors are not treated as personal failures, but as opportunities to improve the system and prevent harm (Kohn, Corrigan, & Donaldson, 2000; Page, 2004). A poor work culture is known to contribute to the occurrence of errors and accidents (Aiken, Sloane, & Klocinski, 1997; Clarke, Rockett, Sloane, & Aiken, 2002; Page, 2004). Assessing and managing risks to patient safety are important factors of clinical practice and patient care.

GOVERNANCE

Work culture is influenced by the health care organization's governance structure. The type of governance is important to the nurse work culture and nursing satisfaction and may be a determinant of nurse turnover and retention (Stumpf, 2001). The management structure of an organization determines the authority and accountability of employees as well as the pathway of communication and coordination (Rowland & Rowland, 1997).

Traditional Governance

One kind of governance, traditional governance, involves a chain of command where work is coordinated by orders from superiors to subordinates, reaching from the top to the bottom of the organization. With traditional governance, decision making takes place above the level of the direct patient care staff. Authority and responsibility are clearly defined, which leads to efficiency and simplicity of relationships. Standardized policies and procedures replace individualized care, and management replaces leadership (Rowland & Rowland, 1997). Nurses and other direct patient caregivers may feel a lack of power and control with this governance approach.

Shared Governance

One of the characteristics of a profession is shared governance. Nursing in institutional settings has predominantly been governed by the institution, instead of by the profession. Medicine, on the other hand, is governed by the profession while practicing in the institution (Dochterman & Grace, 2001). Shared governance is often described as a flat type of organizational structure. Shared governance is decentralized leadership, providing nurses with a work culture that gives them authority for decisions, autonomy to make decisions, and control over the implementation and outcome of those decisions (Marquis & Huston, 2000). In shared governance, health care organizational governance is shared among board members, nurses, physicians, and managers (Hess, 1995). Shared governance shifts power to nurses and other direct patient care providers and reflects their professional stature within a health care setting while building trust in managerial decisions (Baker, Beglinger, King, Salyards, & Thompson, 2000).

In an ex post facto correlational study investigating the influence of governance type on organizational culture, nurse work satisfaction, nurse retention, and patient satisfaction, analysis revealed overall positive findings in the shared governance groups. Comparing shared governance and traditional governance, the researchers found that the traditional governance group had a passive-defensive culture, low work satisfaction, and low patient satisfaction (Stumpf, 2001). This work supported earlier studies that found dissatisfied nurses negatively influenced patient satisfaction and nurse turnover rates (McDaniel & Patrick, 1992; Hinshaw, Smeltzer, & Atwood, 1987).

Historically, decision making has involved minimal input from the nursing staff, particularly when it involves institutional policy. Nurses have also been limited in regard to their professional autonomy (Swansburg & Swansburg, 2002). The goal of shared governance is to empower people within the decision-making system. In health care organizations, empowerment is directed toward increasing nurse authority and control over nursing practice (Mass & Specht, 1994). There is no single model of shared governance, although all models share an underlying theme of the empowerment of staff nurses (Hess, 1995).

The National Health Service (NHS) is the largest organization in Europe and provides health care to citizens of England, Northern Ireland, Scotland, and Wales. The Clinical Governance Model, a form of shared governance, was introduced in the NHS due to a perceived decline in clinical standards, service provisions, and delivery of care. This was reinforced with media coverage of major clinical failures resulting in a lack of public confidence in the NHS. Successfully implemented, the Clinical Governance Model ensures that all the efforts of an organization, including those who work in it, are focused and coordinated to deliver high-quality care and continuously improve standards of care and service (McSherry & Pearce, 2002).

STRATEGIES TO IMPROVE THE NURSE WORK CULTURE

Strategies to improve the nurse work culture are key components of the Magnet Recognition Program and the Clinical Governance Model. The Magnet Recognition Program identifies a positive work culture, excellence in nursing care and demonstrates its importance to quality patient outcomes and the success of the entire organization. Magnet hospitals recognize nursing as an essential part of the health care institution and not as an isolated entity (American Nurses Credentialing Center [ANCC], 2002). The Clinical Governance Model is the framework through which NHS organizations are accountable for continuously improving the quality of their health care services and safeguarding high standards of care (Department of Health [NHS], 1997).

Magnet Recognition Program

Research presented by McClure and Hinshaw (2002) provides substantial evidence that health care facilities achieving magnet status provide an exemplar work culture of care for both nurses and patients. By recognizing the importance of nurses in patient outcomes, involving nurses in the decision-making process, and providing nurses with the resources necessary to care for patients, optimal patient outcomes including safe and competent nursing care are achieved.

In the early 1980s, recognizing a critical national shortage of nurses, the American Academy of Nurses (AAN) embarked on a study to identify hospitals that attract and retain professional nurses in their employment and to identify factors that seem to be associated with their success. These hospitals were called "magnet hospitals" (McClure, Poulin, Sovie, & Wandelt, 1983). In 1994, a decade after the original magnet study was published, the American Nurses Credentialing Center (ANCC) developed the Magnet Recognition Program. This voluntary program recognizes environments that not only attract nurses, but also acknowledge nursing excellence and the role professional nurses play in the delivery of quality patient care (ANCC, n.d.). In 1998 the program was expanded to include long-term care facilities, and in 2002 the first health care facility outside of the United States was awarded magnet status (ANCC, n.d.).

The American Nurses Association's (ANA) "Scope and Standards for Nurse Administrators" provides the evaluative framework upon which the program is based (ANA, 2003). How the nurse administrator functions within the organizational framework and the role of research and its impact on nursing practice are important criteria for magnet status. Magnet recognition criteria categories include assessment, diagnosis, identification of outcomes, planning, implementation, evaluation, quality of care, administrative practice, performance appraisal, education, collegiality, ethics, collaboration, research, and resource utilization (ANCC, 2003a). Specific items for each of these factors influence the nursing work culture, work environment, patient safety, and outcomes.

In a 2001 study entitled "Staff Nurses Identify Essentials of Magnetism," 279 staff nurses working in 14 magnet hospitals were given a list of 37 items and asked to select the ten items most important in giving quality care. From this study eight factors emerged and are referred to as the Essentials of Magnetism (Kramer & Schmalenberg, 2002). These eight factors identified as essential to providing quality care are shown in Table 7.1 along with the percentage of nurses responding to each factor. Each is discussed below, along with strategies for their implementation.

Working With Other Nurses Who Are Clinically Competent

Competence is the state of possessing qualities and abilities that are important for a specific role or task. Nurses value competency, as it is crucial for safe practice (Hamilton, 1996). Competency in health care has received significant interest because it is thought to represent a method to identify

TABLE 7.1   Essentials of Magnetism

Factor	Percent Responding as Important to Productivity
Working with other nurses who are clinically competent	80.1%
Good RN-MD relationships and communication	79.2%
Nurse autonomy and accountability	73.5%
Supportive nurse manager, supervisor	69.8%
Control over practice and practice environment	68.9%
Support for education (inservice, continuing education)	66.2%
Adequate nurse staffing	62.5%
Concern for the patient is paramount in this organization	62.0%

Staff nurses identify essentials of magnetism, by M. Kramer & C. Schmalenberg. In M. L. McClure & A. S. Hinshaw (Eds.) 2002, *Magnet hospitals revisited: Attraction and retention of professional nurses* (pp. 25–59). Reprinted with permission of American Nurses Publishing.

caregiver characteristics that can predict or contribute to successful job performance and ultimately to positive patient outcomes (Dochterman & Grace, 2001). Competence is an essential component of professional nursing. Nurses must frequently update their knowledge and skills, to be competent in an ever-changing field (Hamilton, 1996). Competency is expected of all nurses and is more than just being able to perform a task. Competence also promotes a positive work culture because confidence that one's colleagues are competent promotes teamwork. Nurses utilize technical, critical thinking, and interpersonal relationship skills. Ways to increase competency include:

- Encouraging advanced education, including certification (Kramer & Schmalenberg, 2002)
- Building the value of advanced education and certification into the organizational culture through rewards, recognition, and the salary structure (Kramer & Schmalenberg, 2002)

Good Registered Nurse–Physician Relationships and Communication

Communication is one of the most important processes in a health care organization. Good communication builds productive relationships among health care workers and between health care workers and their patients. Nurses do not work in isolation. In addition to relationships with their peers, relationships with their medical colleagues are an important aspect of the nurse work culture (Adams & Bond, 2000). Ways to improve nurse-physician relationships and communication include:

- Fostering development of collegial relationships between nurses and physicians (Kramer & Schmalenberg, 2002)
- Continuing research to assess the impact of nurse-physician relationships on patient outcomes (Kramer & Schmalenberg, 2002)

Nurse Autonomy and Accountability

Autonomy and accountability are reflected through the ability of a nurse to assess and provide nursing actions as appropriate for patient care (Ritter-Teitel, 2002). It is not a nurse providing medical care without medical supervision. Nursing care complements and often overlaps medical care. Actions that foster autonomy and accountability include:

- Development of autonomy through decentralization (Kramer & Schmalenberg, 2002)
- Participation in decision making affecting professional practice

Supportive Nurse Managers and Supervisors

A strong commitment to nursing, recognition of professional nursing practice, leadership visibility, and support of nursing autonomy are factors that influence nurse leadership. Nurses at magnet health care facilities feel supported from administrators more often than nurses in nonmagnet health care facilities (Upeniecks, 2002). Effective leadership is essential to the establishment of a unified and competent work force and ultimately to the success of quality care (Scott, Sochalski, & Aiken, 1999). Methods to recruit and retain supportive nurse management include:

- Creating a positive culture for competent nurse managers who understand the complexities of health care
- Supporting nurse managers in their leadership role (Kramer & Schmalenberg, 2002)
- Providing continuing education opportunities relative to the continually changing health care environment and leadership
- Rewarding and recognizing nurse managers for empowering and assisting staff

Control over the Practice Environment

Control over practice is the freedom to shape policies and procedures in professional practice. When nurses have limited control over patient care they feel their expertise is not valued (The Change Foundation and the Canadian Health Services Research Foundation, 2001). Ways to achieve control over practice include:

- Creating and supporting shared governance or a similar organizational structure (Kramer & Schmalenberg, 2002)
- Guiding and educating staff nurses and nurse managers in activities that promote empowerment and emphasize shared governance structures (Kramer & Schmalenberg, 2002)

Support for Education (Inservice, Continuing Education)

Due to the restructuring of health care, the advancement of medical technology, and the aging of the population, there are now multiple career opportunities for nurses from diverse backgrounds. Nurses want to know that they will be supported in their interest to advance, to learn, and to grow. Magnet facilities emphasize the importance of education, teaching, and professional growth. In a comparison study of two groups of magnet hospitals, over 50% of RNs were baccalaureate prepared (Aiken, Havens, & Sloane, 2000). This is in contrast to about 34% of RNs working in hospitals in general (Moses, 1997). Actions to increase support for education include:

- Acknowledging the value of educational support to nurse effectiveness and quality patient outcomes (Kramer & Schmalenberg, 2002)
- Encouraging and promoting both formal and informal education
- Developing and providing staff development programs
- Providing mentoring programs
- Offering tuition reimbursement programs.

Adequacy of Nurse Staffing

Sufficient staffing levels allow nurses the time they need to complete patient assessments, perform nursing duties, and respond to health care emergencies (see chapter 6). Vacancy rates, nurse patient ratios, turnover rates, use of staffing agencies, number of applicants for available positions, and staff perception of adequate staffing are routinely used to measure nursing shortages (Kramer & Schmalenberg, 2002). Many hospitals are relying on nurses from temporary staffing agencies. While temporary nurses are typically well-educated and experienced, there are risks to patient safety involved in employing nurses who are unfamiliar with hospital policy and procedures. The *Chicago Tribune* reported that in Illinois, state disciplinary records show that temporary nurses have increasingly been the focus of medical error investigations. Many cases are linked to a lack of knowledge related to hospital procedure or unfamiliarity with patient diagnoses (Berens, 2000). Strategies to achieve adequate nurse staffing include:

- Implementing nursing care delivery systems based on the needs of specific patient populations and characteristics of health care workers (Kramer & Schmalenberg, 2002)
- Monitoring the usage of agency nurses, and the practice of "floating" nurses from their scheduled work area to work in chronically under-staffed units
- Supporting continued research on the relationship between adequacy of staffing and skill mix on patient outcomes (Kramer & Schmalenberg, 2002)

Chapter 6 discusses nurse staffing and patient outcomes in detail.

Concern for the Patient Is Paramount in the Organization

The essence of nursing is helping people. As the health care industry strives to be more business-like, health care leaders need to remember that quality patient care is essential for success. Nurses want to work in organizations in which they can provide good, safe patient care. Researchers have demonstrated that nurses in magnet health care facilities provide higher-quality care (American Nurses Publishing, 2002). Several studies have shown that better outcomes are achieved in magnet health care facilities. Table 7.2 lists positive outcomes realized at magnet health care facilities for patients, nurses, and health care organizations. Actions showing that concern for the patient is paramount include:

- Establishing adaptive organizational cultures in the work setting (Kramer & Schmalenberg, 2002)
- Establishing evidenced-based practice (see chapter 4)
- Implementing strategies to improve processes of care

TABLE 7.2   Positive Outcomes Achieved at Magnet Facilities

For Patients	For Nurses	For Health Care Facility
Lower mortality rates (Aiken, Smith, & Lake, 1994; Aiken, Sloane, Lake, Sochalski, & Weber, 1999)	Increased satisfaction (Aikens, Havens, & Sloan, 2000)	Higher JCAHO scores (Havens, 2001)
Increased patient satisfaction (Aiken, Sloane, Lake, Sochalski, & Weber, 1999)	Lower incidence of needlestick injury (Aiken, Sloane, & Klocinski, 1997)	Lower vacancy and turnover rates (Kramer & Schmalenberg, 2002; McClure, Poulin, Sovie, & Wandelt, 1983)
Shorter length of stay (Aiken, Havens, & Sloane, 2000)	Lower rates of nurse burnout (Aiken, Havens, & Sloane, 2000)	National recognition (ANCC, n.d.)

The Nurse Reinvestment Act (P.L. 107-205) authorizes the establishment of vital programs designed to help address the nursing shortage. Title II of the Act, Nurse Retention, emphasizes the role of the workplace in retaining and advancing the educational and professional development of nurses. The new law provides best practice grants that are designed to encourage health care facilities to implement nursing best practices, such as the Magnet Recognition Program (Library of Congress, n.d.). The Joint Commission on Accreditation of Healthcare Organizations (JCAHO) supports the Magnet Recognition Program because of the positive impact it has had on implementing workplace cultures and nursing practices that support patient safety and high-quality care (JCAHO, 2002). Magnet hospitals are also exemplars that exhibit implementation of the recommendations of the 2003 IOM report on *Keeping Patients Safe: Transforming the Work Environments of Nurses* (Page, 2004).

The decision to pursue Magnet Recognition is a substantial undertaking, and starts with a thorough assessment of both the organizational and nursing environment. The program application itself is a thorough self-evaluation of the nursing service by the chief nurse executive and the nursing staff. The review of the current situation compared with magnet standards provides guidance for the development of an exemplary nursing work culture, if it is not already in place. Magnet health care facilities demonstrate that creating a professional, positive nurse practice environment is a viable solution to the exodus of nurses by lowering nurse turnover, increasing nurse and patient satisfaction, and increasing nurse and patient safety. The Magnet Recognition Program also provides health care consumers with valuable information to help them select health care facilities known to give competent, safe care (ANCC, n.d.).

Clinical Governance Model

The Clinical Governance Model is the framework through which NHS organizations are accountable for the continuous improvement of the quality of health care services. This is accomplished by creating an environment in which excellence in care will occur (Scally & Donaldson, 1998). The Clinical Governance Model incorporates both quality improvement and accountability by identifying problems early, analyzing and correcting them, and replacing a blame culture with a culture of openness (see chapter 1). The Clinical Governance Model is about both patients and health care workers receiving the proper care in a safe environment. The core organizing principles are those of efficiency and excellence (Crinson,

1999). Health care provision and delivery is complex in nature and is dependent on effective teamwork, positive leadership, and sound management drawing together both the nonclinical and clinical aspects of governance.

Key Components of the Clinical Governance Model

The key components of the success of the Clinical Governance Model are safety, culture, quality improvement and maintenance, and professional and organizational accountability. Clinical quality and continuous improvements in health care can only be achieved in a culture that supports, values, and develops its staff (McSherry & Pearce, 2002).

The Clinical Governance Model develops a work culture that encourages and supports improvements in practice and patient care. Developing the right work culture is a huge undertaking that requires commitment from all levels of the organization. A proactive culture of learning that is open and participative, where education and research are valued, where ideas and good practices are shared, and where blame is rarely used are key for the implementation of the Clinical Governance Model. This model receives national support through two agencies.

The National Institute for Clinical Excellence (NICE) was established in 1999 by the NHS to provide a single reference point to front-line clinicians on clinical standards and cost-effectiveness of selected technologies and other health care interventions. NICE also provides information on lessons learned following investigations of deaths and serious adverse occurrences. NICE accomplishes this through independent review, commissioning clinical guidelines, and funding clinical auditing at a national level (Lugon & Secker-Walker, 2001).

The Commission for Health Improvement (CHI) was established to improve the quality of patient care in the NHS. It accomplishes this by reviewing the care provided by the NHS in England and Wales (Scotland has its own regulatory body, the Clinical Standards Board). CHI addresses unacceptable variations in NHS patient care by identifying both evidence based practice and areas that need improvement (CHI, 2002). Acting independently, CHI assesses every NHS organization and makes its findings public.

NURSE RETENTION

Currently the United States is experiencing a shortage of qualified nurses and over the next 20 years the shortage is expected to worsen. According to current projections a shortage of more than 800,000 registered nurses (RNs) is expected by 2020 (AHA, 2002).

The current nursing shortage has emphasized the fact that having a sufficient number of qualified nurses is paramount for patient safety and for the success of our nation's health care system (see chapter 6). Results of the American Health Care Association (AHCA) Nursing Position Vacancy and Turnover Survey (AHCA, 2002) found that national population-adjusted vacancy and turnover rates for staff RNs was 18.5%, and that 25,555 staff RN positions were vacant. The AHCA survey also found that state vacancy and turnover rates varied widely. North Dakota's staff RN vacancy rate was lowest at 11.7%, whereas Utah's staff RN vacancy rate was highest at 24.8%.

A satisfying work culture is key to the retention of nurses. Nurse turnover is routinely viewed as a sign of dissatisfaction. Employees leave organizations for numerous reasons, but most often because their personal needs are not being met. Their needs may be as basic as compensation and benefits, or more complex. Poor working conditions, lack of recognition, poor supervision, lack of potential for professional growth and advancement, and nonaccommodating scheduling are examples of factors that may not meet personal needs. If each employee's contribution to the workplace is not appreciated and recognized it is likely they will leave the organization (AHA, 2003).

Statistics compiled from magnet health care facilities reveal the RN vacancy rate was 9.58% and the average length of employment was 8.92 years for the years 2001–2002 (J. Moran [ANA], personal communication, March 11, 2003). This vacancy rate is lower than the lowest state vacancy rate in the United States (AHCA, 2002). Magnet nursing facilities originally selected for their ability to successfully recruit and retain nurses in the midst of high vacancy and turnover rates are often referred to as "cultures of excellence" and as "setting the gold standard" for working environments (McClure, Poulin, Sovie, & Wandelt, 1983). Not only do nurses experience professional satisfaction at magnet health care facilities, but a stable, experienced nursing staff promotes patient safety and improved patient outcomes.

Nurse Satisfaction

Job satisfaction can be described as the difference between how much a person wants or expects from a job and how much the person actually receives (Steers, 1988). Nurse retention is related to how an organization does or does not value its employees. The most important correlate of work satisfaction is retention. Workers who are satisfied with their work have a tendency to remain in their jobs. Work satisfaction has been studied in a variety of acute care units (Tumulty, Jernigan, & Kohut, 1994; Irvine & Evans, 1995; Blegen, 1993; Lucas, Atwood, & Hagaman, 1993; Shader, Broome, Broome, West, & Nash, 2001) and has been found to affect retention. In a national American Nurses Association staffing survey, 54.8% of respondents stated that they would not recommend the nursing profession as a career for their children or friends, and 23% expressed that they would "actively discourage" someone close to them from entering the nursing profession (ANA, 2001). Nurses in the United States are more likely to be dissatisfied with working conditions rather than with their wages according to a study conducted by the International Hospital Outcomes Research Consortium (Aiken, et al., 2001).

Nurse and patient satisfaction are important issues for nurse executives and nurse managers. Nursing administrators want employees that are productive, dynamic, innovative, and pleased with the work they do. Nursing administrators want patients who feel their nurses have provided them with good care. Nurses' job satisfaction is the key to creating work environments that meet these goals (Kangas, Kee, & McKee-Waddle, 1999). The nurse work culture both reflects and fuels the problems of workforce shortages and turnover (Seymour & Buscherhof, 1991).

Reward and Recognition Programs

Reward and recognition programs, whether formal or informal, economic or personal, create motivation and job satisfaction. External rewards may draw a person to a job, but internal rewards are what keep them there (McCoy, 1999). Although pay may be an incentive to recruit nurses, clinical advancement and recognition by peers and supervisors will retain them. The top motivator for employee performance is recognition for a job well done (Nelson, 1994). Although recognition takes many forms, the motivational value of recognition does not last very long, and frequent reinforcement is necessary for it to be of continuing relevance (Costley & Todd, 1987).

CONCLUSION

The feature that distinguishes health care organizations is their work culture (Scally & Donaldson, 1998). The nursing work culture is known to influence the occurrence of adverse events and errors in health care. A positive nursing work culture is crucial to a stable nursing staff, quality of patient care, and patient safety (Page, 2003). Assessing and managing risks to patient safety are important factors of nursing practice and patient care. Concern for the nursing workforce and the safety of patients in the United States health care system has escalated. Registered nurses, hospital administrators, quality professionals, other health care providers and consumers must come together to create a health care system that supports quality care and the workers who provide that care. The strategies to improve the nurse work culture contained in this chapter are those acknowledged by the Institute of Medicine, the Magnet Recognition Program and the Clinical Governance Model as contributing to a positive work culture that can attract motivated job candidates, and produce better patient, nurse, and organizational outcomes.

WEB RESOURCES

Name of Resource/URL	*Description*
ANCC Magnet Recognition Program *http://nursingworld.org/ancc/ magnet.html*	Magnet Recognition Program information
Commission for Health Improvement (CHI) http://www.chi.nhs.uk/eng/ index.shtml	Established to improve the quality of patient care in the NHS
Controls Assurance Support Unit http://www.casu.org.uk	Created in 2000 to assist NHS organizations improve risk management and the quality of services
Keeping Patients Safe: Transforming the Work Environments of Nurses http://books.nap.edu/books/ 0309090679/html/index.html	Institute of Medicine Report— readable online
National Center for Nursing Quality http://www.nursingquality.org/	Project of the ANA Safety & Quality Initiative addressing issues of patient safety and quality of care arising from changes in health care delivery

NHS Modernisation Agency
http://www.modern.nhs.uk

Information regarding clinical governance

National Institute for Clinical Excellence (NICE)
http://www.nice.org.uk

NICE is associated with and collaborates with organizations concerned with quality improvement within the NHS

University of Michigan Health System Employee Reward & Recognition Program
http://www.med.umich.edu/mchrd/recognition/

Web site offering tips, articles, strategies, and guidance for the design and implementation of recognition programs

REFERENCES

Adams, A., & Bond S. (2000). Hospital nurses job satisfaction: Individual and organizational characteristics. *Journal of Advanced Nursing, 32*(3), 536–543.

Aiken, L. H., Clarke, S. P., Sloane, D. M., Sochalski, J. A., Busse, R., Clarke, H., et al. (2001). Nurse's reports on hospital care in five countries. *Health Affairs, 20*(3), 43–52.

Aiken, L. H., Havens, D. S., & Sloane, D. M. (2000). The magnet nursing services recognition program: A comparison of two groups of magnet hospitals. *American Journal of Nursing, 100*(3), 26–35.

Aiken, L. H., Sloane, D.M., Lake, E. T., Sochalski, J., & Weber, A. L. (1999). Organization and outcomes of inpatient AIDS care. *Medical Care, 37*(8), 760–772.

Aiken, L. H., Sloane, D. M., & Klocinski, J. L. (1997). Hospital nurses' occupational exposure to blood: Perspective, retrospective, and institutional reports. *American Journal of Public Health, 87,* 103–107.

Aiken, L. H., Smith, H. L., & Lake, E. T. (1994). Lower Medicare mortality among a set of hospitals known for good nursing care. *Medical Care, 32*(8), 771–787.

American Health Care Association (AHCA). (2002). *Results of the 2001 AHCA Nursing Position Vacancy and Turnover Survey.* Retrieved April 5, 2003, from http://www.ahca.org/research/vacancysurvey_020207.pdf

American Hospital Association (AHA). (2003, January). *Workforce ideas in action: Case examples.* Retrieved March 18, 2003, from http://www.hospitalconnect.com/aha/key_issues/workforce/content/case_ex.pdf

American Hospital Association (AHA). (2002, November). Workforce. In *Trends affecting hospitals and health systems* (chapter 5). Retrieved April 4, 2003, from http://www.hospitalconnect.com/ahapolicyforum/trendwatch/content/ cb2002chapter5.pdf

American Hospital Association (AHA). (2001). *Patients or paperwork? The regulatory burden facing American hospitals.* Retrieved February 4, 2003, from http://www.hospitalconnect.com/aha/advocacy-grassroots/advocacy/advocacy/content/FinalPaperworkReport.pdf

American Nurses Association (AHA). (2001, February 6). *Analysis of American Nurses Association staffing survey.* Retrieved March 19, 2003, from http://nursingworld.org/staffing/ana_pdf.pdf

American Nurses Credentialing Center (ANCC). (2003). *ANCC Magnet Recognition Program—Recognizing excellence in nursing services.* Retrieved August 16, 2003, from http://nursingworld.org/ancc/magnet.html

American Nurses Credentialing Center (ANCC). (2002). *Credentialing News, 5*(2), 1. Retrieved January 23, 2003, from http://www.nursingworld.org/ancc/news/CredNewsSF.pdf

American Nurses Credentialing Center (ANCC). (n.d.). *Magnet nursing services recognition program.* Retrieved February 23, 2003, from http://www.nursecredentialing.org/ancc/magnet/About.htm

American Nurses Credentialing Center (ANCC). (2003a). *2003/2004 Health care organization magnet instructions and application process manual.* Washington, DC: Author.

American Nurses Publishing. (2002, Summer/Fall). Magnet hospitals revisited: Attraction & retention of professional nurses. *ANCC Credentialing News, 5*(2), 6.

Baker, C., Beglinger, J., King, S., Salyards, M., & Thompson, A. (2000). Transforming negative work cultures. *Journal of Nursing Administration, 30*(7/8), 357–363.

Berens, M. H. (2000, September 10). Dangerous care: Nurse's hidden role in medical error. *Chicago Tribune.*

Blegen, M. A. (1993). Nurses' job satisfaction: A meta-analysis of related variables. *Nursing Research, 42*(1), 36–40.

The Change Foundation and the Canadian Health Services Research Foundation. (2001). *Commitment and care: The benefits of a healthy workplace for nurses, their patients and the system.* Retrieved January 2, 2003, from http://www.chsrf.ca/docs/finalrpts/pscomcare_e.pdf

Clarke, S. P., Rockett J. L., Sloane, D. M., & Aiken, L. H. (2002). Organizational climate, staffing, and safety equipment as predictors of needlestick injuries and near-misses in hospital nurses. *American Journal of Infection Control, 30*(4), 207–216.

Commission for Health Improvement (CHI). (2002, July). *What is CHI?* Retrieved January 29, 2003, from http://www.chi.nhs.uk/eng/about/whatischi.shtml

Costley, D. I., & Todd, R. (1987). *Human relations in organizations.* St. Paul, MN: West Publishing Company.

Crinson, I. (1999). Clinical governance: The new NHS, new responsibilities? *British Journal of Nursing, 8*(7), 449–453.

Department of Health (DOH). (1997). *The new NHS: Modern and dependable.* London: Department of Health.

Disch, J. (2001). Supply is not the only answer. *Journal of Professional Nursing, 17*(2), 72.

Dochterman, J. M., & Grace, H. K. (2001). *Current issues in nursing* (6th ed.). St. Louis: Mosby.

Erlen, J. A. (2001). The nursing shortage, patient care and ethics. *Orthopedic Nursing, 20*(6), 61–65.

Gillies, D. A. (1994). *Nursing management: A systems approach* (3rd ed.). Philadelphia: W. B. Saunders Company.

Greenberg, M. (2002, January 28). *Hailing one of health care's priceless resources—nurses*. Retrieved February 27, 2003, from http://www.ama-assn.org/sci-pubs/amnews/amn_02/edca0128.htm

Hall, K. (2001, February 13). *Testimony of the American Nurses Association on the nursing shortage and its impact on America's health care delivery system before the Subcommittee on Aging, Committee on Health, Education, Labor, and Pensions*. Retrieved February 23, 2003, from http://www.nursingworld.org/gova/federal/legis/testimon/2001/shortage.htm

Hamilton, P. M. (1996). *Realities of contemporary nursing* (2nd ed.). Menlo Park, CA: Addison-Wesley Publishing Company, Inc.

Hamric, A. B. (2001). Ethics development for clinical faculty. *Nursing Outlook, 49*(3), 115–117.

Havens, (2001). Comparing nursing infrastructure and outcomes: ANCC magnet and nonmagnet CNEs report. *Nursing Economic$, 19*(6), 259–266.

Havens, L. H., & Aiken, L. H. (1999). Shaping systems to promote desired outcomes: The magnet hospital model. *Journal of Nursing Administration, 29*(2), 14–20.

Hess, R. G., Jr. (1995). Shared governance: Nursing's 20th century tower of Babel. *Journal of Nursing Administration, 25*(5), 14–17.

Hinshaw, A., Smeltzer, C., & Atwood, J. A. (1987). Innovative retention strategies for nursing staff. *Journal of Nursing Administration, 17*(6), 8–16.

Irvine, D. M., & Evans, M. G. (1995). Job satisfaction and turnover among nurses: Integrating research findings across studies. *Nursing Research, 44*(4), 246–253.

Joint Commission on Accreditation of Healthcare Organizations (JCAHO). (2002). *Health care at the crossroads: Strategies for addressing the evolving nursing crisis*. Retrieved February 22, 2003, from http://www.jcaho.org/news+room/on+capitol+hill/health+care+at+the+crossroads.pdf

Jones, K. R., DeBaca, V., & Yarbrough, M. (1997). Organizational culture assessment before and after implementing patient-focused care. *Nursing Economic$, 15*(2), 73–80.

Kangas, S., Kee, C. C., & McKee-Waddle, R. (1999). Organizational factors, nurses' job satisfaction, and patient satisfaction with nursing care. *Journal of Nursing Administration, 29*(1), 32–42.

Kohn, L. T., Corrigan, J. M., & Donaldson, M. S. (2000). *To err is human: Building a safer health system*. Washington, DC: National Academy Press.

Kramer, M., & Schmalenberg, C. (2002). Staff nurses identify essentials of magnetism. In M. L. McClure & A. S. Hinshaw (Eds.), *Magnet hospitals revisited: Attraction and retention of professional nurses* (pp. 25–59). Washington, DC: American Nurses Publishing.

Library of Congress. (n.d.). *THOMAS: Legislative information of the internet*. Retrieved March 10, 2003, from http://thomas.loc.gov/cgi-bin/bdquery/z?d107:HR03487:@@@L&summ2=m&

Lugon, M., & Secker-Walker, J. (2001). *Advancing clinical governance*. London: Royal Society of Medicine Press.

Lucas, M. D., Atwood, J. R., & Hagaman, R. (1993). Replication and validation of anticipated turnover model for urban registered nurses. *Nursing Research, 42*(1), 29–35.

Marquis, B. L., & Huston, C. J. (2000). *Leadership roles and management functions in nursing: Theory and application* (3rd ed.). Philadelphia: Lippincott.

Mass, M. L., & Specht, J. P. (1994). Shared governance in nursing: What is shared. Who governs, and who benefits? In J. McCloskey & H. K. Grace (Eds.), *Current issues in nursing*. St. Louis: Mosby Yearbook.

McClure, M. L., & Hinshaw, A. S. (2002). *Magnet hospitals revisited: Attraction and retention of professional nurses*. Washington, DC: American Nurses Publishing.

McClure, M. L., Poulin, M. A., Sovie, M. D., & Wandelt, M. A. (1983). *Magnet hospitals: Attraction and retention of professional nurses*. Kansas City, MO: American Academy of Nursing.

McCoy, J. M. (1999). Recognize, reward, retain: Start a program to raise morale and retain staff. *Nursing Management, 30*(2), 41–43.

McDaniel, C., & Patrick, T. (1992). Leadership, nurses and patient satisfaction: A pilot study. *Nursing Administration Quarterly, 16*(3), 72–74.

McLean, A., & Marshall., J. (1983). *Intervening in cultures*. London, England: University of Bath.

McSherry, R., & Pearce, P. (2002). *Clinical governance: A guide to implementation for healthcare professionals*. Oxford: Blackwell Science.

Moses, E. (1997). *The registered nurse population: Findings from the national sample survey of registered nurses, 1996*. Rockville, MD: U.S. Department of Health and Human Services Administration.

Murphy, E. C., Ruch, S., Pepicello, K., & Murphy, M. (1997). Managing an increasingly complex system. *Nursing Management, 28*(10), 33–38.

Narrow, B. W., & Buschler, K. B. (1982). *Fundamentals of nursing practice*. New York: John Wiley & Sons, Inc.

Nelson, B. (1994). *1001 ways to reward employees*. New York: Workman Publishing.

Nursing's Agenda for the Future Steering Committee. (2002, April). *Nursing's agenda for the future: A call to the nation*. Retrieved December 13, 2003 from http://www.nursingworld.org/naf/Plan.pdf

O'Neil, S. (2001). Clinical governance in action. *Professional Nurse, 16*(5), 1074–1075.

Page, A. (Ed.). (2004). *Keeping patients safe: Transforming the work environments of nurses*. Washington, DC: National Academies Press.

Ray, M. A., Turkel, M. C., & Marino, F. (2002). In workforce redevelopment. *Nursing Administration Quarterly, 26*(2), 1–14.

Ritter-Teitel, J. (2002). The impact of restructuring on professional nursing practices. *Journal of Nursing Administration, 32*(1), 31–41.

Rowland, H. S., & Rowland, B. L. (1997). *Nursing administration handbook* (4th ed.). Gaithersburg, MD: Aspen Publishers, Inc.

Scally, G., & Donaldson, L. J. (1998). Looking forward: Clinical governance and the drive for quality improvement in the new NHS in England. *British Medical Journal, 317*(7150), 65.

Seymour, E., & Buscherhof, J. R. (1991). Sources and consequences of satisfaction and dissatisfaction in nursing: Findings from a national sample. *International Journal of Nursing Studies, 28*(2), 109–124.

Schein, E. H. (1992). *Organizational culture and leadership* (2nd ed.). San Francisco: Jossey-Bass.

Scott, J. G., Sochalski, J., & Aiken, L. H. (1999). Review of magnet hospital research: Findings and implications for professional nursing practice. *Journal of Nursing Administration, 29*(1), 9–19.

Shader, K., Broome, M. E., Broome, C. D., West, M. E., & Nash, M. (2001). Factors influencing satisfaction and anticipated turnover for nurses in an academic medical center. *Journal of Nursing Administration, 31*(4), 210–216.

Sovie, M. D. (1993). Hospital culture—why create one? *Nursing Economic$, 11*(2), 69–75, 90.

Steers, R. M. (1988). *Introduction to organizational behavior* (3rd ed). Glenview, IL: Scott, Foreman and Company.

Stumpf, L. R. (2001). A comparison of governance types and patient satisfaction outcomes. *Journal of Nursing Administration, 31*(4), 196–202.

Swansburg, R. C., & Swansburg, R. J. (2002). *Introduction to management and leadership for nurse managers* (3rd ed.). Sudbury, MA: Jones and Bartlett Publishers.

Taft, S. (2001, January 31). The nursing shortage. *Online Journal of Issues in Nursing, 6*(1). Retrieved February 23, 2003, from http://www.nursingworld.org/ojin/topic14/tpc14ntr.htm

Thomas, L. (1983). *The youngest science: Notes of a medicine-watcher.* New York: Viking Press.

Tumulty, G., Jernigan, I. E., & Kohut, G. F. (1994). The impact of perceived work environment on job satisfaction of hospital staff nurses. *Applied Nursing Research, 7*(2), 84–90.

Upeniecks, V. V. (2002). Assessing differences in job satisfaction of nurses in magnet and nonmagnet hospitals. *Journal of Nursing Administration, 32*(11), 564–575.

Chapter 8

Using Technology to Improve Patient Safety

Debra S. Roach, Susan V. White, and Jacqueline Fowler Byers

OVERVIEW

Patient safety involves myriad factors, and each time human intervention is involved, the opportunity for error is increased. Technology provides leverage for improving patient safety by offering solutions that exceed human capabilities such as vast stores of information, speed of retrieval, the ability to make complex calculations, and the capability of providing alarms, alerts, and decision support. This chapter presents an overview of general human factors principles that are critical in using technology. Major barriers to using technology are described, and factors that support implementation will be presented. Then, major technologies that are available to promote safe patient care will be discussed. There are numerous technologies and equipment integrated with computerization that is used in health care. The range of technologies includes a) molecular, cellular, genetic, and pharmaceutical; b) patient administered technologies; c) robotic and remote technologies (remote intensive care unit monitoring, telemedicine); d) Internet-based systems; and e) expert systems (Ball, Garets, & Handler, 2003). Only selected technologies that have been linked to patient safety will be discussed. A full discussion of all types of equipment that promote patient safety is not within the scope of this book.

HUMAN FACTORS AND APPLYING PRINCIPLES TO WORK WITH TECHNOLOGY

Humans have many strengths including a large repertoire of skills and responses, flexibility in responding, and the ability to think creatively (Kohn, Corrigan, & Donaldson, 2000). However, as presented in chapters 1 and 3, there are a number of limitations due to human nature that increase the opportunity for errors to occur. For example, humans have limited problem-solving capacity, which creates difficulty when they are faced with multiple issues at a single time. Humans also have limited recall of information. In 1998 the Food and Drug Administration (FDA) approved 90 new drugs, 30 new molecular entities, and 124 new uses for already approved drugs. In 1990 there were only 3,000 drugs on the market; in 2000 there were over 17,000 (Ball, Garets, & Handler, 2003). It is impossible to maintain a working knowledge of all of these medications and products, so technology can provide ready access to necessary information with the stroke of a key or the push of a button.

Humans have limitations in their experiences, and when encountering a new or unfamiliar situation, they look for a recognizable pattern (Reason, 1990). If the individual practitioner is not familiar with a particular condition, medicine, or treatment, then he/she will not be able to deal with it using existing knowledge or skills. The result is to either spend time in research for the right information, or possibly make a wrong decision based on past experiences. In 1995 over 10,000 articles were published on random clinical trials (RCT), 100 times as many as in 1966; in the past year the National Library of Medicine added over 460,000 references, so expecting practitioners to always be aware of the best practices is extremely challenging, if not impossible, without rapid access to the best research in a manner that is easy to assimilate (Ball, Garets, & Handler, 2003; Agency for Healthcare Research and Quality (AHRQ), n.d.). Knowledge is growing exponentially and technology provides access to large databases of research and evidence-based practices so clinicians can quickly respond to new situations with a sound scientific base and reduce risk of errors in planning.

Humans also have a limited attention span, can only attend carefully to a few things at once, and are subject to distractions and interruptions

(Reason, 1990). Technology, through computers or other devices (such as clinical monitors), can continue to function without regard to fatigue, distractions, interruptions, or forgetfulness. The value of automating repetitive, time-consuming, error-prone tasks is extremely important to improve patient safety and it also improves performance in an industry faced with shortages of clinical personnel (see chapter 6).

Finally, most humans have limited computational skills and technology provides the tool to compute complex problems, calculate dosages, and follow complicated algorithms. Technology provides key resources, that when combined with human creativity and critical decision making, create powerful leverage for safer patient care (Ball, Garets, & Handler, 2003).

TECHNOLOGY ADDS NEW CONCERNS

Technology has grown exponentially and has often been introduced rapidly into health care settings without a full appreciation of how clinicians use and interface with the various technologies. As a result, technology can contribute to system complexity and create unanticipated problems or new opportunities for errors (Ball, Garets, & Handler, 2003; Berwick & Leape, 1999; Kohn, Corrigan, & Donaldson, 2000; Spath, 2000). While technology offers solutions to many problems, it is not a panacea. For example, unanticipated effects may include work-around solutions by staff when the technology does not match the routine workflow. In some cases technology is not used as it was intended, thereby increasing the opportunity for new errors. In one report of bar-coded medication administration studied after implementation, the nurses did not use the scanner at the patient's bedside as intended. This group of nurses scanned a collection of patient bar codes at the medication cart in order to save time. Investigation revealed that introduction of the technology created "automation surprise" and did not account for changes in the workflow and the time constraints related to administering and documenting medications (Patterson, Cook, & Render, 2002).

Technology needs to be designed to support real workflow and processes. This requires adequate planning for how the technology will be used by those who actually use it so that it will be congruent with clinical practice. Some software forces physicians to document in a particular pattern and this changes the way physicians practice (Rogoski, 2003). To create acceptance of a new technology, a balance must be achieved between flexibility and imposed structure. When key users are not involved in the planning and implementing of new technology solutions, then there is a greater likelihood that it will be used incorrectly with errors resulting. The other possible scenario that occurs when users are not involved in planning is that users may sabotage the project, overtly or covertly, as the immediate value may not be evident in the early stages of use. Technology changes the tasks and activities that people do by shifting or modifying work, and by changing decision-making processes. For example, decisions may be changed regarding chemotherapy dosage parameters, type of antibiotic for pneumonia, or reduced nephrotoxic drug dosage due to laboratory values. Technology can also create new work. For instance, bar-coded medication administration requires bringing additional equipment into a patient's room for verification (Shojania, Duncan, McDonald, & Wachter, 2001; Borel & Rascati, 1995). The new work may prompt additional work-around solutions in order to manage time and still use the new technology appropriately (Patterson, Cook, & Render, 2002).

Automated technology inserts a filter between the person and work, so users may encounter information or data overload, or perhaps not the needed data. Massive amounts of data require new management skills to rapidly sift or sort through data and transform it into meaningful information that will be useful in clinical care. Without this new skill, clinicians may not have the right information and could make mistakes in patient care. While we often envision technology as "paperless," interim automated systems actually may increase the amount of paperwork, with a report for each patient, work lists, alerts, and laboratory values. This increased paper flow usually occurs when a full electronic medical record (EMR) is not yet in place and the paper is used as documentation in the medical record. Since only a small handful of health care organizations have a complete EMR at this time, the paper record is still prevalent (First Consulting Group, 2003).

Automated systems usually have back-up systems that rarely fail: however, this means that users do not practice certain skills, so they become less proficient if failure does occur. For example, if a major health information system loses power and a paper back-up system is required, staff often forget how to revert to a paper-based system and paper forms may not be readily available. In fact, in 2002 at Beth Israel Deaconess Medical Center in Boston, a major computer system disruption periodically blocked access to laboratory reports, patient records, prescriptions, and other information, forcing the hospital to revert to the paper-based systems, which impacted care for three and one-half days (*Modern Healthcare*, 2002).

BARRIERS TO TECHNOLOGY IMPLEMENTATION

The barriers to implementation of technology are many, but one of the most significant is cost. Both chief executives and clinician executives at health care facilities cite the lack of financial support as the biggest barrier to implementing information technology, according to a Healthcare Information and Management Systems Society (HIMSS) survey (2003). Twenty-five percent of chief executives and 21% of clinical officers said lack of financial support was the most significant barrier to information technology. Another 17% of chief executives and 15% of clinical officers said proving quantifiable benefits and return on investment was too difficult. Ten percent of chief executives and 17% of clinical officers cited vendors' inability to provide satisfactory products or services as the biggest barrier to information technology adoption (HIMSS, 2003).

The cost of technology covers a huge range, depending on the type of technology, size of organization, and level of interface/integration required. Practically all patient safety technology requires information from existing core foundation applications. Examples of these foundation applications are patient registration, patient billing, laboratory, pharmacy, and clinical documentation. If the new patient safety technology is an integrated module of the foundation applications, the cost of integration may be minimal. However, if the new patient safety technology is not an integrated module of the foundation applications, interfaces will be required. Interfaces are usually costly and can be labor intensive to develop and maintain. Additionally, data needed by the new patient safety technology may not exist in the foundation applications. This will cause interruptions in optimal user workflow. There is usually an initial capital outlay, which can range from hundreds of thousands of dollars to millions depending on the technology. As technology is maintained over time, system upgrades are required. For large systems, a system administrator is usually needed to ensure proper function, maintenance, and performance, thus requiring additional resources. The system administrator usually ensures system functioning but does not focus on patient safety issues. That responsibility often falls to another individual or team.

Another limitation to technology implementation is the lack of standardization with integration and interfaces. There are a number of organizations committed to advancing standardization, however there is no single universally embraced standard for all areas of health care technology. The President's Information Technology Advisory Committee (PITAC) was developed in the 1990s to outline the role the federal government must play in using information technology to transform health care. Health Language 7 (HL7) health care information communication standards are also a major attempt to achieve consistent data transfer across multiple information systems, but there are still difficulties when using several vendors. The National Alliance for Health Information Technology (NAHIT) was created in 2002 to focus specific attention on standards in health care (NAHIT, 2002).

The lack of standardization for interfacing products raises the issue of whether an organization should choose the best functionality in a product ("best of breed" concept) or whether the organization should choose the best integrated system that has several products that work well together but may not be the best individually. There are benefits and risks for either approach, and the individual organization must do a thorough evaluation to make the best decision for their specific situation. Regardless of the approach selected, most organizations still need to have interfaces due to legacy systems, a combination of multiple sites, and stages of system age/replacement. Newer systems are wireless, which requires a radio frequency (RF) backbone structure to be installed in the facility. Depending on the age of the facility this may already exist or may be a costly installation.

Another limitation in technology is the level of system evolution needed to meet current demands for health care and all of the variations for different patients, practitioners, and settings. The medical record institute (MRI), under the leadership of Peter Waegemann has advocated for EMR systems for over 20 years, but there has been limited pressure from the health care industry to develop them until recently (The Leapfrog Group, 2000b). Systems that may appear to offer the full level of functionality in demonstrations, but do not actually have the functionality, are often termed *smoke and mirrors* or *vaporware* since the functionality is not real. More than one organization has been misled into purchasing a system that did not meet expectations. After the Institute of Medicine (IOM) reports (Kohn, Corrigan, & Donaldson, 2000; Aspen, Corrigan, Wolcott, & Erickson, 2003) and with the urging of other agencies (The Leapfrog Group, 2000b; California Senate, 2000) the pressure has intensified for technology resources to provide safer care.

There are other regulations that impact the implementation of technology. For example, the use of telemetry for clinical monitoring is affected by other users of radio signals. One such interference resulted in major loss of service with potential risk to many patients. As a result, regulations have been passed to address this issue. In June 2000, the Wireless Medical Telemetry Services (WMTS) worked to ensure that medical telemetry equipment operates without interference from other sources. The Federal Communications Commission (FCC) set aside bi- or unidirectional electromagnetic signals in the 608–614MHz, 1395–1400MHz, and 1429–1432 MHz frequency bands [American Hospital Association (AHA), 2002]. Other technologies may be affected in the future, but it is not yet known what the effects may be until they occur.

The last technology barrier is related to people. The barriers to success include user acceptance, team participation and ownership, and adequate training of all users. The human component may be the most critical. If a good technology product is selected but not accepted by the staff of a particular organization, it is not likely to be used. A case that illustrates the importance of acceptance took place at Cedars Sinai Health System in California in 2003. Physician dissatisfaction with the product prompted a deinstallation of an estimated $34 million system, illustrating the importance of physician involvement from the start of a project (Benko, 2003). Practitioners, especially physicians, want a technology product that adapts to their practice, not the other way around (Rogoski, 2003).

In summary, the human component of technology deployment and process improvement should not be underestimated. If a multidisciplinary team is not involved to create critical mass for acceptance and adoption, then the technology is not likely to be maximized in serving patients. If users are not trained in the technology then it may not be used correctly, potentiating the risk for errors. Training must involve all users and requires time in training, time away from patients, and a cadre of trainers. "Medical device misuse is an important cause of medical error" (Shojania, Duncan, McDonald, & Wachter, 2001, p. 463). Therefore, to minimize user errors, it is important to understand human factors in the design of devices. The FDA has several regulatory mechanisms to ensure compliance with guidelines for usability and device design.

BENEFITS OF TECHNOLOGY

The benefits of technology are many and have been documented in time savings and efficiencies, but research on the impact on patient safety is limited. There are few studies on computerized provider order entry (CPOE), clinical decision support systems (CDSS), and bar coding that demonstrate improved drug safety. Despite the fact that research is limited related to patient safety, technology continues to demonstrate time savings, access to information across multiple settings, and easier documentation.

Patient and practitioner satisfaction is increased with the speed of online information and time savings from manual documentation (AHRQ, n.d.; Ball, Garets, & Handler, 2003; Bates, 2000). Technology eliminates duplicate work and provides legibility. Online access to information reduces fragmentation in patient care and allows better clinical management. Theoretically, the time savings should allow more time for other activities, but the research is not clear that this time is converted to direct patient care. With personnel shortages, the time savings may actually translate into more focused attention on activities and reduction in opportunities for mistakes. The reduction in paper records depends on the stage of the EMR development. Usually the organization can determine which reports or worksheets need to be printed and thereby control the paper flow.

The technologies that improve medication delivery and provide decision support for medication therapy offer some of the greatest benefits and are in various stages of development. For example, while CPOE has been discussed for years it is not at a mature stage of development, nor is it widely used. Bar coding of medications has only recently been implemented in health care, and the use of robotics, handheld computers, and smart pumps are still first-generation technology. Considerable attention will be given to these technologies since almost 20% of medical errors are medication errors (Leape, et al., 1991). The technologies that support medication safety include computerized provider order entry (CPOE), clinical decision support systems (CDSS), bar coding at point of care (BPOC), automated dispensing machines (ADM), robotics, smart infusion pumps, and handheld computers (HHC). Use of these technologies improves patient safety by:

- Intercepting medication ordering errors
- Providing decision support for new or unfamiliar conditions
- Alerting providers to potential problems, contraindications, or modifications
- Creating clinical efficiency by automating best practice protocols and reducing unnecessary tests
- Providing clear, legible orders
- Standardizing abbreviations
- Limiting formularies and increasing orders for appropriate medications
- Retrieving resource information rapidly
- Reducing risk of dispensing errors
- Simplifying ordering and administration processes

- Reducing reliance on memory and vigilance in medication delivery
- Creating safe modes for high-risk infusions
- Providing alerts for preventive care (such as vaccinations)

The discussion of technologies related to medication safety will be based on the four medication phases identified in chapters 1 and 3. Each phase and the primary technology that affects safety at that phase are outlined below:

Medication Delivery Phases

Ordering	CPOE, handheld computers
Dispensing	Pharmacy systems, robotics, ADM
Administration	BPOC
Monitoring	CPOE, BPOC, ADM, and pharmacy system reports

IMPLEMENTING TECHNOLOGY FOR PATIENT SAFETY

Implementing technology so that patient care is improved or made safer requires specific attention. The most important ingredient to successful implementation is leadership support, and commitment to the technology and to safe care. Leadership is also key in providing the resources that will be needed such as teams, education, and equipment. Without leadership support, the technology may not be implemented in a way that creates the expected clinical benefits. While administrative leaders are critical to successful implementation of technology, medical staff leaders must also be involved.

It is important to ensure that early involvement of staff includes participation in the selection process to establish ownership of the technology, increase satisfaction of users, and verify that the technology actually works in a similar setting. The culture of the organization and philosophy regarding patient safety will affect staff receptivity to change and set the tone for implementation in a way that will minimize risk to patient care and optimize patient safety.

One of the first considerations in implementation strategies is to have users involved at the onset of a project and to have the right users. The right users include a representative mix of staff that will be using the new technology and can identify how processes need to be changed. This will involve a flow or process diagram of the new process (see tools in chapter 3) using the technology so that workflow can be incorporated into the process redesign. The team can help design out potential failures, using tools like health care failure mode and effects analysis (HFMEA™) (see chapter 3). Even though the best approach is to design out failures, it is not possible to identify every eventuality, so expect the unexpected after implementation. A continuous evaluation process will help identify unexpected problems after implementation, and if errors occur, then using root cause analysis (RCA) will be helpful in preventing additional errors.

Another important point to implement technology safely is to be sure that "bad processes," i.e., those which are not working well, are not automated. They just become faster "bad processes." Processes need to be redesigned so that technology will provide efficiencies and benefits. Many organizations are quick to take existing paper forms and processes and try to replicate them in an automated fashion with new technology. These organizations often find that this approach does not work and they then face rework problems.

Other considerations to implement technology safely include selecting or designing technology to default to a safe mode. This is more common in clinical patient technologies such as infusion devices and heat generating devices. It is important that the variety of technology and equipment models be standardized with consistent location of knobs and buttons so that users are able to easily perform work in multiple sites. The principles of standardization, simplification, and having access to the right information can be applied to technology to reduce risk of error (Kohn, Corrigan, & Donaldson, 2000; Leape, Kabcenell, Berwick, & Roessner, 1998; Spath, 2000).

COMPUTERIZED PROVIDER ORDER ENTRY (CPOE)

Technology Overview

CPOE is an electronic information system that provides clinical guidance during the ordering process and intercepts potential errors or variances at the point of order origination. Almost all CPOE systems include or interface with CDSS that provide alerts and triggers as part of the clinical guidance. According to the Harvard Medical Practice Study (Leape, et al., 1991) 38% of medication errors occur at the ordering phase, and Bates and colleagues (1997), found this could be as high as 48%, so the reduction of errors at the point of order origination is a significant improvement over conventional manual processes. (Many sources refer to CPOE as physician order entry. However, with the increase in advanced practitioners who initiate orders the newer concept is to consider all providers at the order entry phase, so the term Computerized *Provider* Order Entry may also be used.) There is pressure to implement CPOE from the Leapfrog Group and certain legislation. For example, in California legislation stipulates that acute-care hospitals must implement information technology to reduce medication-related errors (California Senate, 2000).

Since there is no such thing as a stand-alone CPOE, all CPOE applications come with additional clinical applications and databases (Kilbridge, Welebob, Classen, & The First Consulting Group, 2001; Metzger, Turisco, & The First Consulting Group, 2001). CPOE utilizes data from the foundation applications of the information system as an essential component of the CPOE decision processes. Examples of these additional applications are clinical data repositories, rules and alert engines, reminders and organizational tools, third-party clinical databases, health notes, and clinical documentation. Additionally, CPOE is dependent on the organization's core information system applications as the data foundation. Administrative applications such as registration, medical records, billing, and case management provide CPOE information to frontline managers and users. Ancillary applications such as laboratory, pharmacy, radiology, and emergency department provide the clinical baseline data that are needed. Documentation applications, such as patient documentation, vital signs, assessment and activity charting, and medication administration documentation also supply critical baseline data.

Whereas CPOE incorporates many aspects of ordering, such as treatments and diagnostic testing, the medication ordering process is the most complex and is a very large part of patient safety. There are multiple CPOE applications on the market today. Each one has a different mix of capabilities. What differentiates one CPOE system from another is the level of embedded CDSS and the sophistication of rules, alerts, algorithms, and other support to assist clinicians in making decisions (Metzger, Turisco, & The First Consulting Group, 2001).

An Agency for Healthcare Research and Quality (AHRQ) Technology Report team found five studies related to CDSS in evaluating safety practices. Evans, Classen, Pestotnik, Lundsgaarde, and Burke (1994) studied computerized alerts to physicians and found lower numbers of severe adverse drug events. McDonald (1976) studied alerts to outpatient physicians and found that physicians increased in performing recommended tests and changes in therapy. Rind and colleagues (1994) studied computer alert systems regarding creatinine levels in patients receiving nephrotoxic drugs and found the dose was adjusted or medication was discontinued sooner than without an alert (cited in Shojania, Duncan, McDonald, & Wachter, 2001).

Assessment and Evaluation of Current Systems

CDSS includes any functionality within the application that provides guidance and/or incorporates knowledge to assist the clinician in entering complete, accurate and appropriate patient care orders (Leapfrog Group, 2000a, 2000b; First Consulting Group, 2003). This definition covers a broad range of CDSS tools, which can be categorized based on two interrelated characteristics: (1) the scope of the data used by the tool, and (2) the complexity of the logic that is applied to the available data. CDSS tools can be ranked in nine categories as depicted in Figure 8.1 (Metzger, Turisco, & The First Consulting Group, 2001; Kilbridge, Welebob, Classen, & The First Consulting Group, 2001).

The logic component of the CDSS tool can assimilate more information as the scope of data expands from what is contained within an individual order to information about the patient's condition, as well as information from data repositories and third-party knowledge bases. Descriptions of the nine CDSS levels and their major role in error reduction are provided in Table 8.1.

Benefits of CPOE

A major safety benefit of CPOE is medication error reduction. Organizations that have successfully deployed CPOE report adverse drug event reductions of 70% and greater (Bates, et al., 1999; Bates, et al., 1998). This occurs via several mechanisms. First, with CPOE, orders are structured, legible, complete, and appropriate (as guided by CDSS). Illegible handwriting is virtually eliminated as a source of errors. Feedback is provided to the person ordering during the process so any errors can be identified and intercepted immediately.

Standardization of care with CPOE has improved relative to evidence-based recommendations. Examples of improvements are increased use of histamine (H_2) blockers from 15.6% to 81.3%, reduction of inappropriate

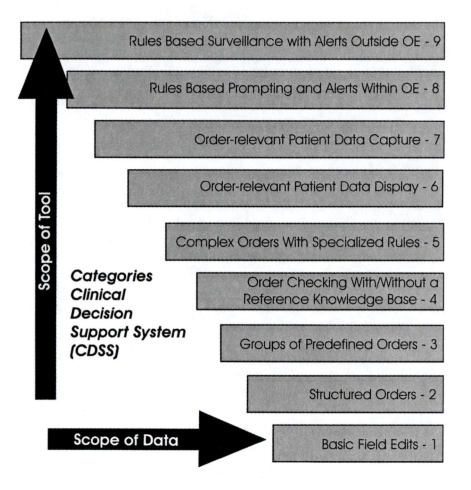

FIGURE 8.1   Levels of CPOE.

OE = Order Entry

Kilbridge, Welebob, Classen, & The First Consulting Group, 2001; Metzger, Turisco, & The First Consulting Group, 2001.

Vancomycin® orders by 75%, and an 80% increase in troponin orders for myocardial infarction patients (Teich, et al., 2000).

Improved efficiencies are achieved not only to CDSS, but also the inherent benefits of automating manual processes. Significant examples of improved efficiencies are a 60% decrease in time to first dose of newly ordered medications; 40% reduction in medication orders being labelled "stat" (an

TABLE 8.1   CDSS Levels, Descriptions, and Error Reduction

Level	Description	Error Reduction
Basic Field Edits	Field edits for dosage amounts, numeric or text entry, decimal format, and required versus nonrequired data entry in a field.	Errors reduced due to elimination of blatant erroneous information in order fields.
Structured Orders	Order templates that specify required data fields and guide data choices with lists of available values and defaults.	Reduced errors of omission or commission through entry of appropriate information as to the type of medication being ordered, such as route of administration. Orders are complete and actionable.
Groups of Predefined Orders	Groupings of orders that are predefined and can be selected as a starting point for specific patient orders. (Examples are order sets and clinical pathways). This level also supports corollary orders, where the clinician is automatically prompted to consider an additional order based on a previously ordered item (e.g., a medication order that should be accompanied by a lab order to determine therapeutic serum levels).	Errors are reduced because information is complete with appropriate fields and field contents. There is increased compliance with recommended care at the diagnosis, procedure, and phase of management level.
Order Checking With/Without a Reference Knowledge Base	Drug order interaction and contraindication checking (e.g., drug-allergy, drug-drug, drug-food, drug-alcohol, duplicate therapeutic overlap, and min-max dosing).	Errors reduced due to alerts to potential contraindications. Duplicate therapies are flagged and drug information and monographs are available.
Complex Orders With Specialized Tools	Tools such as dose calculators that assist with proper dosing, taper dosing, sliding scales, and alternate day dosing.	Errors reduced with more accurate medication dosing and dose calculations.
Order Relevant Patient Data Display	Relevant patient informational display that automatically indicates data such as lab values that should be considered before ordering the medication.	Errors are reduced due to review of relevant patient information that might influence another medication choice or dose.

(continued)

TABLE 8.1 *(continued)*

Level	Description	Error Reduction
Order Relevant Patient Data Capture	Automatic prompting for the clinician to verify or enter patient specific data needed to screen the appropriateness of the mediation being ordered and to perform necessary calculations (e.g., body weight and body surface area). Also includes prompting regarding clinical appropriateness and documentation of relevant clinical indications	Errors are reduced due to more appropriate use of targeted medications and the capture of additional relevant information for subsequent review and analysis of clinical appropriateness.
Rule-Based Prompting and Alerts Within Order Entry	Automatic, real-time prompting and alerting during the order process based on rules and a range of patient specific information (e.g., dosage calculators, suggested dosing)	Errors of omission and commission are reduced.
Rule-Based Surveillance With Alerts Outside of Order Entry	Automatic alerting and prompting to reconsider medication and order interventions based on new patient information, with clinician notification outside of electronic order entry.	Patient management strategy is enhanced due to reduced delays in reevaluating patient condition and needs.

Metzger, Turisco, & The First Consulting Group, 2001.

emergency order) due to improved delivery; and an 85% reduction in unsigned orders (Teich, et al., 2000). CPOE can use constraints and forcing functions to automatically attach provider signatures with the sign-on process creating compliance for medical records with an invisible process to physicians. CPOE has demonstrated other benefits such as reductions in length of stay by 0.89 days and lower hospital charges by 12.7% (California Healthcare Foundation & First Consulting Group, 2000). As length of stay is reduced the patient has fewer exposures to potential errors and nosocomial infections.

CPOE provides benefits at all levels of CDSS. Even the lowest level of sophistication provides value and error reduction. The patient safety and quality benefits that can be achieved at each level of CDSS are listed in Table 8.1. Table 8.2 lists the research supporting the benefits of CPOE with specific examples (Shojania, Duncan, McDonald, & Wachter, 2001).

Organizational Readiness

Organizations must make a serious commitment to the successful deployment of CPOE. CPOE requires significant clinical process redesign, which in turn requires extraordinary commitment by physicians, other clinicians, and executives.

Executive leadership and sponsorship are critical to fostering an organizational culture for CPOE readiness. A critical role of executive leaders is to send a clear message that CPOE is important and to provide unwavering support as the project evolves. Executives should visibly link CPOE to organizational strategies in terms the hospital community can understand, and should position CPOE as part of the culture of quality improvement and patient safety. In addition to the Chief Information Officer, the Chief Executive Officer and the Chief Medical Officer need to take a formal and active role in the CPOE implementation. New processes should be adopted as medical policy. More important, executives need to promote measurement of progress, accountability for implementation, and celebration of success (American Society of Health System Pharmacy, n.d.; California Healthcare Foundation & First Consulting Group, 2000; First Consulting Group, 2003).

In addition to executive leadership, executive sponsorship is an absolute requirement for organizational and cultural readiness. The executive sponsors must be dedicated clinical champions with a strong drive for success. The champion's position as a well-respected, active clinician is far more important than any experience with, and knowledge of, information systems. Executive sponsors must also be committed to planning and supporting significant workflow and process changes that affect not only physicians, but all other caregivers and ancillary departments (Consensus Workgroup on Health Information Capture and Report Generation, 2002).

Physician Acceptance

To understand physician acceptance of CPOE, one must first understand traditional physician values. When introducing a patient safety, care qual-

TABLE 8.2   CPOE Examples and Results

Organization	CPOE safety benefit
Brigham and Women's Hospital (BWH) in Boston, MA	88% drop in serious medication errors; 55% reduction in error rates; CPOE with CDSS at BWH showed 55% decrease in nonintercepted serious medication errors; 17% decrease in preventable ADEs (Bates, Leape, Cullen, Laird, Petersen, Teich, Burdick, Hickey, Kleefield, Shea, Vander Vliet, & Seger, 1998). CPOE with CDSS at BWH and showed 81% decrease in medication errors; 86% decrease in nonintercepted serious medication errors (Bates, Teich, Lee, Seger, Kuperman, Ma'Luf, Boyle, & Leape, 1999). CPOE with CDSS at BWH and found improvement in 5 prescribing practices (Teich, Merchia, Schmiz, Kuperman, Spurr, & Bates, 2000).
Latter Day Saints (LDS) Hospital in Salt Lake City, UT	70% reduction in adverse drug events; use of computerized antibiotic selection consultant at LDS in Utah found 17% greater pathogen susceptibility to an antibiotic regimen suggested by computer vs. physician (Evans, Classen, Pestotnik, Lundsgaarde, & Burke, 1994). Computer based anti-infective management program for ICU patients at LDS found 70% decrease in ADE caused by anti-infectives (Evans, Pestotnik, Classen, Clemmer, Weaver, Orme Jr., Lloyd, & Burke, 1998).
Ohio State University Medical Center, Columbus, OH	Average length of stay (LOS) down by 2 days; turnaround for pharmacy orders 2 hours faster; pharmacy charges down $910 per admission (Shojania, Duncan, McDonald, & Wachter, 2001).
Montefiore Medical Center, New York, NY	Medication errors down 50%; turnaround for pharmacy orders 2 hours faster (Shojania, Duncan, McDonald, & Wachter, 2001).
Wishard Memorial Hospital, Indianapolis, IN	Average LOS down .9 days; average hospital charges down 13% (Shojania, Duncan, McDonald, & Wachter, 2001).
Regenstrief Institute for Health Care, Indianapolis, IN	Studied the impact of faculty and physician reminders using CPOE at Regenstrief—25% improvement in ordering of corollary medications by faculty and residents (Overhage, Tierney, Zhou, & McDonald, 1997).
Multiple inpatient and outpatient settings	CDSS in multiple inpatient and outpatient settings; 6 of 14 studies showed improvement in patient outcomes; 43 of 65 studies showed improvement in physician performance (Hunt, Haynes, Hanna, & Smith, 1998).
Multiple inpatient settings	CDSS for drug dosage advice in multiple inpatient settings found absolute risk reduction with CDSS (Walton, Harvey, Dovey, & Freemantle, 2001).

Shojania, Duncan, McDonald, & Wachter, 2001.

ity, or information technology initiative, many executives wonder why physicians may resist the apparently obvious benefits of CPOE. If physicians choose to enroll in the change initiative and to actively participate, they must believe their efforts will result in benefits that they and patients value as individuals. Values are a physician's reference point when making choices and decisions. When physician choices or decisions are not aligned with their values, then they feel conflict and resist the change (Gaillour, 2003).

Physicians' Values

According to Gaillour (2003), the resistance point most often heard from physicians regarding CPOE is "It will slow me down." And for physicians time equals money. With insight into the physician's personal values, we see why resistance to change is so strong. How does CPOE support these values or create conflict? Table 8.3 illustrates physician values relative to how they perceive CPOE. While there are physicians that have embraced CPOE, others are slower to make the transition. To overcome the potential

TABLE 8.3   Physician Values and Perception of CPOE

Physician Value	CPOE Recognition of Value
Autonomy	Disregarded: I am required to standardize
Integrity	Neutral: On the one hand, I would be "doing the right thing" for patient safety. But on the other hand, any lapse in my ability to concentrate or quickly access information is a threat to patient care.
Achievement	Disregarded: This decision may negatively impact my time, and therefore my own productivity. Also, I may not be competent with new technology.
Service	Disregarded: I am not personally contributing anything new to the patient community.
Creativity	Disregarded: The decisions have been made and I wasn't asked to provide input.
Recognition	Disregarded: This decision is not my brainchild.
Emotional health	Disregarded: This decision will add to my day and will keep me from my family.

Gaillour, 2003.

conflicts and create a culture of physician acceptance, the organization must have a strong, credible physician to champion the CPOE project.

Physicians are the best people to initiate dialogue with their colleagues regarding CPOE acceptance. Dialogue should encourage meaningful change concepts that align physicians' personal and professional values. Understanding how CPOE can support most, if not all, of the physicians' core values is the ultimate goal.

Central to physician acceptance is the CPOE workflow. Physician involvement during the early CPOE design and implementation process is critical in addressing workflow issues. Medical staff leaders must demonstrate commitment and communicate a clear sense of direction, and they must support involvement of a cross-section of physicians prior to implementation to ensure attention to the operational realities of CPOE. Alerts and prompts in the CDSS must be meaningful, they must improve decisions, and they must enhance completeness in order for physicians to value CPOE. Redundant messages and certain prompts can eventually become background noise and a hindrance, thus taking more time and slowing the physician. Efforts to avoid this type of screen flow in CPOE are critical (Gaillour, 2003; First Consulting Group, 2003; Metzger, Turisco, & The First Consulting Group, 2001).

Implementation Issues

Organizations need to evaluate the level and mix of CDSS tools needed to meet overall patient safety goals and objectives (Joint Commission for Accreditation of Healthcare Organizations [JCAHO], 2002b; Centers for Medicare and Medicaid Services, 2003), as well as the ability of the organization to implement and deploy CDSS. It is necessary to consider the work required to implement each type of CDSS, including:

- How many rules can be set up in master files versus how much the organization is required to write rules?
- How difficult is it to write and maintain the rules?
- What tools are available in the vendor's product for managing CDSS, such as audit trails and reports of exception documentation?
- What is the approach to testing CDSS rules before general release?
- What is the availability of vendor "starter sets" and knowledge bases?
- Does the vendor support sharing of CDSS rules among customer hospitals?

- What CDSS features are planned for the next release of CPOE?
- How does the research and development agenda for the product fit with the hospital's safety and quality agenda?
- What are the successes of the vendor's current implementation sites?
- How has staff responsible for CPOE in the current sites rated the ease of setting up and managing CDSS?
- Is the CPOE system interfaced or integrated with the core foundation system? If it is interfaced, the cost and maintenance of interfaces must be considered, as well as data integrity passing from system to system.
- Will the hospital's wireless network need to be upgraded to ensure performance?
- Will foundation systems have to be upgraded and/or replaced to accommodate CPOE and if so, at what cost, in dollars, time, and staff?

Some legacy pharmacy systems are not capable of taking an inbound medication order from a CPOE system or any other ordering application. If this is the case, most likely the legacy pharmacy system will have to be replaced with a new pharmacy system to accommodate CPOE (First Consulting Group, 2003; California Healthcare Foundation & First Consulting Group, 2000).

There are several clear implementation requirements relative to CPOE technology. The design of the user interface should be consistent across CPOE modules. This will simplify and minimize training efforts. System response times need to be fast, preferably displaying subsecond response time. Application availability needs to be around the clock, seven days a week, and adequate numbers and types of workstations need to be in place. The workstations should be located for physicians' as well as other practitioners' convenience. Areas to consider for workstation location are physician lounges, oncall rooms, clinics, and work areas on the inpatient units. Mobile devices should also be considered. There are a variety of mobile devices, and user input into selection should be obtained so that devices support workflow and patient care processes to reduce unnecessary work and risk for error.

Data integration requirements across different systems can represent significant challenges. Two major areas should be addressed. First, it is essential that the medication formularies for the CPOE system and the pharmacy system be the same. In a CPOE-pharmacy interfaced environment, the CPOE system's medication order contains data fields that must map exactly to the pharmacy data fields. Second, data must be imported through real-time interfaces, and data definitions must be standardized sufficiently to permit use with a rules engine or other decision support logic. Frequently the databases containing patient-specific data critical to CPOE, such as laboratory results, pharmacy data, vitals signs, weight, and body surface area, are independent of the CPOE product. So the data transmission is critical.

Workflow and change management policies, and procedures for implementation and ongoing operations need to be defined well in advance of CPOE deployment. Workflow changes must be planned carefully or redesigned to address operational transitions during CPOE rollout. Transition issues to expect include:

- Workflow operations as each care environment goes from paper to CPOE
- Workflow as patients are transferred from CPOE operational units to non-CPOE units
- Workflow as providers/staff go from a CPOE operational unit to non-CPOE units
- Workflow as ancillary departments migrate from paper-based orders to electronic orders.

Inconsistency due to patient or caregiver transition creates increased opportunity for errors to occur by moving back and forth between systems. Other issues may evolve from the CPOE deployment such as lack of standardization in procedures from one nursing unit to the next, and among clinical services. Identifying these variations and developing standards for terminology, procedures, and protocols can be a very time-consuming task, yet important to minimize problems.

Training leads to successful CPOE implementation. The training process should reflect the actual tools, screens, and processes used in the care setting. Training for clinicians should be offered at times most conducive to physician participation. Clinicians who are familiar with the various nuances of patient care should offer CPOE instruction. System design and screen flow should be intuitive, making training a positive experience. Training time should be kept to a minimum, and coaches should be available during the first days and weeks to provide help and assistance as needed.

User support needs to be available around the clock. Neglecting user support can cause significant damage to an otherwise successful implementation. In addition, CPOE changes in response to problems or requests must be made rapidly, or users will not trust that their needs will be met and may begin to find ways to work around or "short circuit" the system, thus derailing a successful implementation. CPOE redesign and support should be ongoing and evolutionary in nature. It is highly recommended that a group of users form a task force and convene regularly to address issues and problems that may arise. This group should comprise physicians and members of all patient care and ancillary areas to ensure an interdisciplinary team addresses issues.

BAR CODING AT POINT OF CARE (BPOC)

Bar Codes

Bar codes are a system of machine-readable codes that uniquely identify an item. Bar codes are a way of encoding numbers and letters by using a combination of bars and spaces of varying widths. A bar code typically has identification data encoded in it that are used by a computer to correlate all specific information associated with the data. A bar code doesn't contain descriptive data, just as a social security number doesn't contain a person's name or address. A bar code is simply a reference number that a computer uses to look up an associated record that contains descriptive data and other important information (Symbol Technologies, Inc., 1999; Bridge Medical Inc., 2001). Bar codes were first used over 30 years ago in laboratories and blood banks. However, they have been used more in materials management rather than the clinical arena. The value of bar codes is that they have very few misidentification errors, with error rates ranging from 1 in 15,000 to 1 in 36 trillion (Wald & Shojania, 2001, p. 491).

Symbology is a language used in bar code technology, just like French or Spanish. Symbology allows a scanner and a bar code to "speak" to each other. Most people are familiar with the bar codes seen in grocery or retail stores, but there are many others that are used as standards in various industries. Health care, manufacturing, and retail industries all have symbologies unique to their industry and typically these are not interchangeable. The reason there are so many different symbologies is that bar codes have evolved to solve specific problems. For example, the Universal Product Number (UPN) is the symbology used on items destined for the checkout line in retail and grocery stores. The Health Industry Business Commissions Council (HIBC) has also developed a standard symbology for the health care industry (Symbol Technologies, Inc., 1999). Characteristics of the HIBC symbology are:

- Alphanumeric capability
- Variable length of the product identification field
- Smaller symbol than a similar mass-market bar code

Whereas HIBC symbology is considered a standard, there is no single uniform standard symbology in the health care industry and no single standard for labeling medications. Unlike most other industries, health care products have special human safety requirements and are routinely monitored by government regulators (Symbol Technologies, Inc., 1999). As a consequence, labels must be as error free as possible, they must contain additional information, and they must satisfy greater needs than those commonly found in point-of-sale environments such as grocery stores. This helps to explain why the technology from retail does not exactly translate to health care. Additionally, in health care three bar codes are needed for a single transaction in medication administration: The bar-coded medication, the bar-coded patient identification band, and the bar-coded caregiver. This ensures that the medication, the patient, and the person who administered it are all captured and documented with scanning of all bar codes.

Unit-of-Use Bar Codes

An important part of deploying a bedside bar-code-enabled medication administration system is to ensure that medications dispensed from pharmacy contain a bar code. While most pharmaceutical manufacturers place bar codes on packaging that contains many single unit-of-use medications, the manufacturers fall short on placing a bar code on the actual unit of use label. It is estimated that only 20%–35% of the unit-dose medications currently contain a machine-readable bar code that could be effectively utilized with bedside technologies (Bridge Medical, Inc., 2001; Chester & Zilz, 1989; *Federal Register*, 2003). For example, there may be a bar code on the outside of a box of pills; however, there is no bar code on the label of the individual pill. The pill is what is carried to the patient's bedside for administration. The bar-coded box of pills never reaches the nursing unit, much less the patient. Achieving 100% unit dose packaging with bar code labeling will challenge health care organizations until drug manufacturers and wholesalers take responsibility for this task.

The FDA issued a rule in February 2004 to require bar codes on prescription drugs, over-the-counter drugs packaged for hospital use, and vaccines by 2006. The proposal would require the National Drug Code (NDC) number, which uniquely identifies the drug, strength, and dosage form. This proposal means that unit dose medications would have a bar code. The proposal would require machine-readable information on blood and blood products as well. The FDA estimates that complying with the rule could cost drugmakers $53 million (*Federal Register*, 2002; *Federal Register*, 2003).

Organizations that are serious about advancing safe medication delivery now are already using bar-coded medicines and scanners. Taking on the challenge may seem daunting, but can be achieved. Solutions ranging from robotics to less expensive packagers, along with appropriate resource allocation, can get the job done. Unless the drug manufacturer labels unit doses of medication, this burden falls to the health care organization. While there are a number of technology solutions for this labeling process, it introduces one more opportunity for an error with mislabeling. Several major drug manufacturers have already committed to bar coding their products (Abbott, 2003; Hammergrenm, 2003; Pfizer, 2003).

If automated packagers or robotics are not used, the pharmacy will need to use resources to either over-wrap or affix a bar code label to medications at the unit dose level. The over-wrap devices on the market require rolls of clear plastic bags that run through a thermal transfer element to place label information on the bag. After the bag passes through the labeling process, a medication is dropped into the bag and it is sealed.

Affixing a bar code label can be a simple, low-cost option since there are many label programs on the market. A label-generating program in tandem with a bar code-generating printer will accomplish the packaging task. Labels may contain medication names (generic and trade), strength and volume, container size, expiration date, lot number, and manufacturer and NDC numbers. Medication wholesalers and hospital information system vendors offer over-wrapping services with a bar code. Wholesalers and vendors that provide this service may charge a nominal fee, so it may be worthwhile for an organization to compare prices for in-house implementation and outsourcing this task.

Scanners and Scanning

A special scanner reads bar codes by focusing a small spot of light across the printed bar code symbol. The user only sees a thin red line emitted from the laser scanner. The scanner's light source is absorbed by the dark bars and reflected by the light spaces. A device in the scanner converts the reflected light into an electrical signal. There are several types of bar code scanners on the market today, including fixed, portable batch, and portable wireless (Symbol Technologies Inc., 1999).

Fixed scanners remain attached to their host computer or terminal, and transmit one data item at a time as the bar code is scanned. A keyboard wedge reader is attached to a computer through a port called the keyboard interface. When a bar code is scanned, the information is transmitted as though it were entered from the keyboard. These are referred to as wedge readers because they are physically wedged between the keyboard and computer and attached as a second keyboard. Another way to transmit data from a bar code reader to a computer is to connect it to the computer's RS-232 serial port. The bar code information will be transmitted in ASCII format and look just like keyed data to the computer. The terminal that this type of scanner is attached to will most likely be a wireless terminal on a cart. The cart is taken to the patient's bedside so the caregiver can scan medications directly at the patient's bedside. Advantages of scanners attached to wireless computers are that the user is working with a full screen application user interface and most likely can access other applications other than medication administration. Disadvantages of wireless terminals on carts is the crowding that occurs when patient rooms are small, making it difficult to move the cart to the patient bedside for scanning. Overcrowding creates an environment in which the nurse or other caregiver does not have sufficient space to adequately reach the patient or all needed items, and thus creates opportunities for something to go wrong.

Wireless portable batch scanners are battery operated and store data in memory for later batch transfer to a host computer. A portable batch reader contains a bar code scanner, a liquid crystal display (LCD) to prompt the user to perform a task, and a keyboard to enter data. Data are transmitted to the host computer via a cradle. Portable batch scanners are ideal when mobility is a must and collected data isn't needed immediately.

Wireless portable scanners can store data in memory or can transmit data to the host computer in real time. Real time data transmission allows for instant data access. A wireless scanner, typically a handheld device, uploads data in real time to the host computer as it is scanned instantly and accurately. Wireless scanners let the user scan the information at the point of activity, which makes this scanner ideal for health care. Advantages of wireless portable scanners are that the caregiver can easily scan at the patient's bedside, and the small size and portability of the device. Disadvantages may arise in the user interface. The screens are much smaller than the full terminal screen display and may be difficult to read and navigate. The possibility of theft is becoming less of a disadvantage, as the application software and the device itself become nonfunctional beyond the range of the hospital's wireless network.

POINT OF CARE SYSTEMS (POCS)

While CPOE systems assist in building safety defenses to prevent errors at the *blunt end,* POCS assist in preventing errors at the *sharp end,* where harm occurs to patients. This is based on the point at which errors are intercepted. With CPOE, errors are intercepted at the ordering phase while with POCS errors are intercepted at the administration phase. If one thinks of nurses as tightrope walkers without a net in the medication administration process, POCS are the safety net.

As with CPOE, POCS medication administration systems have varying levels of capability and sophistication. Generally speaking, there are three levels of application functionality (Grotting, Yang, Kelly, Brown, & Trohimovich, 2002). The most advanced and complete functionality occurs at the fourth level. The first level of application includes checking of the five "rights" of administration (right patient, right drug, right dose, right route, right time), the online medication record administration, and the work lists that assist the nurse in gathering the medications to be administered to a patient at specific times.

The second level of application includes the elements found in level one plus drug reference information. Drug reference information is typically third-party databases that are incorporated into the application. Drug monograph information is made available to the nurse at any time during the medication administration process. Patient medication education sheets and other nursing tools are also available. Finally, this level includes formulary information.

The third level includes level-two capabilities as well as dose checking, usually performed with the use of third-party drug databases. Alerts and messages for look-alike and sound-alike medications, and high-risk warnings are provided through the use of third-party databases. Reporting of "potential medication errors avoided" or near misses are also provided for use with root cause analysis as well as documentation of the system's effectiveness in reducing errors. Some order reconciliation capabilities are available, but the workflow within the application may be cumbersome (Grotting, Yang, Kelly, Brown, & Trohimovich, 2002).

The fourth level of applications includes everything in level three plus integration with other systems that support applications. For example, level-four applications integrate medication administration information with other nursing documentation such as vital signs. Level-four applications of order reconciliation are less cumbersome than level three, because there is a higher level of integration with the CPOE and/or ordering application. In level four, alerts and messages for look-alike and sound-alike medications are modifiable by authorized users, instead of being hard coded messages in level three. Additional functionality for complicated medication delivery, such as sliding scale insulin calculations, are found at the fourth level. Automatic reminders for reevaluation of pain after administration of pain medication are available and integrated into nursing documentation. Level-four applications also perform allergy checking throughout an entire episode of care. While POCS have varying capabilities now, the future is likely to bring integration with new products such as smart pumps and clinical monitoring devices. Organizations should recognize the need to research capabilities of different products in order to purchase systems that will meet their needs and offer flexibility to expand applications. By reviewing each level of application, an organization can identify criteria that should be met by the respective system.

There are obvious patient safety benefits at each system level, but as with CPOE, the higher the system sophistication, the higher the system cost. Organizations must identify specific goals and outcomes desired from point-of-care system deployment in order to determine the level of sophistication needed. As mentioned previously, technology can create changes in workflow and unexpected problems. Table 8.4 identifies examples of issues associated with POCS implementation and suggested solutions to resolve them. Research on POCS for medication administration has been conducted within the Veterans Affairs medical centers. After bar-coded medication administration at the bedside was implemented, researchers initially found an increase in the number of errors, especially late medications. They also found that automatic stop orders created confusion, and resulted in omissions or double dosing errors. Another finding was that nurses were so focused on administering medications on time to avoid a late error, that they did not attend to other patient care activities (Patterson, Cook, & Render, 2002). In the North Colorado Medical Center, use of a bar-coded POCS demonstrated a 71% reduction in errors over 2 years; a 33% reduction in wrong drug errors; a 43% reduction in wrong time errors; and a 52% reduction in omitted dose errors (Bridge Medical Inc., 2001). The benefits of POCS are primarily documented for medication safety at

TABLE 8.4   Side Effects When Technology Adds New Issues

Issue	Solution
Increased reports of medication errors due to lateness	Organization alters the late medication parameters if appropriate
Confusion with automatic stop orders for certain medications (opiates, antibiotics) creating an omission or double-dose error	Provide education about automatic stop orders and/or redesign the system
Communication of orders between physician and nurses, especially on new and stat orders	Use interfaces or assess software capability to ensure orders are communicated in the system
Nurses dropped some activities during high work loads	Ensure software design and set-up accommodates these activities based on user input
Complex orders, such as taper orders and sliding scales, are challenging in an automated system	Ensure software design and set-up accommodates complex orders before implementation

the administration phase. There are other uses of bar coding with specimen handling, supply usage, documentation of standard activities, billing, and tracking of reports or charts that should be explored as organizations evaluate the purchase of BPOCs and various uses.

Implementation of POCS

Successful implementation of POCS requires a dedicated team of individuals to keep the project on track. The success of the project is dependent on this team. Resources for successful deployment include several major roles. The first role is the executive sponsor who is the primary champion and point person for issue escalation. The executive sponsor has authority for allocating resources, setting priorities, and providing funds. The second role is the core implementation team, which is a multidisciplinary management team to establish goals, drive policy changes, and ensure that hospital wide communications take place. Finally, the project manager is the individual responsible for managing the project with the team members and the corresponding vendor project members. This person needs to have a strong positive attitude, a successful track record in project management, and the respect of managers and peers. This person should also be knowledgeable of operations in all hospital departments. The project manager usually has other system responsibilities including:

- Primary hospital contact for the vendor
- Development of project plan with vendor
- Management and monitoring of project progress
- Assurance of completion of implementation activities and adherence to implementation schedules
- Assurance of execution of system design outcomes
- Reporting project progress regularly to the executive sponsor and vendor project manager
- Assurance that the project is completed within budget and schedule.

Most clinical projects, especially those that focus on patient care activities, should include a nurse analyst or liaison who coordinates activities with nursing personnel. The nurse should have an understanding of organizational operations and be familiar with current information systems installed in organization. Experience in project management along with good leadership and communication skills is important for successful implementation (Marthinsen & Scott, 2003).

Since most POCS focus on medication delivery, a pharmacy analyst is a key member of the team. This person is the liaison with pharmacy personnel and is responsible for coordinating policies and procedures for all pharmacy related activities. Additionally, this person coordinates system validation of the configuration of the bar code and interface requirements. Similar qualities of project management and knowledge of operations and information systems are critical.

Finally, an information technology (IT) analyst is essential to manage IT activities, file development, system integration or interface into the IT platform, and system testing. This person must have excellent knowledge of IT systems and the authority to make decisions about the project. Each of these roles is important for a successful project. Patient safety concerns must be incorporated into policy development, system design, and workflow processes as the project is developed or potential for errors can occur.

AUTOMATED DISPENSING MACHINES

Automated dispensing machines (ADMs), automate the access, distribution, management, and control of medications, fluids, and sometimes supplies. Our focus on ADMs is medication distribution. ADMs can increase efficiency and productivity of the process of medication delivery as long as defined policies and procedures are developed for ADM use. The benefits of ADMs include:

- Timely access to controlled substances, as-needed (PRN) medications, and first doses of medications
- Interface to hospital admission/discharge/transfer and billing systems
- Display of approved orders for a selected patient
- Ability to track inventory of medications
- Secure controlled access to medications
- Elimination of narcotics counts and keys
- Reduction of potential drug diversion

Additionally, when ADMs are used with pharmacy robotics, the ADM system can monitor par levels and automatically activate the robot to pick bar-coded medications for restock purposes. Other optional features include a detachable scanner that can be used to scan bar-coded medications upon restocking to verify that the right medications are placed in the right drawer and pocket.

ADMs focus on the drug dispensing phase, not administration, so it is still possible to have medication administration errors. Workflow policies and procedures are key to the effective use of ADMs. Best practices for ADMs include policies identifying the window of time allowed for removal of a medication and the subsequent administration to the patient. Also, policies should define the number of patient medications a nurse can remove for the next scheduled dose. Ideally, the nurse should retrieve medications for one patient at a time, and only those medications due for the scheduled dose time, but this may not be the most efficient method. ADM policies should reflect safe practice but should not increase work or inefficiencies. The method of medication transport to the patient is also important. Procedures should include a standardized closed system such as clear plastic bags or zipped pouches with transportation note. The transportation note validates the medications that were removed and provides a double check of the medications removed in conjunction with the medication administration record. The transportation note should be destroyed or shredded after use to ensure compliance with Joint Commission for the Accreditation of Healthcare Organizations (JCAHO) patient confidentiality standards and Healthcare Insurance Portability and Accountability Act (HIPAA) requirements.

ADM configuration and location should be appropriate for patient populations being served and the number of nurses accessing the ADM. Nurses should not have to wait in line to retrieve medications. If waiting in lines takes a long time, nurses may take shortcuts to circumvent the system, which may increase the risk of errors. As with all technologies, sometimes users embark on inappropriate practices if workflow policies are cumbersome. Access to multiple drugs at one time can be one such pitfall. Just because the nurse retrieved a medication for patient "A" does not ensure that patient "A" received the medication. To help avoid such practices, most ADMs offer cabinet drawer options that allow access to only a single medication at a time.

Other considerations with ADMs are interfaces to the pharmacy system, CPOE, and point-of-care medication administration systems for order accuracy and discrepancy resolution. Interfaces to the pharmacy system are common and provide streamlined order, inventory, and charging control. However, typically CPOE and point-of-care medication administration interfaces are very challenging as these systems may be disparate systems from multiple vendors. If there are no interfaces, organizations must create policies and procedures to account for accurate medication retrieval and administration. Patient safety is enhanced by the cabinetry design of drawers so that slippage of medications from one drawer to another does not occur. Secure access is another feature that is important so that the patient's medications are available when needed. Timely filling of the medication drawers is essential so that new orders and first-dose medications can be delivered on time for maximum benefit.

An Agency for Healthcare Research and Quality Technology Report team analyzed three ADM devices and found no real evidence that ADMs reduce medication errors and no evidence to suggest that outcomes are improved with these devices. Human intervention may prevent these systems from functioning as designed, especially if clinicians can override safety features. Errors may occur during cabinet filling and medications may shift from one drawer compartment to another. However, research is limited and other benefits have been reported such as better control of medications. Other benefits of ADMs may include reduced personnel and drug waste (Shojania, Duncan, McDonald, & Wachter, 2001).

ROBOTIC STORAGE AND RETRIEVAL SYSTEMS

Robotics technology has been advanced to the point that robots are being used for a variety of functions from dispensing medications to assisting in surgery. The focus in this discussion is the robotic drug distribution system that automates the storage, dispensing, returning, restocking, and crediting of bar coded, unit-dose medications. These robotic systems are primarily used in acute care settings or large pharmaceutical distribution centers. The benefit of robotics in enhancing patient safety is that robotics ensure that the right medication is dispensed for the right patient. Robots work faster and tirelessly, 24 hours a day, to reduce dispensing errors. Using robots frees up pharmacists for clinical activities such as patient rounds, consultation with physicians, and patient education. The reduction of time-consuming activities such as dispensing, checking, and distributing medications, allows pharmacists more time for safety interventions. Researchers (Scarsi, Fotis, & Noskin, 2002) have found that having clinical pharmacists making rounds on the unit reduced medication errors by 51%.

Robotics use also positions the organization for accurate bedside administration of medications. Since most pharmaceutical companies do not currently provide medications bar coded at the unit-dose level this burden falls to the health care organization. Robotics is another technology that can provide bar-coded medications to be scanned at the bedside by the nurse. Robots do not just work in the pharmacy. Some robots actually transport medications or other supplies from one location to another. This saves time for a busy staff and allows clinicians to focus on direct patient care activities.

AUTOMATED CLINICAL DEVICES

Smart Infusion Pumps

Intravenous (IV) medications pose the greatest risk of medication harm due to the rapid pharmacologic action, and the drugs most frequently cited as causing serious errors are often given by this route (opiates, insulin, heparin) (Cohen, 1999). Bates and colleagues (1997) found that medication administration is the phase most vulnerable to error and that serious or life-threatening adverse drug events (ADE) were most often related to IV therapy. IV therapy errors have a severe impact on the patient, and it is difficult to intercept them before they reach the patient. Smart infusion pumps can be an effective technology that prevents these errors.

Traditional infusion pumps rely on the settings the nurse enters for flow rate and dosage. There is no test of reasonable, safe dosage and flow rate. Unfortunately, if the settings are incorrect then errors can be fatal.

Examples of programming errors on infusion pumps that resulted in patient death include:

- Morphine drip reset to 90 mL/hr instead of 9.0 mL/hr
- Infusion pump programmed with 100 mg/L, was actually 1000 mg/L
- Infusion pump rate increased to remove air, but infusion rate was not reset
- Neonatal nurse resets infusion pump to 304, intended to be 3.4
- Nitroglycerin infusion programmed as mcg/kg/min, but the dose was ordered as mcg/min (Schneider, 2002)

Smart pump technology contains computerized medication software to make sure dosage and flow rates are appropriate based on parameters for safety. The software contains data sets at the drug and nursing unit level. Appropriate drug ranges for an adult unit may be different from the ranges in a pediatric unit, so customization by patient type takes place. These data sets define the appropriate flow rate and dosage that a nurse can program into the pump when hanging an IV solution. The nurse is alerted when IV programming is outside the defined parameters and the specific medication order, thereby intercepting any errors. The smart pump then displays information to assist the nurse in correct programming. Figure 8.2 depicts an example of the smart pump logic.

Smart infusion pumps benefits can be summarized in the following ways:

- Protection against patient harm at the point of infusion
- Promotion of best practice guidelines, customized by care area and population
- Tracking and documentation of events outside best practice guidelines, and providing data to analyze trends to make clinical practice improvements
- Future benefits of integration with documentation applications.

HANDHELD COMPUTERS

Doctors and nurses move from room to room and unit to unit, frequently practice in more than one location, and occasionally visit patients at home. These practitioners work in a mobile environment, and handheld computers (HHCs) provide data access at every point of care. The HHC and the less complex counterpart, Personal Digital Assistants (PDAs) are an adjunct

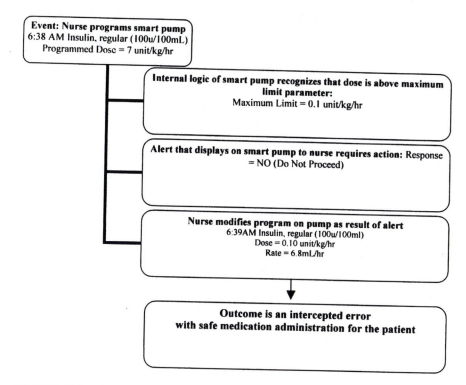

Event: Nurse programs smart pump
6:38 AM Insulin, regular (100u/100mL)
Programmed Dose = 7 unit/kg/hr

Internal logic of smart pump recognizes that dose is above maximum limit parameter:
Maximum Limit = 0.1 unit/kg/hr

Alert that displays on smart pump to nurse requires action: Response = NO (Do Not Proceed)

Nurse modifies program on pump as result of alert
6:39AM Insulin, regular (100u/100ml)
Dose = 0.10 unit/kg/hr
Rate = 6.8mL/hr

Outcome is an intercepted error
with safe medication administration for the patient

FIGURE 8.2   Smart pump logic.

to previously discussed technology by providing health care providers access to critical information. Some HHCs and PDAs have wireless network ability and therefore can access and transmit data in real time. Newer HHC versions include cell phone, electronic mail, and digital camera capabilities. In 2001, 26% of physicians used HHCs, and 50% are estimated to use them by 2005 (Larkin, 2001). In addition to the business applications of HHCs and PDAs for scheduling, dictation, and coding, the use of the database information and communication capabilities of the HHC fosters patient safety by promoting evidence-based practice (see chapter 4), safe medication ordering, accurate dosage calculations, and critical value alerts. Specific patient safety promoting capabilities of HHCs are described in Table 8.5.

Since HHC and PDA technology is fairly new, research on their efficacy is minimal, but anecdotal and descriptive information supports the benefits

TABLE 8.5   Handheld Computer Capabilities That Promote Patient Safety

Clinical Content	Decision Support	Patient Data*	Healthcare Education
• Pharmaceutical database, formulary and costs • Medical reference materials (textbooks, differential diagnoses guides, therapeutic manuals) • Clinical listserv e-mails	• Disease management guidelines • Clinical practice guidelines • Drug and food interactions database • Dosage calculations • Wireless electronic prescribing	• Current patient list/patient tracking • Appointment schedule • Digital pictures of wounds, etc. • Access to patient data • Critical alerts (laboratory values, patient emergencies, bioterrorism) • Clinical documentation	• Tracking student experiences and competencies • Student reference materials • Case studies • Patient education resources

Brewin, 2003; Larkin, 2001; Skolnik, Willyard, & Cohen, 2001.
*Limited by current technology capabilities and confidentiality issues.

of HHCs and PDAs in promoting quality of care and patient safety (Fischer, Stewart, Mehta, Wax, & Lapins, 2003). One use of HHCs and PDAs clearly demonstrated to promote patient safety is electronic prescribing. In a paper world, 30% of prescriptions have to be rechecked. This decreases by 55% with electronic prescribing (Houck, 2001).

Barriers to the use of HHCs include the limitations of HHC memory, infrared transfer speeds, screen size, patient confidentiality issues, and resistance to the use of technology. Due to the portability of HHCs and PDAs, either biometric access or passwords and encryption are critical if patient data are available (Blanton, 2001). Facilitators include relatively low cost, ease of use, portability, and the plethora of available, medically related HHC downloads. See sample download links in the Web Resources section at the end of this chapter.

GENERAL SYSTEM VULNERABILITIES

Technology systems usually have alarms, alerts, back-up systems, and override capabilities. A discussion of these vulnerabilities as they apply broadly to technology will be presented.

Alarms

Recent attention to alarms was raised in the JCAHO Sentinel Event Alert on ventilator deaths (JCAHO, 2002a, 2003). The *Alert* communication based on the number of adverse incidents was the impetus for one of the national patient safety goals to address the "full spectrum of alarm systems that are triggered by physical or physiologic monitoring of the individual. In other words, any alarm that is intended to protect the individual receiving care or alert the staff that the individual is at increased risk and needs immediate assistance would be within the scope of this goal" (JCAHO, 2002b). An example would include infusion pumps. Technologies such as CPOE, BPOC, and ADMs don't fit into the JCAHO definition, but alarms in these technologies are important to identify potential problems and warn users.

There are several features of alarms that should be assessed for safety. These features include audibility, visibility, and distinction. There are no standards related to decibel levels for alarms, so loudness and tone must be considered in each patient care setting. When multiple alarms are used in a clinical setting, caregivers often have difficulty recognizing multiple alarms at one time, i.e., the inability to distinguish high-priority versus low-priority alarms. Multiple alarms can then become background noise and lose their effectiveness. The occurrence of false positive alarms prompts caregivers to become less sensitive to alarms or to ignore them. For instance, false alarms may occur during patient movement. In many cases it is not the device that fails but the user, who can manipulate parameters to reduce false alarms. Organization policies should define the management of alarms and any disablement.

Alerts

Alerts are found in CPOE, CDSS, BPOC, and smart infusion pumps. Alerts notify the practitioner of specific information to provide clinical guidance and assist the practitioner in decision making. As with audible alarms, too many alerts can become background noise and after a while are not even seen. If alerts change behaviors in practice then they may not be needed because the behavior has been learned. If there are too many alerts, or many complex alerts, ordering physicians may become overwhelmed and frustrated, so a balance of types of alerts is needed. Alerts can be provided directly on a screen during the ordering process and may also be transmitted by other modalities such as e-mail or automatic pages of laboratory panic values. A process for continual reassessment of alerts is needed so that the right information is provided to clinicians at the right time in the right way.

Back-ups

Every major information technology system should have redundant systems for dealing with emergencies, power failures, and other disruptions of service. Once systems are in place, staff become dependent on them for patient care. Any failure of CPOE, BPOC, pharmacy systems, or ADMs can cause numerous opportunities for errors as staff revert to alternative methods and have limited access to information. In most cases, health care organizations have contracted for off-site storage of files for disaster recovery as a safeguard so valuable patient data are not lost.

Overrides

Many technologies have default modes and parameters. For example, a formulary may limit antibiotic orders or dosages. Policies should be established with the medical staff that define parameters and when or if a physician can override the parameters. The rationale should be thoroughly discussed since the parameters serve a function for safe care and overriding them may contribute to an error. If there are special situations that should allow an override then an additional monitoring process should be in place to review these situations and determine any modifications to the parameters.

CONCLUSION

Technology is a strong enabler for patient safety. It usually comes with a large price as well as the necessity for major organizational changes. Critical analysis and evaluation of the organization's culture, resources, and stakeholders must be performed to create the most successful implementations. The future of health care and technology is a constantly changing field and new technologies will present opportunities, challenges, and risks for patient safety. As each new technology is introduced, assessment and evaluation must be performed to ensure that these technologies enable patient safety.

WEB RESOURCES

Name of Resource/URL	*Description*
Agency for Healthcare Research and Quality http://www.ahrq.gov/data/informatics/informatria.htm	Medical Informatics for Better and Safer Health Care report on technology and safety
American Hospital Association www.aha.org www.hospitalconnect.com/hhnmostwired/archives/forward_progress.html	White paper on CPOE, costs, benefits; list of most wired hospitals; pathways for medication tool that contains bar coding readiness tool
American Society of Health System Pharmacists www.ashp.org	Provides an overview of CPOE issues and barriers
Arizona Health Sciences Library Healthcare PDA Applications http://educ.ahsl.arizona.edu/pda/hlth.htm#g	Numerous excellent health care PDA resources for many disciplines
Bridge Medical Inc. www.bridgemedical.com/pdf/whitepaper_barcode.pdf	Two white papers on bar coding of medication
California Health Care Foundation www.chcf.org/documents/ihealth/UseAdoptionComputerizedPatientRecords.pdf	Use and adoption of computer-based patient records
CPRI Toolkit www.himss.org/asp/cpritoolkit_toolkit.asp	Computer-based patient record system toolkit with all aspects of implementation
Epocrates http://www.epocrates.com	Widely used desktop and HHC drug reference that is customizable to most commonly used medications and periodic e-mail "DocAlerts" (fee based)
Evidence Based Medicine to Go http://www.ebm2go.com/	Free, regularly updated HHC evidence-based information including medications, guidelines, tools, and research summaries

Health Information Management Systems Society www.himss.org	Multiple resources, conference proceedings, and white papers on all aspects of technology including CPOE, bar coding, ADMs, and patient safety
The Leapfrog Group www.theleapfroggroup.org	Evaluation tool for CPOE and a tool on CPOE vendors to get started
Joint Commission on Accreditation of Healthcare Organizations www.jcaho.org	Sentinel Event Alert on clinical alarms, national patient safety goals
Medical Record Institute www.medrecinst.com/	Private organization that sponsors annual conference, Toward an Electronic Patient Record (TEPR)
PDAMD http://www.pdamd.com	Case studies and PDA software reviews
PDA Cortex http://pdacortex.com	Specialty listservs, PDA software (fee), and news.
President's Information Technology Advisory Committee http://www.itrd.gov/	Reports to the president including transforming health care through information technology

REFERENCES

Abbott Laboratories. (2003, March 27). *Abbott Laboratories completes initiative to bar code 100 percent of its hospital injectable pharmaceuticals and IV solutions.* Retrieved June 10, 2003, from http://abbott.com/news/press_release.cfm?id=541

Agency for Healthcare Research and Quality (AHRQ). (n.d.). *Medical informatics for better and safer health care.* Retrieved June 1, 2003, from www.ahrq.gov/data/informatics/informatria.htm

American Hospital Association (AHA). (2002). *FCC updates WMTS rule.* Retrieved June 10, 2003, from www.hospitalconnect.com/ashe/currentevent/wmts/wmtsupdate2_19_02.html

American Society of Health System Pharmacy (ASHP). (1993). ASHP guidelines on preventing medication errors in hospitals. *American Journal of Hospital Pharmacy, 50,* 305–314.

Aspen, P., Corrigan, J. M., Wolcott, J., & Erickson, S. M. (Eds.). (2003). *Patient safety: Achieving a new standard for care.* Washington, DC: National Academies Press.

Ball, M. J., Garets, D. E., & Handler, T. J. (2003). *Leveraging IT to improve patient safety.* Retrieved June 1, 2003, from www.himss.org

Bates, D. W. (2000). Using information technology to reduce rates of medication errors in hospitals. *British Medical Journal, 320*(7237), 788–791.

Bates, D. W., Leape, L. L., Cullen, D. J., Laird, N., Petersen, L. A., Teich, J. M., et al. (1998). Effect of computerized physician order entry and a team intervention on prevention of serious medication errors. *Journal of the American Medical Association, 280*, 1311–1316.

Bates, D. W., Spell, N., Cullen, D. J., Burdick, E., Laird, N., Petersen, L. A., et al. (1997). The costs of adverse drug events in hospitalized patients. *Journal of the American Medical Association, 277*(4), 307–311.

Bates, D. W., Teich, J. M., Lee, J., Seger, D., Kuperman, G. J., Ma'Luf, N., et al. (1999). The impact of computerized physician order entry on medication error prevention. *Journal of the American Medical Informatics Association, 6*, 313–321.

Benko, L. B. (2003, January 27). *Back to the drawing board: Cedars-Sinai physician order entry system suspended.* Retrieved June 9, 2003, from www.modernhealthcare.com/article.cms?articleId=28431

Berwick, D. M., & Leape, L. L. (1999). Reducing errors in medicine. *British Medical Journal, 319*, 136–137.

Blanton, S. H. (2001). *Securing PDAs in the health care environment.* Retrieved June 9, 2003, from http://www.sans.org/rr/paper.php?id=256

Borel, J. M., & Rascati, K. L. (1995). Effect of an automated, nursing unit-based drug-dispensing device on medication errors. *American Journal of Health-System Pharmacy, 52*(17), 1875–1879.

Brewin, B. (2003). HHS tests Palm PDAs for bioterror alerts to doctors. *Computerworld.* Retrieved June 9, 2003, from http://www.computerworld.com/industrytopics/healthcare/story/0,10801,79660,0.html

Bridge Medical, Inc. (2001, April). *The effect of barcode-enabled point of care technology on medication administration errors.* Retrieved January 2, 2003, from www.bridgemedical.com

California Healthcare Foundation & First Consulting Group. (2000, September). *A primer on physician order entry.* Retrieved June 8, 2003, from http://quality.chcf.org/view.cfm?itemID=3315

California Senate (2000). California Senate Bill No. 1875. Chapter 816, September 28 Statutes of 2000.

Centers for Medicare and Medicaid Services (CMS). (2003). Hospital conditions of participation: Quality assessment and performance improvement. *Federal Register, 68*(16), 3435–3455.

Chester, M. I., & Zilz, D. A. (1989). Effects of bar coding on a pharmacy stock replenishment system. *American Journal of Hospital Pharmacy, 46*, 1380–1385.

Cohen, M. R. (Ed.). (1999). *Medication errors.* Washington, DC: American Pharmaceutical Association.

Consensus Workgroup on Health Information Capture and Report Generation. (2002). *Healthcare documentation: A report on information capture and report generation.* Retrieved June 7, 2003, from www.medrecinst.com/resources/infoCap/FinalReport.pdf

Evans, R. S., Classen, D. C., Pestotnik, S. L., Lundsgaarde, H. P., & Burke, J. P. (1994). Improving empiric antibiotic selection using computer decision support. *Archives of Internal Medicine, 154*, 878–884.

Federal Register. (2002). Bar code label requirements for human drug products: Notice of public meeting. *Federal Register, 67*(117), 41360–41361.

Federal Register. (2003). Bar code label for human drug products and blood. *Federal Register, 68*(50), 12499–12534.

First Consulting Group. (2003). *Computerized physician order entry: Costs, benefits and challenges.* Retrieved June 1, 2003, from www.aha.org

Fischer, S., Stewart, T. E., Mehta, S., Wax, R., & Lapins, S. E. (2003). Handheld computing in medicine. *Journal of the American Medical Informatics Association, 10*, 139–149.

Gaillour, F. (2003). Healthcare transformation, part III: Enrolling physicians through a values dialogue. *HealthLeaders News.* Retrieved June 11, 2003, from www.healthleaders.com/news/feature1.php?contentid=44777

Grotting, J. B., Yang, M., Kelly, J., Brown, M. M., & Trohimovich, B. (2002). *The effect of barcode-enabled point-of-care technology on patient safety.* Retrieved June 1, 2003, from www.bridgemedical.com

Hammergrenm, J. (2003). *Scanning for safety: FDA announces proposed bar code regulations.* Retrieved June 10, 2003, from www.mckesson.com/feature_031703.html

Health Information Management Systems Society (HIMSS). (2003). *14th annual HIMSS leadership survey.* Final report, April 7. Retrieved June 10, 2003, from www.himss.org/2003survey/docs/Healthcare_CEO_final_report.doc

Houck, J. B. (2001). *GM, Medscape prescribe PDAs for MDs.* Retrieved June 9, 2003, from http://www.newsfactor.com/perl/story/7015.html

Joint Commission for the Accreditation of Healthcare Organizations (JCAHO). (2002a). *Sentinel event alert: Preventing ventilator-related deaths and injuries.* Retrieved June 7, 2003, from www.jcaho.org/about+us/news+letters/sentinel+event+alert/print/sea_25.htm

Joint Commission for the Accreditation of Healthcare Organizations (JCAHO). (2002b). *2003 national patient safety goals.* Retrieved January 12, 2003, at www.jcaho.org/accredited+organizations/patient+safety/npsg/index.htm

Joint Commission for the Accreditation of Healthcare Organizations (JCAHO). (2003). *Questions about goal #6 (alarm systems).* Retrieved June 7, 2003, from www.jcaho.org/accredited+organizations/patient+safety/npsg/faqs+about+national+patient+safety+goals.htm#goal6

Kilbridge, P., Welebob, E., Classen, D., & The First Consulting Group. (2001). *Overview of the Leapfrog Group evaluation tool for CPOE.* Retrieved June 10, 2003, from www.leapfroggroup.org/CPOE/CPOE%20Evaluation.pdf

Kohn, L. T., Corrigan, J. M., & Donaldson, M. S. (Eds.). (2000). *To err is human: Building a safer health system.* Washington, DC: National Academy Press.

Larkin, M. (2001). Can handheld computers improve the quality of care? *Lancet, 358*, 1438.

Leape, L. L., Brennan, T. A., Laird, N. M., Lawthers, A. G., Localio, A. R., Barnes, B. A., et al. (1991). The nature of adverse events in hospitalized patients: Results from the Harvard Medical Practice Study II. *New England Journal of Medicine, 324*(6), 377–384.

Leape, L. L., Kabcenell, A., Berwick, D., & Roessner, J. (1998). *Reducing adverse drug events*. Boston, MA: Institute for Healthcare Improvement.

The Leapfrog Group. (2000a). *Computer physician order entry (CPOE)*. Retrieved June 6, 2003, from www.theleapfroggroup.org

The Leapfrog Group. (2000b). *Leapfrog initiatives to drive great leaps in patient safety.* Retrieved January 12, 2003, from www.leapfroggroup.org/safety1.htm

Marthinsen, J., & Scott, M. L. (2003). Enhancing medication safety and efficiency: The critical role of nursing in automating the medication management process. *Voice of Nursing Leadership, 1*(3), 5–6.

McDonald, C. J. (1976). Use of a computer to detect and respond to clinical events: Its effects on clinician behavior. *Annals of Internal Medicine, 84,* 162–167.

Metzger, J., Turisco, F., & The First Consulting Group (2001). *Introduction to CPOE clinical decision support in CPOE: A look at the vendor market place and getting started.* Retrieved June 10, 2003, from http://www.leapfroggroup.org/CPOE/CPOE%20Guide.pdf

Modern Healthcare. (2002). *Hospital's computer crash a lesson to industry.* Retrieved June 10, 2003, from www.modernhealthcare.org

National Alliance for Health Information Technology (NAHIT). (2002). *About us.* Retrieved June 8, 2003, from www.nahit.org

Patterson, E. S., Cook, R. I., & Render, M. L. (2002). Improving patient safety by identifying side effects from introducing bar coding in medication administration. *Journal of the American Medical Informatics Association, 9* (5), 540–553.

Pfizer. (2003). *Pfizer introduces unit dose bar coding.* Retrieved June 10, 2003, from www.pfizer.com/download/do/barcode_standard.pdf

Rind, D. M., Safran, C., Phillips, R. S., Wang, Q., Calkins, D. R., Delbanco, T. L., et al. (1994). Effect of computer-based alerts on the treatment and outcomes of hospitalized patients. *Archives of Internal Medicine, 154,* 1511–1517.

Reason, J. T. (1990). *Human error.* Cambridge: Cambridge University Press.

Rogoski, R. R. (2003). EMRs/CPRs: Having it your way. *Health Management Technology, 24*(5), 12–14, 16.

Scarsi, K. K., Fotis, M. A., & Noskin, G. A. (2002). Pharmacist participation in medical rounds reduces medication errors. *American Journal of Health-System Pharmacy, 59*(21), 2089–2092.

Schneider, P. J. (2002). *FMEA on IV medication delivery. Identifying the gaps in drug administration.* Presentation at the November Inter-Professional Conference at the ALARIS™ Center for Medication Safety and Clinical Improvement in San Diego. Retrieved December 8, 2003, from www.alarismed.com/alariscenter/pdf/RoundTable_Selected_Slides.pdf

Shojania, K. G., Duncan, B. W., McDonald, K. M., & Wachter, R. M. (2001). *Making health care safer: A critical analysis of patient safety practices* (Publication 01-E058). Rockville, MD: Agency for Healthcare Research and Quality.

Skolnik, N. S., Willyard, K., & Cohen, H. (2001). Handheld computers: Revolutionizing clinical data management. *Family Practice Recertification, 23*(6), 23–26.

Spath, P. L. (2000). *Error reduction in health care.* San Francisco: Jossey-Bass.

Symbol Technologies, Inc. (1999). *Bar coding for beginners.* Holtsville, NY: Author

Teich, J. M., Merchia, P. R., Schmiz, J. L., Kuperman, G. J., Spurr, C. D., & Bates, B. W. (2000). Effects of computerized physician order entry on prescribing practices. *Archives of Internal Medicine, 160*, 2741–2747.

Wald, H., & Shojania, K. G. (2001). Prevention of misidentifications. In K. G. Shojania, B. W. Duncan, K. M. McDonald, & R. M. Wachter (Eds.), *Making health care safer: A critical analysis of patient safety practices*. Rockville, MD: Agency for Healthcare Research and Quality.

Chapter 9

The Role of Risk Management in Patient Safety: The Needs, Benefits, and Reasons to Disclose Errors

Monica C. Berry

P atient safety and health care errors have become a major concern of consumers, providers, policymakers, and manufacturers of health care products. Since the inception of the role of risk management, the profession has been inextricably entwined in dealing with health care errors and patient safety issues (Berry, 2002). In reality, the current interest in patient safety has provided risk managers an opportunity to showcase what the profession can offer health care organizations as well as the community of patients and providers by being a member of a multidisciplinary team that collaborates to improve patient safety by building safety nets around patients (Berry, 2002).

HISTORICAL ROLE OF RISK MANAGEMENT

It is important to understand the terms *risk* and *risk management*. Webster defines risk as the possibility of loss or injury. Risk management is an organizational function that heightens the level of awareness of possible risks that could threaten the financial stability of the organization or that are potentially harmful to patients, visitors, or employees.

In order to build safety nets for the present and the future, it is important to understand how health care providers and organizations in the past handled an error or adverse event that threatened patient safety. The role of risk managers in patient safety reflects the training and experience of the individual risk manager as well as the philosophy and culture of the organization in which the risk manager works.

Risk managers handle a significant amount of confidential information, including facts related to medical errors and adverse events. When a lawsuit is filed citing an adverse event or error as the cause of injury, concerns about the confidentiality of the information are heightened due to the fear of discoverability by the defendant. Because of fear of litigation and discoverability, health care organizations, through risk managers, may attempt to withhold facts about the error or event to prevent the information from being introduced at trial and risking a substantial jury verdict against an individual provider or health care organization. Risk managers are trained to, and bear the responsibility of, protecting the financial assets of the health care organization and protecting information about medical errors or adverse events is one method commonly used to accomplish this goal. While this self-protective model of risk management is, at least in part, a common model, it is by no means the universally accepted model.

Our litigious society, in conjunction with excessive jury verdicts or settlements, has contributed to creating an environment in which reporting of events and disclosure of facts has resulted in deeply entrenched webs of secrecy. In March 2002, a circuit court jury in Florida determined that Orlando Regional Healthcare System was liable for $78.5 million in total damages as a result of a misdiagnosed tumor that resulted in permanent brain damage (McDonald, 2002). Such an unpredictable and extreme jury verdict can be very unsettling to organizations, especially from a financial perspective and seems to support the self-protective model. A conflict of interest for the risk manager may arise as the risk manager attempts to serve competing interests, those of the organization and those of the profession. In addition, there may be circumstances where personal ethics may further compound the situation.

While the role and responsibilities of risk managers may vary significantly depending on the structure of the organization's risk management program, there are some generalizations that will be discussed. Prior to the 1999 Institute of Medicine (IOM) Report *To Err is Human*, adverse events or medical errors were frequently touted as an extremely rare situation or an aberrant outcome (Kohn, Corrigan, & Donaldson, 2000). It was not uncommon for information or knowledge about an adverse event or medical error to be kept secret by providers and health care organizations. The error may not have been reported to any of the internal (such as risk management, administration, or medical staff department chair) or external (such as the insurance carrier, Joint Commission on the Accreditation of Healthcare Organizations [JCAHO], or state licensing board) stakeholders. If the error was reported to an internal stakeholder, such as the department chair, it often remained a well-kept secret unless a lawsuit was filed. There was a tendency to "sweep it under the carpet." Under this cloak of secrecy there was little or no opportunity to work with the patient or family to resolve the matter. Neither was there an opportunity to attempt to understand how the event happened while it was still fresh in the minds of the involved individuals in order to prevent future occurrences.

There were a limited number of health care organizations that did not fit the "sweeper" model. Rather, these organizations acknowledged an error or adverse event when it occurred, but it generally was not publicized and was handled in a private manner. Settlement agreements frequently contain a confidentiality clause that prohibits either party from disclosing any of the facts, especially to the media. If there is no prohibition, some progressive organizations share the information with the media, but it is rare. What has been learned is that although organizations that share information with the media may suffer a temporary and short-lived setback, the overall rewards and community support for the organization is amplified. Duke University Medical Center is an example of an organization that acknowledged an error when it publicly accepted the responsibility, at least in part, for a donor mishap in February, 2003 (Snyderman, 2003).

In the past, neither the *sweeper* nor the *acknowledger* organizations shared the event in a public forum for the benefit of identifying the lessons learned and providing other health care organizations the opportunity to learn from another's mistake. The concept of developing best practices in a public forum did not previously exist.

The Duke Event

Jesica Santillan, a 17-year-old with restrictive cardiomyopathy and secondary nonreactive pulmonary hypertension, came to the U.S. for a heart-lung transplant in May, 2002. On February 6, 2003 Carolina Donor Services (CDS), the organ procurement agency in North Carolina, communicated with Duke University Hospital regarding the availability of organs. The initial call was to an adult transplant surgeon and subsequent calls were made to a pediatric transplant surgeon. The pediatric surgeon mentioned Jesica Santillan by name to CDS, discussed height, weight, and size of the organs being offered, and then accepted the offer of the organs for Jesica. The surgeon does not recall a conversation with CDS regarding the blood type of the donor. The harvest team traveled to the donor site and called back to Duke University Hospital reporting the condition of the organs to be of good quality. The donor organs were then harvested for transport.

The donor organs were implanted in Jesica and functioned well for approximately 30–40 minutes. At about the time the organs began to fail, the clinical transplant immunology lab at Duke reported that the organs were Blood Type A and Jesica was Blood Type O, and that this was an incompatible transplant. Jesica underwent another transplant but ultimately died.

Immediately after learning about the error, Duke University Hospital notified the family and launched an intensive review of the organ procurement process. The review revealed a lack of redundancy in the verification process as a significant weakness. Duke and CDS pulled together to identify meaningful ways to build safety nets into the various stages of the organ procurement process. Internal as well as external communication and a better understanding of individual responsibilities were a significant focus of the safety nets created.

Duke University Hospital publicly took responsibility for their part in the error and handled the media exposure in a very professional, kind, and warm manner. They created a specific Web site where letters from various Duke University medical and administrative leaders were posted that were open, honest, and forthright. In addition, they posted on the Web site all of the changes that were made to the organ procurement process so that other health care organizations could learn from the experience. To view various articles about this event, go to http://www. dukemednews.org/news/index.php?view=all

---

ROLE OF BEING A TEAM MEMBER

The IOM report challenged the idyllic belief that adverse events were rare occurrences and even suggested that they are much more common than traditionally believed (Merry & Brown, 2001). The IOM report gave the health care industry the opportunity to acknowledge these occurrences and the opportunity to learn from them, thus revolutionizing how the health care industry perceives adverse events and medical errors. The report put patient safety in the spotlight and provided risk managers the opportunity to move away from the reactive, self-protective model towards a more proactive response model by collaboratively designing systems that build safety nets around patients.

Reducing and preventing medical errors and improving the safety of the health care delivery system does not take place in a vacuum and neither does it belong to one person or one department. Rather it requires the building of new partnerships among all stakeholders to learn from mistakes and improve processes. The literature is replete with information stating that only in organizations where the culture of safety is embraced, supported, and promoted by the board and executive leaders will a clear culture of safety emerge and thrive (Minnesota Alliance for Patient Safety [MAPS], 2002). Patient safety is a complex, multidisciplinary topic that requires a team approach. While the hierarchical structure of medicine and health care (physicians viewed as the top and nurses viewed as the bottom) may create a gap in which it will be challenging to have true teamwork at the point of care, the collaborative efforts of a team are essential for the patient safety initiative to be successful. Members of the team might include the chief executive officer, chief operating officer, chief medical officer, chief nurse executive, pharmacist, performance improvement staff, physicians, managers of patient care areas, biomedical staff, human resources personnel, risk managers, staff development personnel, and members of the community.

The Duke University Medical Center donor mishap is a recent example of how the efforts of organized teamwork can showcase professionalism in responding to a sentinel event. On February 7, 2003 the Chief Executive Officer of the Duke University Health System disclosed to the public in a very caring manner the results of the investigation, identified its part in the tragic result, and provided information on changes made in the process (both internal and external processes were scrutinized and modified) so that other health care organizations could learn from the medical error (Snyderman, 2003).

The root cause of the mishap was identified as a failure to communicate. The most important safety tool that all members of the health care team have at their immediate disposal is communication, yet it is the tool that is utilized the least. Of the six JCAHO National Patient Safety Goals, improving communication is believed to be the most difficult. Dr. Peter Pronovost (2003) found in research that the lack of communication among team members is the basis of most medical errors. In the following section, the importance of the team concept as well as the contribution of the various team members will be discussed.

REPORTING EVENTS THAT THREATEN PATIENT SAFETY

The IOM report demonstrated to internal and external stakeholders the importance and impact of adverse events on patients that result from medical errors. The report encourages health care organizations to identify errors, analyze causes, and take appropriate action to improve performance. The first step in identifying errors requires that there be a reporting process from which the organization can understand the underlying causes of an adverse event and then translate those causes into corrective actions. The success of a reporting system is directly related to a sense of mutual trust between care providers and the executive leadership of health care organizations. If care providers in the trenches are willing to identify the system vulnerabilities, then the executive leadership must be willing to listen and to make changes that are sustained over time.

The IOM report recommends both a mandatory and voluntary reporting system for medical errors, both of which will be addressed. The IOM report challenges health care organizations to work collaboratively with federal legislative initiatives to design reporting systems that promote the goal of finding the most effective approaches to improve patient safety while promoting public trust. The intent of such reporting systems is that improvement is to be based on understanding the adverse event in the context of systems or processes that have failed and not on punishing those individuals involved in the event (see chapters 1 and 3).

What to Report

The literature abounds with various terms used to describe events that may or may not cause harm to patients in the health care setting (Thomas, et al., 2000). The JCAHO uses sentinel events and unanticipated outcomes, while literature from other industries may use such terms as errors, mistakes, untoward events, serious or potentially serious events, critical incidents, mishaps, as well as near misses, close calls, or good catches (Rasmussen, 1982). In addition, terms used to define the culture may include blame-free, nonpunitive, or just positive culture (Spath, 2000). Two concerns that are raised as a result of the variety of terms used to explain the event or the culture include the following: (1) perceptions are created by the use of certain words while the same connotation does not apply to other terms, and (2) while the literature may suggest the presence of a common nomenclature, in many respects, the names are not synonymous but are used interchangeably, thereby creating confusion for the individual attempting to apply a policy.

At the 2002 National Patient Safety Foundation (NPSF) Annenberg Conference, attended by clinicians as well as experts in the patient safety field, a series of clinical vignettes was presented and the audience was asked to respond whether the situation constituted an error (NPSF, 2002). The significant disparity in responses raises concern that if health care experts cannot define by example what is meant by an error, how can one expect to appropriately educate the public, the media, health care workers, patients, or potential jurors. A common nomenclature is needed to promote patient safety learning and to create an even playing field for providers. At a minimum, organizations should establish a process to promote reporting of the following:

- Those events that fit the JCAHO definition of "sentinel event"
- Those events that do not meet the sentinel event definition, but may be bad or perhaps unanticipated outcomes that threaten patient safety
- Those events that cause patient harm
- Those events that do not cause harm to the patient, but indicate latent system errors, commonly termed "near misses" or "close calls."

While it is helpful to understand the plethora of possible terms, each organization should select the terms to be used in that organization and provide an acceptable definition to ensure reporting of events that impact patient safety.

Barriers to Reporting

Every organization has barriers to reporting adverse and sentinel events to both internal as well as external stakeholders. The role of managers, directors, and other administrative leaders is to search out and remove these barriers. Some barriers are obvious while others are not so obvious. The complexity of the environment in which health care is provided only adds to the difficulty in identifying existing barriers. Common barriers to reporting events that impact patient safety are outlined below.

A "We Have Always Done It This Way" Philosophy

- Ingrained traditions in the culture of health care
- No scientific data to suggest a better way until recently
- Health care profession has learned to tolerate mistakes
- Lack of sufficient resources to make changes
- Absence of true accountability
- Denial that even the most well-trained and competent practitioner can make mistakes

A "Blame and Shame" Culture

- Finger pointing after an event with the intent of identifying *who did it* rather than *what happened*
- Defensiveness that blocks possibility of learning from the event
- Profession demands perfection that creates an impediment to acknowledging error
- Fear of legal liability
- Fear of loss of credibility and reputation
- Fear of punishment by the practitioner or organization
- Fear of loss of license to practice
- Webs of secrecy and attempts to cover up a mistake creates victims of all involved

Internal Reporting

The leadership and cultural support provided to practitioners will determine the degree of accuracy and completeness of an organization's internal reporting process. If the culture is one in which the staff are punished when errors happen and the patient is harmed, be assured the number and kind of reports will grossly underrepresent the activities in the organization. A punitive environment tends to drive reporting of errors underground for fear of punishment, and managers and leaders do not know what the true error rates are (Larson, 2000). A punitive environment negatively impacts the ability of the organization to make positive changes and improve patient safety. The staff must feel safe to report events and protected from potential negative ramifications, such as being counseled or fired, if they report near misses, adverse events, and sentinel events. If the culture is one in which staff do not feel secure from reprisals, then one can expect minimal reporting of errors.

It is generally recognized that most health care organizations have had, at least in part, a punitive culture or what is perceived as a negative culture. Studies now provide evidence to demonstrate the need to actively change old paradigms of "blame and shame" (Bagian, et al., 2001). An organization-wide commitment is required to change the culture through education (MAPS, 2002). Results will occur when cultural theory is converted into practice. A culture of safety is challenged with each near miss, or adverse/sentinel event, as ingrained ways of thinking compete with systems thinking about health care errors. This challenge to create and sustain a nonpunitive culture mandates that clinical leaders be alert to the possibility of reverting to a punitive approach. The staff must feel that it is safe to report events and that they are protected from potential negative ramifications (such as an angry physician who may make the life of a nurse miserable because of a previously reported event) if they report such events. If the culture is one in which the staff do not have this safety net, you can expect to see victims—the patients, the staff, and the organization. The role of the executive leadership is to actively drive the organization towards a system and process approach of understanding the underlying cause(s) that must be identified before actions can be taken to improve patient safety.

To encourage the staff to participate in building patient safety nets, organizations should develop a process that clearly states that the purpose of reporting is to identify the system vulnerabilities as well as to develop action plans that reduce or minimize these vulnerabilities. One component of the reporting process is an amnesty policy. An amnesty policy is one in which the organization states that no disciplinary action will arise out of a safety investigation if the event is reported within 24 hours. Amnesty policies frequently have an exclusion provision, in cases of criminal activity or staff incompetency. The intent is not to suggest that staff can get off the hook if the event is reported, but rather to encourage reporting while allowing the organization to remain accountable for providing safe patient care. However, one must be wary of situations in which a staff member has competency or performance issues; becomes involved in an event that threatens patient safety; reports the event and expects the amnesty provision to apply; or is fired for competency or performance problems and then uses the organization's failure to apply the amnesty policy as the foundation for a lawsuit.

Another recognized component of a quality reporting system is that there is flexibility in terms of how an event is reported. Organizations that have both a formal and informal process are far more likely to be successful in receiving reports. Different health care providers have various thresholds of comfort in reporting events. It is important to allow providers to report based upon their level of comfort. Reporting options may include the following methods: a telephone call directly to staff, use of a hotline (both active and passive), stopping staff in the hall, after a meeting, or during patient safety rounds, completing a report (paper or Web-based), or via e-mail. In evaluating various reporting options organizations should determine whether reporting anonymously is an appropriate methodology for that particular organization. Anonymous reporting has received mixed reviews and may work better in some organizations than others.

The value of an internal reporting system is not in counting numbers or attempting to benchmark with other health care organizations according to the number of reports received. While the measurement and utilization of error rates has been a hot topic in health care for years, comparisons of error rates such as medication errors or falls from one organization to another are not meaningful or useful for several reasons. First, errors must be detected and reported to the organization before they can be included in the error calculation. Organizations vary widely in their ability to detect such errors and in the completeness of the information provided in reporting the error. In addition, the culture of the organization will affect the validity of the reporting. This variability is undetectable in the error rate. Second, there is great disparity among organizations in the nomenclature used to define errors. For example, what constitutes a "fall" may or may not be defined to require that the patient had a body part that touched the floor. Uniform definitions are needed as well as the consistent application of the definitions before benchmarking of this nature will be meaningful.

While it is true that the greater number of reports may suggest that the organization has a greater understanding of the events in the organization, it also may demonstrate that the staff completing the reports are excellent reporters. The real value in an internal reporting system is in the identification of system vulnerabilities that provide the organization an opportunity to evaluate and improve the processes involved as well as to monitor the organizations ability to sustain the changes over time. The tool used for internal reporting, whether it is a paper-based reporting system or a Web-based program, should be aimed at learning rather than focusing on accountability.

Analysis of the data provided in the reporting process is critical to understanding where to focus the learning. Data can be analyzed from many perspectives to provide a foundation upon which to learn. One perspective that is not commonly appreciated in health care when it comes to reporting events is the richness that can be found in the narrative or free-text portion of the report forms. Many health care professionals state that the information in the narrative does not lend well to being displayed in graphs or charts. While this may be true, it is not the reason for collecting the information related to events that threaten patient safety. The point of the narrative is to identify the system vulnerabilities and analysis of the information in the free-text portion of the report may yield the greatest insight to the underlying causes of the event.

The free text or narrative is the section where staff are encouraged to "tell their story". Several leading patient safety organizations have redesigned their report forms to promote telling the story while reducing the focus on the traditionally collected "data" (Knox, 2002). Organizations that are successful at telling and sharing their stories provide educational sessions for staff to learn how to tell their story so as to obtain valuable information related to the event rather than a "blame and shame" saga. Organizations can provide a framework within which to tell a story, such as asking the following questions:

- What happened?
- Has it happened before?
- Could it happen again?
- What caused it to happen?
- Who should be told? (Knox, 2002)

Telling the story captures feelings and thoughts, promotes comprehension as well as suggests an interrelatedness of facts associated with an event, and energizes staff to identify solutions. Telling the story about a health care event that seems unbelievable or implausible shifts the focus from "unexpected" to "expected". To shift the focus to expected does not mean that it is acceptable to have a high rate of error, harm, or death, but rather is intended to demonstrate acceptance that errors will occur in any system, no matter how well managed (Merry & Brown, 2001). Only with the shift to "expected" can health care organizations begin to manage and learn from such events.

Staff that take the opportunity to complete reports have commented that the incentive to continue to do so can be severely limited in organizations where they receive no feedback on the outcome of the report, such as when the reports fall into a "big black hole." For staff to see value in completing reports, organizations must provide relevant and meaningful feedback. Organizations can provide information related to patient safety events such as medication errors to the individual nursing units on a quarterly as well as annual basis. Such feedback is more than numbers—it requires data analysis as to causation and system vulnerabilities. For example, The United States Pharmacopoeia Medication Errors Reporting (MER) program is a voluntary reporting program for health care professionals that has been operational for more than 30 years. The USP publishes an annual report that identifies where errors commonly occur in the medication process, as well as the causes (performance deficit, protocol not followed, and knowledge deficit) and types (omissions, improper dose/quantity, and unauthorized drug) of errors. Organizations can benchmark with the USP and provide meaningful data if they are resourceful. In addition, such benchmarking or comparative data analysis may be helpful in identifying system vulnerabilities that bring about change through education.

External Reporting

The IOM Report launched Congress and the regulatory community into the medical errors arena by recommending that both mandatory and voluntary reporting systems be developed as one mechanism to enhance the understanding of errors and the factors that contribute to such errors (Kohn, Corrigan, & Donaldson, 2000). Specifically, it was recommended that a nationwide, state-based reporting system be developed to provide for the collection of standardized information (Kohn, Corrigan, & Donaldson, 2000). Such information might include essential facts associated with a particular event that have been deidentified, lessons learned from the event, and identification of best practices associated with how to avoid a similar event from happening in the future. Various private and public organizations and associations stepped forward to provide the government with ideas as well as solutions in building the system for reporting medical errors. The National Aeronautics and Space Administration (NASA) offered the Aviation Safety Reporting System (ASRS) as a place to begin, which provides health care with an excellent example of a 25-year history reporting model that is successful, trusted, voluntary, confidential, and nonpunitive (Kaiser Permanente, 2000). This reporting system collects, protects, and uses incident data to improve the National Aviation System. Pilots, air traffic controllers, flight attendants, maintenance workers and other aviation personnel with knowledge of actual or potential hazards to safe aviation operations submit over 36,000 voluntary reports annually. There are three components to the reporting system that essentially drive its success which include:

- Individuals that report the hazards are guaranteed confidentiality and limited immunity
- All identifying information is extracted prior to being entered into the database
- Reports are not used for enforcement if the report is submitted within ten days of the hazard, exclusive of criminal activity.

In addition to evaluating the ASRS to determine the components that may be applicable to health care, Cook, Woods and Miller (1998) suggest 11 other strategies for improving patient safety as part of the reporting process which are presented in Table 9.1.

TABLE 9.1   Strategies for Improving Patient Safety Related to Reporting Process

- Identification of any effective safety practices that were implemented
- Nonregulatory national entity should be the primary vehicle to collect the data
- Recommendation that it be a voluntary system that has strong federal confidentiality protections—to avoid the current patchwork of state protections that currently exist, but are ineffective
- The confidentiality provisions must stipulate that the reports are nondiscoverable as well as inadmissible in a court of law
- Develop incentives for reporting that includes eligibility for consideration in the event of a claim being filed
- Reports are analyzed by experts and effective corrective actions are identified through an understanding of the system vulnerabilities involved
- Pilot testing of the corrective actions is conducted prior to a large scale roll-out of new initiatives
- Exclusion of any events that are found to be intentional acts or grossly negligent acts, i.e., acts resulting from an impaired practitioner, or abusive acts addressed by state laws
- Review of state mandatory reporting systems and encouragement of such systems to focus on licensing violations
- Issuance of routine safety alerts based upon data placed in the repository
- Promote patient safety research

Cook, Woods & Miller, 1998

The IOM report included a recommendation that there be legislation to support the patient safety initiative. To date there have been no less than seven bills introduced in Congress that have in some form addressed the various aspects of reporting of events that threaten patient safety in the provision of health care. Some of the bills support a voluntary reporting system while others strongly urge that the reporting system be mandatory.

Mandatory reporting programs in all likelihood will result in pushing issues underground, which is the complete opposite of what is needed in health care in order to improve patient safety. Issues pushed underground do not give the organization or other health care providers the opportunity to learn from mistakes. In the health care arena there are several examples of mandatory programs that have not been successful in accomplishing the goals that were originally established for the program. There are about 12–15 states that currently have a mandatory reporting program and the success of these state programs has been questionable at best. Another example is the reporting of sentinel events to the JCAHO. The JCAHO has been vocal about the fact that they do not believe that all reportable sentinel events are being reported. This example is one of the primary reasons for which the private and public entities identified as potential repositories specifically exclude bodies such as JCAHO. Another disappointing mandatory reporting model with results suggestive of failure in accomplishing its goals is the National Practitioner Data Bank (NPDB). There are a variety of loopholes in the NPDB as it relates to reporting that are well recognized by providers, health care organizations, and insurance companies. It is not uncommon for the industry to take advantage of the loopholes especially because there have been no significant consequences of doing so.

The last issue with respect to mandatory versus voluntary reporting is that health care providers do not trust or believe that a mandatory program will advance the patient safety initiative. This absence of buy-in may result in failure of any mandatory program. Forcing a mandatory reporting program upon providers will not work, but giving them the opportunity to improve the process might. If given the chance to ease into a voluntary process and see success, health care providers will ultimately embrace this process.

If an externally legislated reporting process is identified for health care organizations to report events that threaten patient safety, organizations will need an internal policy that supports the legislation. Organizations should have a coordinated plan for reporting to external repositories that includes the individual (by title or department, not by name) that bears the responsibility of actually doing the reporting. Having one individual responsible for reporting allows the organization to avoid situations where:

- There is a conflict of interest in reporting
- Everyone who is allowed to report misbelieves that someone else reported
- No one has the final authority to report, or
- The information reported reflects turf battles or other internal organizational problems.

The organizational policy should also include a provision that promotes a team approach to making decisions associated with reporting. The number of team members varies according to the situation and can be as few as two individuals. A team approach is encouraged in situations where there is a conflict of interest or a need to determine the exact language used to report an event. The final decision can be communicated to the individual responsible for reporting, or this individual can be a member of the team. In most instances it would be preferable that the individual who is responsible for reporting be a member of the team so that he/she has full knowledge and understanding of the concerns and their resolution.

LOSS PREVENTION AND REDUCTION

Generally, loss prevention and loss reduction are techniques designed to reduce to the least possible cost the losses that an organization incurs. Specifically, loss prevention is recognizing the possibility of loss and taking measures to reduce its *frequency*, while loss reduction is intended to reduce the *severity* of such losses. Developing an informed consent policy is an example of a loss prevention technique that provides the organization with the opportunity to reduce the number of claims associated with failure to obtain consent for procedures or surgical interventions. Another example of a loss reduction technique is the creation of a policy for handling sentinel events. Loss prevention is proactive while loss reduction is reactive. It is important that all health care organizations have the ability to engage in both reactive and proactive methods to improve patient safety.

Management of Events

How an adverse event is handled may impact not only the outcome of the event but also the financial obligations of the organization. It is not uncommon for staff to inform the risk manager about an event several hours, days, weeks, months, or years after the event. It may also be possible that the risk manager is not informed of the event until such time as a lawsuit summons or complaint is served on the organization. Such late notice reduces the opportunity to work with the patient or family in resolving issues and concerns about the event and the potential impact, both short-term and long-term, on the patient. Late notice puts the staff and the organization in a reactive mode in managing the event and its outcome. It also allows for a multitude of surprises to surface. These surprises may be things discovered about the event that are not shared until late in the discovery or trial process. Surprises are often detrimental to the organization or providers involved. As a matter of fact, one should assume that surprises will be painful and costly. The reason all facts about an event should be identified early in the process is to give the organization the opportunity to know the situation they are facing and determine how to successfully manage the positive as well as the negative aspects of the event.

Organizations that have taken a more proactive approach in managing events have involved the risk manager early in the process and have seen significant differences in event outcomes. The well-known 1995 Ben Kolb story from Martin Memorial Hospital in Florida is an example of such a case (Bridge Medical, 1997). It is advisable for staff to notify risk management as soon as possible about an adverse event. Obviously, the patient should be stabilized first and the environment made as safe as possible prior to notification. The other option is to request that an individual not involved in the care of the patient notify risk management.

The benefit of early notification is that it allows the risk manager to work with staff in investigating the event and understanding the root causes of the event. This was the manner in which the Ben Kolb investigation took place (Bridge Medical, 1997). As a neutral person not directly involved in the event, the risk manager may provide insight that those close to the event may not have. Ben's story, presented in the sidebar, serves to clarify this point.

Ben's Story

On December 13, 1995 Ben Kolb, a seven-year-old avid soccer player, was scheduled to have scar tissue removed from his ear. Twenty minutes after successful anesthesia induction, the scrub technician handed the surgeon a syringe of what should have been lidocaine 1% with epinephrine 1:100,000 for local injection in the tissue surrounding Ben's ear. Ben's vital signs showed an immediate reaction to the medication which required the surgeon to pause until Ben was stabilized at which time the surgeon specifically requested that the involved syringes be saved.

Within 10 minutes Ben experienced cardiac arrest that required significant efforts to resolve. Ben was transferred to the ICU and the surgeon specifically asked to speak with Ben's mother before anyone else. The surgeon and anesthesiologist met briefly with the risk manager then spoke with Ben's mother to gently and thoroughly explain that Ben's heart had stopped and how difficult it was to restart. They explained that he was in a coma and attempted to help her begin to cope with the seriousness of Ben's condition. That evening Ben was transferred to a tertiary care center that specialized in pediatrics where he died the following day.

The local papers and television ran the story. The community was in shock. The risk manager called Ben's mother the following day and promised her that she would exhaust her resources to find an answer to what happened to Ben in surgery that day.

The root cause analysis revealed that topical adrenalin 1:1000 was also on the scrub tech's table, but the staff was adamant about the fact that it was impossible to mix them up based upon their process. Variations in the practice of how medications are transferred to the sterile field started to become more obvious as individuals who were not involved in the event were added to the root cause team. The syringes and vials so possessively guarded by the scrub technician were sent to a forensic lab for testing. The results revealed that the lidocaine syringe actually contained topical adrenalin. Although the coroner initially ruled Ben's death an idiosyncratic reaction to lidocaine, upon further discussion with the risk manager after the laboratory results became available, the cause of death was changed to an overdose of adrenalin.

The risk manager and anesthesiologist met with the Kolb family and their attorney to disclose the findings and apologize again for the error. Mr. Kolb specifically thanked the risk manager for giving them an opportunity to get answers they so desperately needed.

For additional details of this incident, see Beyond Blame, a videocassette produced by Bridge Medical (1997), and Risk Management Reports, Volume 25, Number 12, December, 1998.

Shortly after receiving a routinely prescribed medication, a patient arrests and dies. The staff does not call to report the incident to risk management because "we did not do anything wrong." When the staff was asked if they knew whether the medication received was the medication ordered the answer was not conclusive. By the time the code was finished, the vial of medication along with the syringe had already been destroyed, preventing the organization from determining a potential cause of death.

After an event that has harmed a patient has occurred, a common reaction is that both medical and nursing staff do not want to interface, dialogue, or communicate with the patient or the family. The staff have a tendency to want to avoid the family. This is the time when injured patients need the most support with open communication lines. Especially when harm is significant, and the patient or family must make decisions as a result of the harm, they need compassion, a good listener, and staff that are empathetic. While the interface with the staff may be limited to the hospitalization, the decisions made by the patient and family may have long term effects that reach far beyond the course of treatment at the hospital.

The risk manager can also provide support for the staff as well as participate in decisions that affect the staff or the patient. For example, if a staff member appears to need employee assistance program (EAP) services after an adverse event, or the family might benefit from a visit from their clergy, the risk manager can orchestrate meeting these needs. The risk manager can also assist with determining if any equipment should be sequestered, if there is any possibility of the equipment being involved in the event. The risk manager and the manager of the involved unit may also want to colead a staff meeting to discuss concerns raised by staff. The critical action is to utilize the risk manager as a resource when systems fail, which they are prone to do as long as humans provide care.

The role of the staff in conjunction with the risk manager is to facilitate communication about the event. The communication is with internal as well as external stakeholders. The importance of educating the staff after an event regarding the lessons learned from the event is crucial to the success of the organization's patient safety program, yet the timing of the conversation could be detrimental to the organization if not handled appropriately. The greatest opportunities to learn arise when staff and the risk manager collaborate early in the process in an effort to manage the event.

One concern about engaging the staff after an event that has caused harm to a patient is that the conversation, dialogue, or educational program may be discoverable in a court of law. The laws in various states may not protect the conversation, dialogue, or educational program, and therefore the risk manager and counsel should be consulted to protect the organization in the event of a trial.

Managing the Media

Health care organizations may at some time experience an event that receives media attention. It is important to keep in mind that the media are doing their job to create a story of interest for the public, although unfortunately one with sensationalism. Health care organizations and providers must respect the role of the media and not become antagonistic to the exposure. Generally the events that receive media attention are perceived as a crisis, such as the Duke University Medical Center donor mishap in 2003. How the organization handles both the crisis itself and the media will focus attention on the organization and therefore a policy and plan should be developed to provide guidelines for spokespersons. A well-written crisis plan will serve the organization before and during a crisis situation. The policy should support the philosophy that with media exposure, first impressions are lasting impressions. Rarely will an organization get a second chance to correct a bad impression and therefore the first media exposure is critical in creating a positive impression with the community.

The organizational crisis plan or policy should include a provision that addresses the role of the Chief Executive Officer (CEO), the Chief Operating Officer (COO), and the Chief Medical Officer (CMO). This provision should be descriptive to avoid any questions during a time when there is little opportunity for discussion. For each event that receives media attention, the organization will need to designate a spokesperson to approach the media, and that role may need to be assumed by the CEO, the COO, or the CMO, with advisement from the public relations manager and the risk manager. The individual selected will set the tone and create the first impression of the organization's response to the event. Choosing the hospital lawyer as the spokesperson would not be wise, but choosing a leader in the organization would be smart to convey the message that the organization considers the event significant. It is equally important to ensure that a copy of the plan is readily available for the CEO, the COO, and the CMO. In crisis situations, there is a slim margin of error and if the plan is readily available, the organization reduces the chance of creating a negative image.

In the introductory section of the plan, the organization should provide direction regarding when to remain silent versus making a public statement after an event that could be of interest to the media. Humans have a need to fill in the blanks and will do so if the organization elects to remain silent. Even a short statement is better than no statement and the statement could be one in which the organization expresses concern for the patient or patient's family followed by the fact that the organization is investigating the event.

Another provision in the plan should address a crisis team consisting of various core members as well as ad hoc members where needed for their expertise in a particular subject matter. With a team approach, there is usually no unanimous agreement on damage control measures or what should be communicated to the media. It is more realistic to expect consensus to be difficult to achieve.

The team can participate in preparing the spokesperson for meeting with the media by determining three to five key points and anticipating questions and developing appropriate responses. Another role of team members might include communicating with the family regarding the media interest in the case. In this instance, it is incumbent upon the organization to assure the family that the organization will respect their privacy. One way of addressing the concerns about confidentiality is to call a media conference in which the family and the organization are both represented. Coordination of what is to be discussed is critical to avoid unexpected outcomes. Generally this strategy works exceptionally well because it does not give the public or media much opportunity for sensationalism, and public interest wanes quickly.

In times past it was not uncommon for organizations to respond to media requests for information with "no comment". Today, such a statement is a death knell for the organization. If an organization feels compelled to decline to provide information, it is crucial that the organization provide a rationale. If it is expected that there will be an opportunity to engage the media in the near future, then a date should be provided. Preserving the confidentiality of the patient may be a reason to decline comment and the public generally accepts this response. When the organization fails to provide information without adequate explanation, it can expect the public to speculate, possibly causing greater damage to the organization than revealing the facts.

Prior to communicating with the media, health care organizations must take the opportunity to assess the situation from three different perspectives in order to understand what is at stake:

- Clinical perspective
  - The communication creates a climate that either enhances patient safety or does not

- A greater understanding of the event may prevent the same error from happening again as well as demonstrates the organization's commitment to taking the event seriously
- "Blame and shame" culture vs. nonpunitive culture will impact how the staff respond to this event as well as to future events
- Legal perspective
  - Consider whether the event will result in legal conflict
  - Determine if a settlement offer would best serve the patient or family
  - Consider whether adverse publicity will attract legal action on other issues or event related issues
- Professional perspective
  - Consider whether the event will impact the relationship with physicians or other providers
  - Ask whether the event will harm the reputation of the organization in the community
  - Address whether there will be financial ramifications such as terminating Medicare funding or fines assessed against the organization
  - Consider whether the event will impact the hospital license or the JCAHO accreditation status (Littlejohn, 1999)

The assessment must be completed as quickly as possible and the results delivered to the public in a timely manner. To approach the media without having completed the assessment is not in the best interest of the organization. These are the areas the media will question, and the media and the community will amply note the lack of preparation by the organization.

Many organizations, such as Duke University Medical Center in the donor mishap mentioned above, have a four-point media communication strategy that includes the following:

- Provide as much information to the public as possible in a timely manner
- Maintain public confidence by demonstrating reasonableness of steps taken
- Underscore the organization's sincere concern for those involved
- Demonstrate cooperation with regulatory agencies, law enforcement officers, and the media (Snyderman, 2003)

Another provision of the crisis plan should discuss recognition of, and strategies to respond to, various audiences. There are internal audiences, such as employees, governing body, physicians, other patients—and external audiences, such as regulatory agencies, investigating bodies, media, and the public. One message to the internal staff is the importance of not talking to media personnel. Recognize in the plan the role that the Internet can play. The organization can post information written and controlled by the organization on the Internet, such as changes in practice or policies, an apology letter to the community, a list of lessons learned, or the identification of best practices. The value of providing information on the Internet is that it gives many other health care organizations the opportunity to evaluate their practices or policies in comparison with the one where the event occurred and to learn from the mistakes. This illustrates the proactive aspect of the patient safety initiative in sharing with others to make health care safer.

Informed Consent

The informed consent process has been around since Hippocrates' time but, with the focus on patient safety and disclosure, there is a renewed interest in understanding the implications of the informed consent process in the patient safety context. In its simplest form, informed consent is disclosure of the recommended treatment, risks, benefits, and alternatives prior to the intervention. This is disclosure on the front end as opposed to disclosure after there has been an unanticipated outcome.

The informed consent process was once simple in its execution. The physician engaged in a one-way dialogue in which the patient was given a cursory explanation of the proposed treatment and then the patient gave his/her consent. This process has evolved over time so there is a two-way dialogue where the patient is given the opportunity to raise questions and sign a form to signify agreement. Lawsuits in which a failure to provide informed consent was asserted were not common in times past, and lack of informed consent for the most part was a secondary claim rather than the primary claim. (A primary claim is the major reason for filing a lawsuit, such as failure to diagnose breast cancer, and a secondary claim is one that does not have as much substance as the primary, such as inadequate consent.) Where an informed consent claim was asserted, there was limited success in proving damages.

A new trend in claims and lawsuits substantiates the finding that when patients suffer a bad outcome, injury, or death, they often are allege a failure to obtain informed consent, regardless of what they were told or which forms were signed (Rice, 2000). In addition, allegations in lawsuits asserted that the physician failed to disclose his/her experience, or lack of experience, with a procedure or surgical intervention (Rice, 2000). This trend suggests that providers need to reassess the quality of the conversation as well as the level of understanding of the patient at the time the consent was obtained. Realistically, the trend provides an opportunity to review how the process is executed and the documentation that is generated to support the conversation.

State law regulates the consent process and therefore there may be some differences and distinctions from state to state that make the informed consent process less universal than believed by the general public. For the most part, the informed consent process cannot be delegated and resides with the practitioner performing the procedure, surgical intervention, or providing the care or treatment. Other practitioners should avoid accepting this duty. If the physician does delegate the duty, the physician is bound by the conversation between the patient and the person to whom the duty was delegated. Another part of the process that has been problematic is the misunderstanding that informed consent is only getting a form signed. This is an invalid presumption. Informed consent is a process that involves the exchange of information between a physician or practitioner and the patient, a verification of the patient's understanding, followed by the patient's signature on a form granting the physician the authority to proceed. During the conversation the physician or practitioner is required to identify the risks and benefits of the recommended intervention, the risks and benefits of alternative treatments, and the risks associated with no treatment. Providers other than the individual performing the intervention may not necessarily have all of this information and therefore should refrain from accepting the responsibility of informing the patient. In the event that other providers accept the responsibility, the safety of the patient is compromised.

Equipment Safety and Product Recalls

The vast number and kinds of equipment that are used to deliver patient care are another source of potential harm to inpatients, outpatients, home health patients, and other ambulatory care patients who may use durable medical equipment. The growing technology associated with the various pieces of patient care equipment creates additional demands on health care professionals unlike any that have been seen in the history of medicine.

As health care professionals become increasingly reliant on equipment and technology, the need for standardization of the equipment throughout the organization must be addressed. The greater the number and variety of equipment that perform the same function in an organization, the greater the likelihood of a mishap resulting from confusion or insufficient knowledge that may harm the patient. In addition, it is not uncommon for staff to become too reliant on equipment and fail to recognize signs or symptoms of problems. As reliance on new technology continues to increase, organizations must build infrastructures to recognize device failures and back-up systems to reduce the likelihood of patient or financial harm.

The use of infusion pumps has been associated with so many deaths and tragic events that the JCAHO in 2000 issued a *Sentinel Event Alert* addressing the problem (JCAHO, 2000). In the *Alert* JCAHO identified the most common reason for sentinel events associated with infusion pumps: the lack of protection from free flow. In addition, the use of alarms on patient care equipment such as infusion pumps is one of the six national patient safety goals developed by the JCAHO. Two points addressed in the national patient safety goal on the use of alarms include the importance of setting appropriate parameters for the alarms and the need to ensure that the alarms are sufficiently audible in the environment in which they are used (JCAHO, 2002).

Two critical components of a solid equipment safety infrastructure are the presence of an effective and reliable preventive maintenance program and product recall process. How organizations manage their equipment preventive maintenance program and the product recall process will directly affect patient safety and can possibly save the organization millions of dollars. Flaws in either one of these systems can be exceptionally problematic as noted by *The New York Times* (Altman & Grady, 2002) in the case of 410 patients at Johns Hopkins Hospital in Baltimore who may have been exposed to *pseudomonas aeruginosa* after procedures in which the Olympus bronchoscope was used three months post recall of the bronchoscope. In this incident, there were problems with the manufacturing process as well as the mail routing process at the hospital in the receipt of the recall notice. The recall notification letter was sent to the hospital's loading dock with no specific name attached (*The New York Times*, 2002).

Organizations should have a policy and procedure that defines how recalls will be handled. The product recall policy should be a stand-alone policy that is not hidden in other equipment related policies. The policy should specify one point person, by title and not just by name, who is responsible for managing the process. Last, organizations must ensure that the policy is consistently followed. For example, all recalls should be handled using the same process rather than different processes for different kinds or types of equipment or products. Consistency in the application of the process translates into practices that ensure safe patient care.

DISCLOSURE OF EVENTS THAT THREATEN PATIENT SAFETY

The state of the current health care industry is one in which consumers and the community have lost faith in health care providers (Wu, Cavanaugh, McPhee, Lo, & Micco, 1997). This lack of trust results from providers, practitioners and health care organizations not disclosing adverse events, unanticipated outcomes, medical errors, or care that caused patient harm. The mistrust is based not just on nondisclosure, but on the timing of discovery of the event as well. Patients entrust their safety and well-being to health care providers, and providers have an obligation to the patient community to be worthy of that trust. If a patient or family becomes aware of an error that was not disclosed, they develop mistrust that erodes the physician-patient relationship.

In health care, errors or events that cause patient harm can be benign or they can involve system breakdowns that result in a patient's permanent disability or death. Researchers now believe that most medical errors cannot be prevented by perfecting the technical work of physicians, nurses, and pharmacists (Shojania, Duncan, McDonald, & Wachter, 2001). As described in chapters 1 and 3, a multifactorial comprehensive approach is needed for patient safety. Improving patient safety involves the coordinated efforts of many members of the health care team and starts with providers communicating honestly with patients, families, and colleagues if an adverse event or unanticipated outcome occurs. It is relatively easy to maintain a positive relationship with patients and families when caregivers have good news to share. However, communication assumes a special dimension when providers become the bearers of bad news. Learning to communicate well with patients and their families, especially after a bad outcome, is the best risk management tool providers can use.

Research

A significant amount of research has been conducted on medical errors (Brennan, Leape, & Laird, 1991), disclosure after unintended injuries,

(Witman, Park, & Hardin, 1996), and the likelihood of litigation after such an event (Vincent, Young, & Phillips, 1994). Approximately 92% of health care providers believe more can be done to address and reduce medical errors, such as better communication strategies, modernization of complex procedures, and reduction in workplace distractions (Voluntary Hospitals of America [VHA], 2002). Much of the struggle in recognizing and disclosing medical errors, for both providers and patients, centers on the difficulty in accepting that even the best trained and competent professional is not perfect and can make mistakes (Witman, Park, & Hardin, 1996). The medical profession's demand for perfection creates an impediment to acknowledging errors and may result in health care practitioners distancing themselves from errors by denial, blaming others, and becoming unavailable to the patient or patient's family after an adverse event or bad outcome (Witman, Park, & Hardin, 1996).

Studies have demonstrated that a physician's communication skills often determine whether a patient or patient's family will consult an attorney or file a lawsuit (Kraman & Hamm, 1999). Hickson, Clayton, Githens and Sloan (1992) found that of 127 lawsuits filed against providers after an injury where the patient's or family's perception was one of betrayal:

- 70% said they were not informed about long-term problems
- 48% felt that physicians had attempted to mislead them
- 32% stated that the physician did not talk openly to them
- 13% believed the physician did not listen to them

Patients become dissatisfied with a perceived lack of openness after an unintended injury or error, and negative communication may result in the very action the profession wishes to avoid, that is, litigation (Hingorani, Wong, & Vafidis, 1999). Ninety-eight percent of patients expect physicians to acknowledge error, regardless of the severity of the error (Witman, Park, & Hardin, 1996). Patients who are not informed of the error are significantly more likely to change to a new physician. As the severity of the error increases, patients expect a more substantial explanation about the error (Witman, Park, & Hardin, 1996).

Physicians often question their ability to disclose errors and base their decision on the following potentially conflicting factors:

- Personal ethics
- Professional obligation to prevent a recurrence of the error
- Concern that disclosure could jeopardize their professional relationships

- Patient's right to know
- Concern that disclosure may cause additional distress for the patient
- Fear of damaging the patient's confidence in their physician (Sweet & Bernat, 1997)

Disclosure conversations are unpleasant, difficult, and in many instances painful as practitioners face their own fallibility. Organizations that create systems or protocols for responding to medical errors and provide a forum for the unencumbered discussion of errors enhance the opportunity to understand errors and learn from them (Sweet & Bernat, 1997).

Studies have demonstrated that most physicians who admit their mistakes find patients to be understanding and forgiving, yet appreciate that there are exceptions (Gray, 1990). The most compelling reason to disclose is found in the quote "Honesty lets you carry your head high, regardless of what you did wrong" (Gray, 1990).

Rationale for Disclosure

Two essential building blocks of the physician-patient relationship are honesty and trust. When an error is acknowledged and the patient is informed of the error, the relationship is strengthened. When asked the question "Why disclose?" there are several responses, yet only one of them captures the true essence of disclosure. That response is "Because it is the right thing to do." Research has found that patients expect physicians to acknowledge errors and to inform the patient or the patient's family of the error (Witman, Park, & Hardin, 1996). Disclosure humanizes the physician in the eyes of the patient and provides the patient or family the opportunity to forgive as well as to put closure to the situation. Disclosure promotes healing for all of those affected by an event, which may include the patient, the patient's family, the physician, and other staff.

Another reason to disclose is that it is the responsibility of a professional. According to the National Patient Safety Foundation (NPSF) "healthcare professionals and institutions that accept th(e) responsibility (to disclose) are acknowledging their ethical obligation to be forthcoming about health care injuries and errors" (NPSF, 2000).

In addition, JCAHO requires of accredited organizations that "patients, and when appropriate, their families are informed about the outcomes of care including unanticipated outcomes" (JCAHO, 2002b). JCAHO does not require a written disclosure policy. An excellent way to address the need for communication with the patient or family is through an organizational communication policy that states the philosophy, value, and expectation that all individuals in the organization that interface with patients will communicate in an open, honest, factual, and respectful manner. In the general guidelines section of this communication policy, special circumstances such as complaints, patient's rights, consent, and disclosure can be delineated. In the rationale or purpose section of the policy, one goal may include providing patients or their families with the information needed in order to make decisions about their care, which may include the potential for seeking legitimate compensation.

In the disclosure section of the communication policy, the parameters for when nondisclosure is permissible rather than when it is expected should be defined. To place a disclosure provision in a communication policy avoids the following pitfalls:

- A stand-alone policy implies that the organization does not disclose unless required under the policy, which defeats the concept of shifting to a culture of safety
- Stand-alone policies support disclosure for "substantial harm" without defining the term, or define it very narrowly, which sends a message to staff that the organization does not feel compelled to inform patients about things that do not cause substantial harm
- Stand-alone policies may not address issues associated with providers who do not support the philosophy and therefore enforcement actions are severely limited.

Although organizations are not required to have a written policy that addresses disclosure, leaders should be able to articulate the organization's approach to disclosure. During a JCAHO survey, caregivers at the bedside should expect to be queried on their understanding of the organization's policy on unanticipated outcomes and how to apply the policy. A written communication policy with a disclosure provision will provide staff a tangible product upon which to formulate an understanding of the organization's philosophy and practice.

In the event that disclosure of an error, adverse event, or unanticipated outcome does not take place, the likelihood of a cascade of additional negative events may become an untenable reality. For example, families suspect a mistake has occurred, speculate as to what went wrong, search for answers, create their own answers (which may be worse than the truth), and exhibit anger because they lack information. This situation will only damage the physician-patient relationship and make further communication difficult. Families may consult a lawyer to assist them in finding the truth about an event. Even though the lawyer was not present when the error took place, an answer will be provided or at the very least postulated through the litigation process. In addition, staff who are aware of an error that is not disclosed to the patient or patient's family may feel compelled to discreetly share facts or perceived facts with the patient or patient's family. In this situation, the webs of secrecy that are created erode the relationship between care providers and have a negative impact on staff morale and loyalty to the organization. The reputation of the organization in the community is at stake and it will ultimately suffer.

The notion of disclosure is not without concerns from a variety of perspectives. The most notable concern is whether disclosure will be an admission of guilt or a statement of liability in a court of law. Regardless of the content, most conversations between physicians and their patients generally are not protected under peer review statutes in most states. Other concerns include the fact that disclosure does not always work to avoid a lawsuit. Referring to the earlier discussion of reasons for which it is important to disclose, we recall that the single most important reason to disclose adverse events or medical errors is "because it is the right thing to do". The reason is not to avoid lawsuits. Although this may be a secondary gain from the disclosure, it should not be the primary reason for the conversation with the patient or the patient's family.

Another concern is that meaningful disclosure conversations take practice and skill. Delivering bad news is not easy to do and generally does not come naturally to most practitioners. Rarely has this skill been taught in medical or nursing schools. Some practitioners are better at delivering bad news than others, presumably because of their natural ability to empathize. It is hoped that a particular practitioner does not gain skill because of a high frequency of such conversations. Risk managers can provide the needed practice and skills for a meaningful disclosure conversation and therefore should be used as resources.

Persons Qualified to Disclose

Every event that requires a disclosure deserves its own discussion with a core group of team members to develop a coordinated disclosure plan. In some instances, the team may decide not to disclose any information to the patient or patient's family, but this should be a rare decision. While there may be instances where it is believed to be in the patient's best interest not to disclose, a decision not to disclose occurs most often in organizations that function under the old *sweeper* model. These organizations have not evolved to a patient safety culture.

The individuals that comprise this core group of members will vary according to the situation or event. For example, if the event involves a medication error, it may be advisable to have a pharmacist on the team to discuss the implications of the error, and wrong-site surgery should include operating room staff. This core team should include all individuals who could bring a dimension of content and process expertise for the discussion of communication plan details.

The team decides the best person to break the news to the patient or the patient's family based on the organization's philosophy and the specific situation. JCAHO suggests that a licensed independent practitioner disclose the necessary information to the patient. Presumably, this means the patient's primary care provider (PCP) since this individual, in all likelihood, has the greatest knowledge of the patient and family or the individual in whom the patient or family has the greatest trust. In some instances, however, the PCP may not be the best person. In the event an individual other than the PCP is chosen, the team must carefully reflect on the decision to have someone other than the PCP disclose, as this decision may send an unintended message to the patient or family. Realistically, it is understood that the PCP may not be the best communicator or may be extremely upset about the event such that conversation with the patient or family is too painful or will result in an unintended admission of guilt. If an individual other than the PCP is chosen, it is best for the organization to have selection criteria.

One essential criterion is that the individual chosen must be able to convey sincerity and concern for the patient and family. The individual chosen will need to have a conversation with the PCP prior to meeting with the patient or family to garner knowledge from the PCP about the patient as well as determine whether the event will affect future care of the patient, and if so, in what way.

Another component of the coordinated plan is to determine those persons who will attend the disclosure conversation. The total number of individuals from the organization should be kept to a minimum to avoid overwhelming or intimidating the patient or family. The presence of more than one person will keep the conversation honest and avoid implicating any particular individual. This can be a difficult task if the patient or family asks questions concerning who is to blame. At a minimum, two individuals should meet with the patient or family, including the physician and an individual that represents the organization. Too many administrators at this conversation may unintentionally send an alarming message to the patient or family. Keeping the total number of individuals who participate in the disclosure conversation to three or fewer is the best way to manage the conversation.

What has been noted from a variety of experiences disclosing information to a patient or family is that the difficulty for the individual identified as the primary spokesperson is fairly high. Either the individual struggles with the conversation, can't communicate important information, makes a defensive or insensitive statement, does not convey the message, or delivers a message that is different from what was planned. The presence of another team member in the disclosure conversation is extremely valuable to assist the spokesperson and monitor the patient's responses. The second team member can engage in conversation to allow the primary spokesperson the opportunity to recover, redirect the focus of the conversation, or assist in conveying the message in the manner intended.

The plan should also include the identification of the individual who will be responsible for maintaining continual contact with the patient or family after the initial disclosure conversation. It is not unusual for patients or families to have questions after the disclosure conversation, and it is helpful to have a single staff contact to whom their questions can be directed. It is important that the patient or family be informed of the identity of this individual and given various ways to reach the primary contact person. The primary contact person should be included as part of the team at the initial disclosure conversation.

Usually patients or their families will want to inquire of a variety of staff members what they know or have heard about the error, including agency or temporary staff, and other staff members who were not present at the time of the error. An excellent way to manage the possible array of conversations that could take place is to script for staff their response when approached by the patient or a family member about the event in question. The script should include the name of the primary contact. It is acceptable to inform the patient and family members that the staff will be specifically asked to refer all questions to the primary contact for the exclusive purpose of allowing the information that the patient or family hears to come from an individual who has knowledge, as opposed to those who do not have knowledge. Speculation about the event can be damaging for the patient as well as the organization, especially when it becomes information that could be admitted at trial. Although the overall management of the event is the responsibility of the risk manager, the collaborative efforts of managers and directors in the disclosure follow-up is critical to improving patient safety in a learning organization.

Information to Disclose

Research has revealed that patients believe the following six components are essential to convey after an event:

- Acknowledgement that a mistake or error occurred
- An explanation as to why it happened
- An apology
- Statement that the organization is taking the event seriously and investigating it
- Statement that the organization is taking steps to prevent similar events from happening in the future
- In some cases, punishment and compensation (Vincent, Young, & Phillips, 1994)

When discussing what happened and how it happened, the information provided to the patient or family must be limited only to those verifiable facts that are known at the time of the disclosure conversation. Giving the patient or family misinformation when all the facts are not yet known is harmful, leaving the patient with a wrong impression that may have to be corrected later. Changing stories may cast doubt on the credibility of the information and the physician, as well as further erode the physician-patient relationship. Hedging questions and guessing will erect barriers and the patient or family may perceive that providers are not being honest. If the discussion takes place relatively soon after the event and before a root cause analysis (RCA), the verifiable facts may be limited. It is acceptable practice to tell the patient and family that you do not know, but as facts are discovered during the course of the investigation, they will be shared with the patient and family. This conveys to the patient or family that the organization and physician are not intentionally hiding information, but being honest with the information that is known or can be confirmed.

The role of the primary contact person becomes essential at this time in keeping communication channels open between the patient, the family, and the organization. The primary contact person should identify a specific date and time when the patient or family can expect further communication.

The first follow-up conversation should be soon after the initial discussion. The next day is an ideal time because it provides an opportunity for the patient or family to ask further questions as well as demonstrates the sincerity of the organization in taking the event seriously. If the primary contact misses this first follow-up meeting, there will never be an opportunity to recover. The patient or family already are distrustful of the organization and missing this appointment time will further erode the relationship as well as make further conversation difficult.

In subsequent conversations it is appropriate to provide the patient or family with information regarding the facts of the event as the investigation progresses. It is important for the patient or family to understand that various facts will be shared at different phases of the investigation process, that the variation may be due to the focus of the investigation such as state licensing board, JCAHO, or state department of health, and that one set of factors may influence another set of factors in a manner not previously anticipated. Patients and families should be encouraged to ask questions at any time they need clarification.

If the organization performs an RCA of the event, various perspectives will surface and the core team members may want to determine which facts can or should be shared with the patient or family. It is critical that the risk manager of the organization be included in this discussion and decision so as to protect information from discovery if necessary. Although an RCA is an internal quality improvement tool used to identify contributory causes of events in order to reduce morbidity and mortality, it is not discoverable in most states. Informed patients or families as well as savvy lawyers are now familiar with health care processes and are asking for a copy of the RCA analysis. If the patient or family asks whether the organization performed a RCA, it is best to respond in the affirmative and then state that the RCA is protected information under state laws, if that is true for that particular state. It is acceptable to share with the patient or family some of the action items to be taken by the organization to prevent similar events from happening.

Being able to acknowledge an error, unintended outcome or bad result is an important first step in a disclosure conversation. Of equal importance is an apology made to the patient or family in the disclosure conversation. Previously, apologies made by health care organizations or practitioners were interpreted as an admission of guilt. Fortunately, that is no longer the case. Many states have passed specific laws that make it easier for physicians to apologize without the fear of the apology haunting them in the courtroom (Prager, 2000). Legislatures and courts traditionally perceived benevolent gestures that express sympathy as attempts to reduce unnecessary lawsuits, while patient safety experts view it as an opportunity to improve patient safety (Prager, 2000).

The manner in which an apology is conveyed to the patient or family will set the stage for any future relationship between the patient and the physician. If the physician does not express his regret sincerely, provides an insensitive apology, avoids apologizing in a face-to-face meeting, uses defensive language, or focuses on the patient's reaction rather than the caregiver's apology, the patient or family will not believe the physician and may become angry and confrontational (Veltman, 2002). See Table 9.2 for appropriate language and ways to address patients concerns in a disclosure conversation. A well-articulated apology will humanize the physician in the eyes of the patient as well as diffuse the anger or reduce the insult of the injury. Such an apology may promote forgiveness, or at the very least engender understanding by the patient, as well as allow the physician to forgive himself. This kind of apology can be presented to the jurors as a benevolent gesture that expresses sympathy after an event and not an admission of guilt if it is introduced in a courtroom.

Patients or families may not recall whether an apology was made because they are so distraught over the event itself. It is wise to ensure that an apology is provided several times in the course of the first conversation, but avoid saying it so much that it loses its value. In addition, some patients and families see an apology from the physician and the institution as two separate yet very important components. Both components should be addressed in the initial disclosure conversation or in subsequent conversations if necessary.

A disclosure conversation that includes an apology can convey warmth, kindness, and empathy without admitting fault. In summary, disclosure and apology are always right when an adverse event, sentinel event, or unanticipated outcome occurs, and they can provide strength and credibility for the organization and the physician in building an environment in which to provide safe patient care.

Timing and Location of Disclosure

The first disclosure conversation should take place in the patient's room if possible. Privacy must be assured. If the patient has been discharged from the facility, transferred to another facility, or died, the team should take into consideration the patient's or family's wishes as to the meeting

TABLE 9.2   Things to Say and Ways to Approach a Disclosure Conversation

EXAMPLE ONE:

- I want to go over with you what happened this past {insert time} and to talk through together some of things that we have appreciated that may have led to your {insert event}. Does this make sense to you?
- ALTERNATIVE 1: Start by saying: I am very sorry about the frightening experience that you have had.
- ALTERNATIVE 2: Say: I am sorry you are having this frightening/upsetting uncomfortable experience.

EXAMPLE TWO:

- I wanted to meet with you to apologize for what happened.
- I know that we have disappointed you and I want to let you know that we are disappointed as well.
- Although we may not know what to expect as far as your future, and sometimes not knowing is the hardest part—I sincerely apologize for the anguish that this may cause you.
- We want to hear your concerns—now or those that you think of later.
- What I am asking for is an open and honest dialogue between us.
- We want you to feel comfortable asking us questions—anytime. We also want you to feel comfortable with our answers.
- Sometime the answer is going to be "we do not know at this time." This is a difficult answer to give you and more importantly, I believe this answer is one that is difficult for you to hear.
- We are committed to working with you to work things out as we go along.

EXAMPLE THREE:

- At this time we do not know exactly what happened. Although we could make some guesses, you do not deserve guesses—you deserve the truth.
- We do not know the truth but we are investigating what happened and how it happened.
- I would like your permission to come back and discuss with you our findings.
- We all feel very bad about what happened and appreciate your understanding of us as we take a hard look at our {practices/policy and procedure} to see how we can keep this from happening to anyone else.

EXAMPLE FOUR:

- Dr. {insert name} is devastated about what happened and he asked me to join him in this meeting with you to make sure he doesn't forget anything and to help you understand how serious we are taking this event.
- I am sorry this happened to you. I know it has caused great {pain, harm, anguish, fear}. I think that I would feel the same way too.
- Just like you, I wish that things had not turned out this way. There are some things that we will need to do and I would like to discuss those with you.

location. The home of the patient may or may not be an appropriate location. It is strongly advised that a gift of any kind not be part of the disclosure conversation, no matter what the location, but especially when it takes place in the home because it will likely be perceived as a bribe. Although the gift may be well intended, in reality it is one way to ensure that the patient will file a lawsuit. Furthermore, finding out about the gift in a settlement conference or in the course of a trial is a risk manager's worst nightmare. Therefore, if the disclosure takes place in the home of the patient or family it is wise to specifically inquire if any gifts, including food, accompanied the conversation if the risk manager was not a part of the conversation with the patient.

The decision regarding timing of disclosure in relation to the event itself is an issue to be addressed by the team assembled to discuss the disclosure. The benefits and risks should be weighed by the team in determining to disclose immediately or wait for a period of time. The disadvantage to disclosing immediately is the lack of verifiable facts early in the investigation, which may result in many "we do not know yet" answers to questions raised by the patient or family. The disadvantage of waiting until the facts are verified is that the patient or family may inadvertently hear about the mishap or event from someone other than a team member. The trust that might have existed in the physician-patient relationship will be completely eroded and the opportunity to rebuild this trust will be almost nonexistent. The likelihood that a patient or family who is angry because their trust has been betrayed will then actually hear a sincere apology is slim.

The staff involved in the incident and staff who will be caring for the patient after the event should be informed about the disclosure plan in order for them to assist in the plan. It also provides them with an opportunity to know the event is being addressed, which allows the staff to have closure. Events that are not disclosed to the patient or family affect staff morale and decreases faith that the organization does what is right for the patients. Support for staff involvement in the process also indicates leadership commitment and support for a culture of safety.

Methods of Disclosure

Each situation in which there is a need for a disclosure conversation requires a coordinated plan for successful management of the event as well as the disclosure. In developing the plan the team can expect that there may be some disagreement among members, especially with regard to aspects of the plan that may be disadvantageous to a particular individual or group. It is important to be mindful that there may be personal agendas for some members of the team, especially when the event has been particularly difficult or painful, or when the outcome has been highly disturbing or has evoked strong emotions. Members of the team may not personally agree with the plan or various aspects of the plan, but all members of the team must outwardly support the plan at the conclusion of the discussion. Team members must understand the importance of the collaborative approach and specifically refrain from sabotaging the plan.

The initial disclosure conversation with the patient or family must allow ample time for dialogue as well as questions and answers. The patient and family must understand the specific words chosen and spoken by the physician. The use of medical jargon may make the patient and family feel uneducated, stupid, or degraded, and therefore is discouraged. Those in the room should be seated and make direct eye contact with the patient and family members, if it is appropriate for the patient and family's culture. Gentle consoling touch is acceptable and encouraged, depending on the patient, the provider, and the culture of both. The PCP or other preselected team member should lead the conversation with an explanation that something unexpected has occurred. The provider and organization should then offer an apology, stating that the outcome of the event will be monitored and controlled as well as possible, and that the patient's treatment and care are of the utmost concern (Popp, 2002). By initially focusing the conversation on the treatment and care of the patient, the provider demonstrates the importance the organization places on the patient and away from placing blame.

This format demonstrates to the patient and family that the organization is willingly disclosing the event (i.e., being accountable) and the patient does not have to probe for information. After the explanation, the provider gives the patient or family the opportunity to ask questions. If the patient or family raises questions regarding the process or systems that led to the error, the explanation is limited to the fact that the situation is under investigation according to what is known at that time. The criticality of what is said and how it is said when the patient asks question cannot be overemphasized. This is the linch pin of the conversation and it is important that the team consider ways to respond to various questions that could be raised. One of the roles of the members of the team is to assist in preparing other team members for this part of the conversation. While the response should not be orchestrated to the point that it comes across as sterile, uncaring, unresponsive, or an attempt to hide the facts, it can be rehearsed to provide feedback from team members on how it sounds or ways to improve the communication. Expect this part of the disclosure dialogue to fail if there has been no preparation and the provider goes in unprepared. This is the point where providers often stumble with the explanation and recovery from possible damages may be impossible. In many instances this is the part of the conversation that determines whether the patient or family will sue and whether they are comfortable with the responses provided.

It is unrealistic to think that every disclosure conversation will go as planned, but the better prepared the team, the greater the opportunity to respond in a way that is satisfying to the patient and family. If the conversation does not go well, it is also an opportunity to learn what went wrong, why it went wrong, and identify ways to improve the conversation the next time.

In dialoging with practitioners about the disclosure conversation, many have raised questions about how to handle their own emotions. There is no doubt that these conversations are difficult on providers. Some caregivers will handle the conversation better than others. The personal experiences of the provider affect the ability to deliver bad news. In many respects, how a provider handles being the *recipient* of bad news directly relates to how that same provider *delivers* bad news. Frankly, it never hurts to allow the patient to see that the conversation is painful for the provider. This will only highlight the humane, caring qualities of the provider in the eyes of the patient or family. What has been reported by providers about particularly painful conversations between a patient/family and the provider, where the provider cried with the family, is that it was one of the most valuable, meaningful, and therapeutic conversations in which the individuals have had the privilege of participating (NPSF, 2002).

WEB RESOURCES

Name of Resource/URL	Description
Agency for Healthcare Research and Quality *http://www.ahrq.gov/clinic/ptsafety/spotlight.htm*	Critical analysis of patient safety practices
American Society of Healthcare Risk Management *www.ashrm.org*	White paper on disclosure

Joint Commission for the Accreditation of Healthcare Organizations www.jcaho.org

Policies on sentinel events; safety standards; disclosure policy

National Patient Safety Foundation http://www.npsf.org/html/statement.html

Policy on talking to patients about health care injury

National Coordinating Council for Medication Error Reporting and Prevention www.nccmerp.org

Categorization of medication errors: identification of comparative data related to medication errors

REFERENCES

Altman, L. K., & Grady, D. (2002, March 5). Hospital said faulty recall might have put 400 in danger. *The New York Times*, Section A, pg. 1.

Bagian, J., Lee, C., Gosbee, J., DeRosier, J., Stalhandske, E., Eldridge, N., et al. (2001). Developing and deploying a patient safety program in a large healthcare delivery system. *JCAHO: Journal on Quality Improvement, 27*(10), 522–530.

Berry, M. (2002). The role of risk management in a culture of safety. *Joint Commission Perspectives on Patient Safety, 2,* 6.

Brennan, T. A., Leape, L. L., & Laird, N. M. (1991). Incidence of adverse events and negligence in hospitalized patients. Results of the Harvard Medical Practice Study I and II. *New England Journal of Medicine, 324,* 370–384.

Bridge Medical, Inc. (1997). *Beyond Blame* videocassette.

Cook, R., Woods, D., & Miller, C. (1998). *Tale of two stories: Contrasting views of patient safety.* Retrieved December 8, 2003, from http://www.npsf.org/exec/front.html.

Gray, J. (1990). Should you tell the patient when you mess up? *Medical Economics, 23,* 135–139.

Hickson, G., Clayton, E., Githens, P., & Sloan, F. (1992). Factors that prompted families to file medical malpractice claims following perinatal injuries. *Journal of the American Medical Association, 267,* 1359–1363.

Hingorani, M., Wong, T., & Vafidis, G. (1999). Patients' and doctors' attitudes to amount of information given after unintended injury during treatment: Cross-sectional questionnaire survey. *British Medical Journal, 318,* 640–641.

Joint Commission on the Accreditation of Healthcare Organizations (JCAHO). (2000). Infusion pumps: Preventing future adverse events. *Sentinel Event Alert,* Issue 15, November 30.

Joint Commission on the Accreditation of Healthcare Organizations (JCAHO). (2002a). *National patient safety goals.* Retrieved January 5, 2003, from www.jcaho.org

Joint Commission on the Accreditation of Healthcare Organizations (JCAHO). (2002b). *Comprehensive accreditation manual for hospitals.* Oakbrook Terrace, IL: Joint Commission Resources, Inc.

Kaiser Permanente. (2000, March 16–17). *Reporting as a means to improve patient safety.* Roundtable discussion at the Kaiser Permanente Institute for Health Policy.

Knox, E. (2002). *Patient safety as a way of life.* Keynote address at the American Society of Healthcare Risk Management annual conference, Seattle, Washington.

Kohn, L. T., Corrigan, J. M., & Donaldson, M. S. (Eds.). (2000). *To err is human: Building a safer health system.* Washington, DC: National Academy Press.

Kraman, S., & Hamm, G. (1999). Risk management: Extreme honesty may be the best policy. *Annals of Internal Medicine, 131,* 963–967.

Larson, L. (2000). Ending the culture of blame. *AHA Trustee Magazine, February,* 9–12.

Littlejohn, S. (1999, May). *Communicating during a clinical crisis.* Presentation to Illinois Society of Healthcare Risk Management, Springfield, Illinois.

McDonald, M. (2002). Despite legal headaches, Florida Health System to sell $109 million. *The Bond Buyer, 340,* 28.

Merry, M., & Brown, J. (2001). From a culture of safety to a culture of excellence. *Journal of Innovative Management,* Fall, 122–139.

Minnesota Alliance for Patient Safety (MAPS). (2002). A call to action: Roles and responsibilities for assuring patient safety. White paper, March.

National Patient Safety Foundation (NPSF). (2002). Comment by an anonymous family member attending the Annenberg Conference.

National Patient Safety Foundation (NPSF). (2000). *Talking to patients about health care injury: Statement of principle.* Retrieved December 17, 2002, from www.npsf.org

Popp, P. (2002). How to—and not to—disclose medical errors to patients. *Managed Care, October,* 52–53.

Prager, L. (2000). New laws let doctors say, "I'm sorry." *American Medical News, August,* 8–10.

Pronovost, P. (2003). *Lack of communication is root of errors.* Research findings presented at AHRQ media briefing. Retrieved March 17, 2003, from http://reuters.com/newsArticle

Rasmussen, J. (1982). Human errors: A taxonomy for describing human malfunction in industrial installations. *Journal of Occupational Accidents, 4,* 311–333.

Rice, B. (2002). The new rules on informed consent. *Medical Economics, June 19,* 150–162.

Shojania, K. G., Duncan, B. W., McDonald, K. M., & Wachter, R. M. (2001). *Making health care safer: A critical analysis of patient safety practices.* Rockville, MD: Agency for Healthcare Research and Quality.

Snyderman, R. (2003). *Statement of Ralph Snyderman.* Retrieved February 26, 2003, from http://news.mcduke.edu/news

Spath, P. (2000). *Patient safety improvement guidebook.* Forest Grove, OR: Brown-Spath & Associates.

Sweet, M., & Bernat, J. (1997). A study of the ethical duty of physicians to disclose errors. *Journal of Clinical Ethics, 8,* 341–348.

Thomas, E., Studdert, D., Burstin, H., Orav, E., Zeena, T., Williams, E., et al. (2000). Incidence and types of adverse events in negligent care in Utah and Colorado. *Medical Care, 38,* 261–271.

Veltman, L. (2002). *Disclosure and apology: The physician's perspective.* Lecture to Oregon Society of Healthcare Risk Management March meeting in Portland, Oregon.

Vincent, C., Young, M., & Phillips, A. (1994). Why do people sue doctors? A study of patients and relatives taking legal action. *Lancet, 343,* 1609–1613.

Voluntary Hospitals of America (VHA). (2002). Survey of attendees at a national patient safety symposium, Dallas, Texas.

Witman, A., Park, D., & Hardin, S. (1996). How do patients want physicians to handle mistakes?: A survey of internal medicine patients in an academic setting. *Archives of Internal Medicine, 156,* 2565–2569

Wu, A., Cavanaugh, T., McPhee, S., Lo, B., & Micco, G. (1997). To tell the truth: Ethical and practical issues in disclosing medical mistakes to patients. *Journal of General Internal Medicine, 12,* 770–775.

Part III

Patient Safety in Specific Settings and Populations

Chapter 10

Pediatric Patient Safety

Jacqueline Fowler Byers and Beatrice A. Schafhauser

BACKGROUND

Patient safety is of concern to people of all ages. However, infants and children are more vulnerable compared with their adult counterparts due to several issues. First, their developmental level plays a role in their safety. Ferris and colleagues (2001) concluded that when caring for sick children, developmental needs must be considered in conjunction with their medical needs. Pediatric study findings also suggest increased potential for error based on "changes in patient weight and physiologic maturation; limited capacity for cooperation in young children and high levels of dependency on others; and the relative rarity of most pediatric illnesses and accordant lack of widespread familiarity with their care" (Lannon, et al., 2001, p. 1474). Finally, in addition to medical errors, pediatric patients, especially infants, are also vulnerable to abduction. In this chapter we will discuss some of the challenges of keeping the pediatric patient safe.

Developmental levels are a key factor in understanding a child's ability to cooperate with the treatment plan. Consider, for example, an infant's total dependence on his caregiver, a toddler's need for independence, or an adolescent's desire for peer-group approval. These are just a few of the normal developmental issues that are a factor in safe and effective care. Each age and stage of development has its own unique challenges. For example, it is unreasonable to expect a diabetic toddler to understand that he needs to take his insulin injection and that he should be cooperative during the procedure. In fact, there is a good chance he will assert his independence repeating "no" and doing his best to squirm away from the caregiver. A toddler also lacks the ability to tell his caregiver that the dose in the syringe looks different from the last time he had his medication or what effect the medication has on him after it is given. Thus, it requires more vigilance on the part of the caregiver or parent to deliver the medication correctly, detect potential errors, and identify adverse drug events. Consider this same scenerio with an older child. It is not unreasonable to expect a school-age child to perform his own insulin injection with supervision and to understand why he has to take it. He should also be able to tell someone if the medication is causing him to "feel funny" or if the dose of medicine is different from before. The school age child is developmentally ready to accept some responsibility for his care.

RISKS OF MEDICATION ERRORS

Medication dosing is also problematic for children. Historically, the pediatric population has been understudied due largely to financial and ethical issues involving minor subjects. This has led to a knowledge deficit with regard to the safety and efficacy of pediatric drug administration. There is a lack of clinical drug trials that test the metabolism, excretion, and safety of drugs in infants and children, thus making pediatric pharmacology a practice based on experience, not science. In 1997, Congress passed the first legislation to encourage pharmaceutical companies to test products considered to be therapeutically important in children. (U.S. Food and Drug Administration [FDA], 1997). In 1998 the FDA issued the "Pediatric Rule" to enforce the regulation (FDA, 1998). In January 2002 the FDA enacted the Best Pharmaceuticals for Children Act (BPFCA) to provide incentives to test pharmaceuticals in children (BPFCA, 2002). These rules were enacted to make it more likely that children will receive improved treatment due to the availability of pediatric dosing information. However, there is still controversy as to the statutory authority of the FDA to require testing on children. Consequently, approximately 75% of pharmaceuticals still lack empirical evidence for their use in children (American Academy of Pediatrics, 2002).

Medication errors have been identified in the majority of pediatric studies as the most frequent type of patient safety error (Kaushal, 2001). Kaushal found further that dosing errors were the most common type of pediatric error. Most potential errors occurred at the stage of drug ordering (79%) and involved incorrect dosing (34%). In a subsequent study, Kaushal (2002) found that medication errors occurred three times more frequently in the pediatric acute care setting than in comparable adult settings. Pediatric medication administration is one of the most complex processes in health care today. Compared with adults, the process is much more detailed, requiring increased medication preparation, calculation, and double checking. As we learned in chapter one, complexity refers to both the numbers of steps involved as well as the rules or algorithms used to complete the steps. Take, for example, an intravenous dose of the antibiotic, Claforan®, for an infant. Before the dose can be ordered, the practitioner must have an accurate weight in kilograms and age in days so that the mathematical calculation and the pediatric dosing rules can be applied. Once the dose is calculated, the medication is reconstituted, and the correct volume is determined for administration. The medication requires two calculations, first for the dose and then for the volume of medication to be delivered to the patient. Second, the age of the patient must be known in order to determine if the patient should be dosed every 8 or every 12 hours. An incorrect selection in the dosing algorithm will cause an over- or underdose of medication. In comparison, an adult order for Claforan® would only require that the practitioner use the standard recommended dose. To administer, the practitioner reconstitutes the medication and the content of the entire vial is given. No calculations are required. Due to the increased number of steps in the pediatric process, medication administration for this population is more susceptible to error. There are more opportunities for the caregiver to forget a step, perform a step incorrectly, or select an incorrect decision arm.

The most highly publicized medication error in pediatrics is the "ten fold" error, in which a decimal point is misplaced during dosage calculation, and inadequate or excessive medication is administered (Kaushal, 2001). There are numerous examples cited in the literature that chronicle the devastating effects of this error. Reported in an American Academy of Pediatrics (AAP) summit newsletter, Jose Eric Martinez was an ill, two-month-old who exhibited early signs of congestive heart failure. In order to ameliorate his condition, the physician ordered intravenous digoxin over a hospital stay of several days. However, because of a decimal point error in determining the appropriate dosage, the infant was given a dose that was ten times what was intended and died (AAP, 2003). In 1998, an infant that was born to a mother with a prior history of syphilis had a similar fate. A decision was made to treat the infant with penicillin G. benzathine. Staff, unfamiliar with the medication or the correct dose, administered ten times the recommended amount. In addition, the medication was delivered intravenously instead of the correct route, intramuscularly. After approximately 1.8 mL of the dose, the infant experienced cardiac arrest and resuscitation efforts were unsuccessful (Institute for Safe Medication Practices [ISMP], 1998). In November 1997, a child died in a New Jersey teaching hospital after receiving 204 mg of cisplatin, a chemotherapeutic agent, instead of 20.4 mg. The error was the result of an unseen decimal point. The child, who was on his last chemotherapy dose and had been in remission, died as a result of the overdose (ISMP, 1997).

These tragedies are not the result of a single error, but a system failure. In each of these examples we see how multiple factors contribute to the adverse outcome. In Jose Eric Martinez's case complexity was an issue. The original calculation of digoxin was incorrect. Subsequent double checks either were forgotten or omitted. Consequently, the pharmacy sent the incorrect medication dose and the nurse administered it. In the penicillin example, the staff encountered an unfamiliar situation (in this case, the medication) and as we learned in the chapter 1 discussion of human factors, they compensated by looking for a recognizable pattern. The specific medication, penicillin G. benzathine, was mistaken for a more familiar form of penicillin and therefore the dose was calculated and delivered incorrectly. The last example was the result of an erroneous perception of written communication. There was a transcription error compounded by a lack of patient information. According to the report, the pharmacy staff did not know the medication was for a pediatric patient because that information was not readily available. The dose calculated was appropriate for an adult.

The ISMP and the United States Pharmacopoeia have published specific recommendations to address the tenfold error. They recommend that a trailing zero never be used after a decimal point, and a leading zero always precede a decimal point (USP, 2003; Levine, et. al., 2001). In addition, the ISMP recommends rounding chemotherapeutic agents over 10 mg to the nearest whole number. In the case of the cisplatin overdose, if the dose had been written as 20 mg instead of 20.4 mg, the error would not have occurred (ISMP, 1997). More pediatric medication best practices are included in an exemplar later in this chapter.

The highest rate of medication errors with potential harm was found in neonatal intensive care units (NICUs) (Kaushal, 2001). Preliminary data from the Vermont Oxford Network NIC/Q collaborative found NICU medication errors to be in the following areas: ordering 16%, transcribing 12%, dispensing 25%, administration 31%, monitoring 1%, wrong medication 8%, uncertain 6% (Goldmann, 2003). A relatively small dosage calculation error in this population is much more likely to result in an adverse patient outcome. This is a serious safety concern due to the limited physiologic reserves of premature infants. Their decreased body mass and immature physiologic systems may not be able to buffer an overdose of medication. In addition, dosage forms for neonatal and pediatric patients may not be commercially available, requiring the pharmacist to prepare medications with no standard compounding approach. Thus, an error can be made due to the availability of varying strengths of a particular medication. In recognition of these facts, additional safeguards have historically been in place in the acute care setting to protect this susceptible patient population. Some of these safeguards include "standardizing and simplifying equipment, supplies, and processes" (Lannon, et al., 2001, p. 1474). However, since the attention placed on medical errors in the 1999 Institute of Medicine (IOM) Report, *To Err is Human: Building a Safer Health System* (Kohn, Corrigan, & Donaldson, 2000), even more attention has been placed on protecting the safety of this young patient population.

What is unknown at this point is the frequency and severity of pediatric medical errors outside of the hospital setting. Approximately 70% of pediatric health care is provided in the ambulatory setting (AAP, 2003). Potential errors in this setting may be the result of errors in physician prescribing, pharmacy dispensing, or parental or school medication administration (AAP, 2003). Kaushal and colleagues are currently conducting a pediatric outpatient study to better understand ambulatory pediatric medication phenomena (Goldmann, 2003). With increased understanding of risks for errors, strategies to ensure patient safety can be implemented and evaluated. Medication ordering and administration are the highest priority in this area (AAP, 2003).

PEDIATRIC PATIENT SAFETY PRINCIPLES

In 2001, the AAP published their principles of patient safety in pediatrics (Lannon, et al., 2001). This statement, the AAP's response to the IOM report, provides recommendations for identifying and learning from errors in all settings where children receive health care: child care centers, schools, ambulatory care facilities, and inpatient settings. The general principles include:

- Commitment from pediatricians to provide the best possible health outcomes for children and their families
- Use of a systems approach to improve patient safety and prevent errors
- Development of systems to identify and learn from errors
- Nonpunitive error reporting
- Mandatory reporting of only the most critical errors
- Protection of error reports from discoverability for civil or criminal action
- Anonymity of individuals involved in adverse events
- Recognition that adverse events are not always caused by medical errors
- Organizational leadership focus for system improvements

Further recommendations from the Academy of Pediatrics address ways to tackle the problems of pediatric patient safety across settings (Lannon, et al., 2001). These recommendations include:

- Maximizing use of technology and drug packaging to reduce the potential for medical errors
- Encouraging the inclusion of children in new drug trials to ensure understanding of the drug related to pediatric patient outcomes
- Collaborative, organized efforts to promote patient safety in the pediatric population

PEDIATRIC PATIENT SAFETY IMPROVEMENT BARRIERS AND FACILITATORS

Barriers to patient safety improvement in children include the relatively rare incidence of negative outcomes, the provision of health care outside traditional health care settings (public health services, schools, and child protective services), poor development of outpatient information systems, and limited cooperation of family practice physicians and pediatricians (Ferris, et al., 2001). Lack of competition for tertiary pediatric services also limits the incentives for improving patient safety (Ferris, et al., 2001). This is further complicated by significantly fewer patient safety studies in pediatrics when compared with adult populations.

Ferris and colleagues (2001) performed an integrated review of the literature of children's quality improvement publications from 1985–1997. The most successful strategies in the literature included guidelines/clinical pathways with performance feedback, real-time action prompts (for instance, immunizations or follow up visits), and disease management (e.g., cystic fibrosis, asthma, diabetes). Despite the reported success of these strategies, physician adherence to clinical guidelines is often low (Leape, et al., 2003).

EXEMPLARS

Safe Pediatric Medication Ordering, Dispensing, and Administration

Patient safety in pediatric drug ordering, dispensing, and administration is a life and death issue. There are well-researched and documented ways to decrease the risk of errors in these processes. Key approaches are listed in table 10.1. Use of these strategies in the pediatric setting can decrease the risk of medication errors by over 80% (Kaushal, 2002). Key aspects of these approaches to promote pediatric medication safety are the common patient safety themes of communication, collaboration, and technology optimization. Mechanisms can be instituted to ensure that organizations employ these pediatric medication processes. Beyond organizational commitment and leadership, there are two key teams that can facilitate these safety activities: a pediatric medication performance improvement team and a proactive pediatric pharmacy and therapeutics committee.

Although patient safety is a system responsibility, Levine and colleagues (2001) propose individual health care professional's responsibilities for safe pediatric medication administration. These responsibilities are listed in table 10.2. These responsibilities are similar to those posed by the American Nurses Association (ANA) Code of Ethics for nurses (ANA, 2001) and other professional codes. The list, however, is helpful because it focuses a health care professional's thoughts on the specific medication process, and guides best practice. Lay employees or parents frequently administer pediatric medications outside of the acute care setting, so safe administration in these settings must be addressed as well (see the Parents as Partners exemplar).

Use of Evidence-Based Practice Guidelines

Evidence-based practice (EBP) can be described as health care providers using current best evidence from systematic research and applying it in

TABLE 10.1 Strategies for Safe Ordering, Dispensing and Administration of Pediatric Medications

Goal	Strategies
Decrease reliance on memory	• Computerized Physician/Prescriber Order Entry (CPOE) including electronic prescribing with computerized clinical decision support for drug/disease/nutrient interactions, allergies, and automated dispensing calculations within safe dosage ranges • Guided dose algorithms/dosing cards • Bar coding of medications, staff, and patients (allows an automated medication administration record)
Simplifying	• Restrict choices of drugs, dosages, and concentrations • Automated medication administration record generated from the CPOE • Automated medication dispensing devices with link to pharmacy information system • Minimize variety of medications available on unit; only stock frequently used medications in lowest available dosage amount • All intravenous fluid additives done by the pharmacy
Standardizing	• Prescribing conventions regarding abbreviations (elimination or an approved list) • Consistent use of leading zeros and elimination of use of trailing zeros (to decrease decimal point errors) • Protocols for administration of heparin, insulin, and chemotherapy • Standardized equipment (e.g., intravenous pumps) • Ensure that appropriate measuring devices are available (e.g., oral syringes, pediatric insulin syringes) • Consistent storage in medication rooms on all units
Forced functions	• Individualized lock and key connections (connections for intravenous and gastric tubes cannot be used for the wrong purpose due to physical design) • Eliminating concentrated potassium from patient care units • CPOE requirement of patient weight and allergy information in system for use • CPOE does not allow unacceptable dosages, routes, or frequency of administration orders

TABLE 10.1 *(continued)*

Goal	Strategies
Protocols and checklists—use wisely	• Use as prompts for safe action but do not substitute for active thought • Provide ongoing education and evidence-based updates • Ensure they are easy to use, update and access (online)
Increase information access	• CPOE with links of all current and archived patient information • Internet/intranet access • Personal digital assistant software • Consider color-coded drug allergy wristbands • Access to other organization's medical error and near miss information
Decrease reliance on vigilance	• Double checks for insulin, heparin, narcotic, and chemotherapy administration • Electronic monitors and alarms • Limit long shifts of nurses and physicians • Rotate staff for repetitive tasks that require high vigilance • Low traffic, well-lit area on unit for medication preparation and administration • No "after hours" pharmacy access by nonpharmacists for pediatric medications; have pharmacist "on call" for dispensing and consultation
Reduce process handoffs	• Unit-based pharmacists that interact during physician/patient rounds • Automation • CPOE
Decrease look-alikes and sound-alikes	• Address packaging and drug name similarities
Automating carefully	• CPOE • Automatic medication dispensing devices • Robotics in pharmacy

Kaushal, 2002; Levine, et al., 2001.

TABLE 10.2   Individual Health Care Professional's Responsibilities for Safe Medication Administration

---

- Keep informed about pediatric medical knowledge through review of the literature, continuing education programs, and communication with colleagues
- Actively participate as a member of the patient care team; collaborate and be involved in staff development programs
- Carefully perform and double check dosage calculations
- Consult literature, references, and/or colleagues if unsure of a prescription, preparation, or administration of a drug or a pediatric treatment requirement
- Ensure that all pertinent patient information is current and available so that therapies can be evaluated
- Focus on a single task and avoid interruptions in order to maintain concentration
- Participate in multidisciplinary teams to improve medication administration system functions
- Clarify illegible or vague orders with the prescriber

Levine, et al., 2001.

the prevention, detection, and care of health disorders (Donald, 2002). Guidelines can be defined as a set of rules intended to define appropriate care and to guide practice (Ferris, et al., 2001). Thus, EBP guidelines help practitioners plan the process of care for the correct or best practice. This approach reduces variability in practice and standardizes treatment. This standardization has been shown to improve quality in health care settings. Use of guidelines aid the practitioner in managing complexity, ensuring consistent treatment, and reducing inappropriate care and related costs (Leape, et al., 2003). In some settings, the patient's treatment plan is actually mapped out with interventions and expected patient responses. These "care maps" can then be used to document the patient's progress and determine if the standard treatment is effective (see chapter 4 for further discussion of evidence-based practice).

There are many sources for pediatric practice guidelines. The AAP has published over 40 guidelines for pediatric diagnoses. The National Initiative for Children's Healthcare Quality (NICHQ) partners with practitioners and organizations to produce pediatric guidelines that can be used in both ambulatory and acute care settings. Government agencies such as the Agency for Healthcare Research and Quality (AHRQ) publish both pediatric and adult evidence-based guidelines that can be accessed through the National Guideline Clearinghouse. Many of these resources are available on the Internet (see the Web Resources section at the end of this chapter).

Pediatric Quality Improvement Initiative

The National Initiative for Children's Healthcare Quality (NICHQ) is a not-for-profit organization dedicated to the improvement of children's health care. With a focus on primary care, NICHQ seeks to improve health care for children by providing tools that translate theoretical evidence into real-world practice. Working in close collaboration with key partners such as the AAP and the Institute for Healthcare Improvement (IHI), their strategies include education and training, improvement partnerships, and data management services (NICHQ, 2002).

The backbone of NICHQ's educational service is their "Learning Collaborative." Primary care practice teams learn evidenced-based practice for asthma, preventive services, foster care, attention deficit/hyperactivity disorder (ADHD), and children with special health care needs, over a nine- to twelve-month period. During this time, practitioners test, share, and implement the improvement strategies they have acquired. Utilizing the NICHQ data management system these teams of clinicians also measure their progress as they work toward improving quality in their practices. To date NICHQ has facilitated 30 projects affecting 290 primary practices in 19 states (NICHQ, 2002).

Neonatal Quality Improvement Collaborative

The Vermont Oxford Network (VON) is an international leader in the area of neonatal intensive care quality and safety (see Web Resources). There are over 400 NICU members in the VON, with approximately 35 NICUs participating in their quality improvement and safety initiatives through enrollment in the NIC/Q evidence-based practice quality improvement collaborations (VON, 2002). A confidential shared database for outcomes data and voluntary error reporting for internal and external benchmarking is one component of the program. Other activities include clinical trials, long-term outcome studies, family perception research, and ongoing performance improvement and safety activities. Specific goals of the NIC/Q collaboratives are to obtain measurable improvements in quality outcomes and efficiency for newborn infants and their families, to develop knowledge, resources, and technology that promote evidence-based quality improvement, and to disseminate improvement knowledge to the NICU community (VON, 2003). Similar to the patient safety principles discussed throughout this book, the underlying principles of the NIC/Q collaboratives include change management or theory, evidence-based practice, collaborative learning, and systems theory. The goal is better clinical, operational and organizational practices (VON, 2003). Outcomes of various collaboratives to date include improvement in understanding of NICU errors and a reduction in coagulase-negative staphylococcal infections in infants less than 1500 grams (Goldmann, 2003). Development of pediatric patient safety triggers similar to those developed for adult acute care (see chapter 11 for more about safety triggers) is in progress (Goldmann, 2003).

Developmental, Family-Centered Care in the NICU

In order to best meet the needs of families with an infant in a neonatal intensive care unit (NICU), developmental, family-centered care has been created as a health care delivery model. This model can provide expectations for families that a collaborative approach will be initiated in the NICU and extended beyond discharge. Perhaps the most critical aspect of developmental, family-centered care related to patient safety is the inclusion of the family as part of the team. This promotes increased knowledge, involvement, and empowerment of the parents. Informed, advocating parents can provide an additional safeguard against medical errors in all settings.

Developmental care is a philosophy of care that requires rethinking the relationships among the infant, the family, and the health care providers. Developmental care includes a variety of activities that manage the environment and individualize the care of the premature infant based on behavioral observations (Byers, 2003). The goal is to promote as stable, well organized, and competent an infant as possible in order to conserve energy for growth and development. Family members are partners in the infant's care, not visitors to the NICU. The health care team is there to educate and support the parents and their choices, as well as to provide ongoing assessment and the complex aspects of care. Interventions are used to simulate the in utero environment and to promote normal neonatal development. Caregiving is based on the infant's behavioral and physiologic cues and the nurse's knowledge of normal development and functional maturity from 24–40 weeks gestation as well as age-appropriate interventions. Developmental care strategies include management of the environment (decreased noise and visual stimulation), flexed positioning (to simulate in utero positioning), clustering of care (to promote rest), nonnutritive sucking, kangaroo care (placing infants on the parent's chest with the baby facing the parent), cobedding (placing multiple gestation infants in the same bed), as well as other activities to promote self-regulation and physiological and behavioral state regulation. Research reflects high parental satisfaction with this care approach and a trend towards an improvement in short-term physiological, developmental, and resource utilization outcomes with developmental care for up to 24 months (Byers, 2003).

Parents as Partners as Best Practice

Taking the developmental, family-centered care concept beyond infancy, parents who are involved with their child's care are better equipped to make informed decisions relating to their care. Parents who partner with their child's physician and health care providers also tend to be more cooperative with the treatment plan. Partnership can be defined as a relationship between individuals characterized by shared cooperation and responsibility for the achievement of a specified goal (American Heritage Dictionary of the English Language, 2000). This relationship is based on mutual respect for each other's skills and competencies. In a true partnership information is shared and decisions are made jointly. In the physician/parent partnership, parents should be encouraged to take part in every decision about their child's health care (see chapter 5 for further discussion of this topic). The Agency for Healthcare Research and Quality (AHRQ) calls parental involvement and advocacy the single most important way to help prevent medical errors. The AHRQ patient fact sheet "20 Tips To Help Prevent Medical Errors in Children" provides helpful tips for parents to use across settings to protect their children from errors (see Table 10.3). Knowledge, ongoing communication, and vigilance are proposed across health care settings, and for medication administration. Table 10.4 lists the minimum knowledge and skills that should be demonstrated by parents and other caregivers who administer medications. Knowledge can increase the probability of parental compliance with prescribed therapies and follow-up (Levine, et al., 2001).

Protecting Infants from Abduction

Infant safety is of great concern to parents, health care providers, law enforcement professionals, and accreditation agencies. According to the National Center for Missing and Exploited Children (NCMEC), a total of

TABLE 10.3   20 Tips To Help Prevent Medical Errors in Children

1. Be an active member of your child's health care team
2. Make sure your child's doctor knows all the medications and supplements your child is taking.
3. Make sure your child's doctor knows about any allergies
4. Make sure you can read your child's prescription.
5. When you pick up the medication from the pharmacy, ask: Is this the medication that my child's doctor prescribed?
6. As for information about the medication in terms you can understand
7. If you have any questions about the directions on the medication label, ask.
8. Ask the pharmacist for the best device to measure liquid medication and instructions on how to use the device if you're not sure.
9. Ask for written information about the side effects of the medication.
10. Choose a hospital at which many children have the procedure or surgery your child needs.
11. Ask all health care workers who have direct contact whether they have washed their hands.
12. Ask for an explanation of how to care for your child at home.
13. If having surgery, make sure that you, your child's doctor, and the surgeon all agree and are clear on exactly what will be done.
14. Speak up if you have questions.or concerns.
15. Make sure that you know who is in charge of your child's care.
16. Make sure all health professionals have important health information about your child.
17. Ask a family member or friend to be there with you and be your advocate.
18. Ask why each test and procedure is being done.
19. Ask when test results will be available.
20. Learn about your child's condition and treatments.

AHRQ Publication No. 02–P034.

217 infants (birth through six months) were abducted between the years of 1983–2002. Of these infants, 113 were abducted from health care facilities, 78 from homes, and 26 from "other places" (NCMEC, 2003). Most commonly, abducted infants are seven days old or less. As a response to the problem, accrediting bodies have required institutions that care for infants and children to develop and have security plans in place. Effective security plans incorporate both physical and preventive strategies.

Infant abductions do not appear to be associated with any specific geographical area. Abductions have been reported in 41 states with the

TABLE 10.4   Medication Discharge Counseling

Patients or caregivers should:

- Receive written instructions for administration including the drug's indications
- Demonstrate the measurement of medication doses if dispensed in liquid form
- Use the appropriate measuring device (discourage the use of teaspoons or tablespoons)
- Demonstrate any manipulation of a commercially available dosage form (e.g., dilution required before administration)
- Demonstrate the administration of the medication if special techniques are required (e.g., injection, nebulizer, inhaler)

Levine, et al., 2001.

highest volume reported in California (31) and in Texas (30). While there are no demographic similarities, NCMEC has identified a typical abductor profile from 187 cases occurring from 1983–1999:

1. Female of childbearing age (12–50), often overweight
2. Most likely compulsive: most often relies on manipulation, lying, and deception
3. Frequently indicates that she has lost a baby or is incapable of having one
4. Often married or cohabiting; companion's desire for a child may be the motivation for the abduction
5. Usually lives in the community where the abduction takes place
6. Frequently visits nursery and maternity units at more than one health care facility prior to the abduction; asks detailed questions about procedures and the maternity floor layout; frequently uses a fire exit stairwell for her escape; and may also move to the home setting
7. Usually plans the abduction, but does not necessarily target a specific infant; frequently seizes any opportunity present
8. Frequently impersonates a nurse or other allied health care personnel
9. Often becomes familiar with health care personnel and even with the infant's parents
10. Demonstrates a capability to provide "good" care to the baby once the abduction occurs

Although these characteristics have been described in numerous cases there is no guarantee that an infant abductor will always fit this description (NCMEC, 2003, p. 2).

Some of the physical strategies adopted by health care institutions to keep infants safe include tagging systems, access control, and closed-circuit television. Together these measures serve to document and deter potential abductors as well as record possible abductions as they unfold. Although these devices are reliable tools when installed and maintained properly, they are not infallible and must be checked regularly (NCMEC, 2003).

Preventive strategies to decrease the risk of infant abduction encompass education of parents and staff, and the development of policies and procedures to safeguard infants. Education must include information on the offender profile, unusual behavior, prevention procedures, and a critical-incident response plan. Both staff and patients should be educated about these safety strategies. Table 10.5 summarizes these infant abduction prevention strategies. Critical to prevention of infant abduction is not only the development of policies and procedures, but 100% adherence to them once they are developed.

CURRENT RESEARCH AND FUTURE RESEARCH DIRECTIONS

Safe patient care includes the appropriate use of medications and procedures. Two areas of concern regarding overuse in the pediatric population are the excessive use of psychotropic medications and antibiotics in children. These are priority research areas for the AAP (2003). In other areas, Miller and colleague's (2002) research using discharge codes of pediatric hospitalized patients found a high incidence of birth trauma, postoperative infection, and obstetric misadventures in mothers less than 18 years of age. Therefore, these are additional priority areas for patient safety initiatives and research in the pediatric acute care setting.

The AAP states that research on medical errors should be extended beyond hospitals to the sites where pediatric care is primarily provided, including schools, childcare centers, and ambulatory care settings (Lannon, et al., 2001). Pediatric patient safety research must focus on the highest-risk area, i.e., acute care, and also the areas of highest volume: ambulatory care, childcare centers, and schools. The role of parents' knowledge as a safety net needs to be further investigated.

Recently completed and currently funded projects related to pediatric patient safety by the Agency for Healthcare Research and Quality are

TABLE 10.5   Infant Abduction Prevention Strategies

General	Immediately report persons exhibiting behaviors of potential abductor
	Notify law enforcement, NCMEC, and other birthing facilities of attempted abductions
Proactive Measures	Have identification system for mother/infant with special ID bands or antitheft devices
	Have identification for infant clearly documented within 2 hours of birth (prints, photos, identifying marks)
	Transport infants by authorized staff in bassinets only
	Have infant shirts, gowns, blankets, clearly identifiable as hospital patient
	Mother education on nursery staff and identification process to give/take baby
	Implement staff identification procedures (e.g., photo, uniform, codes, keypads, etc.)
	Nurseries and maternity units away from main lobbies with street access
	Do not post births with identifying last name, address, etc. (e.g., newspapers)
	Have visitor check-in policy, procedure, and identification
	Educate staff and parents on identification process, security measures, lock-down procedure; in addition, educate staff to identify behaviors of abductors
	Provide consistency in staff to reduce unfamiliar personnel to unit and mothers
	Never leave infant unattended (e.g., while mother naps/showers)
Physical Security Safeguards	Limited access to nursery areas—eliminate multiple entries/exits; electronic key card access or similar control, self-closing, locking hardware
	Security cameras, alarmed exits, electronic surveillance systems. Conduct safety rounds regularly.
Plan	Develop lock-down and search procedure if abduction occurs
	Develop notification procedure
	Conduct debriefing if abduction occurs
	Develop media plan if abduction occurs
	Conduct response drills annually

National Center for Missing and Exploited Children, 2003. Reprinted with permission.

TABLE 10.6   Recent Pediatric Patient Safety Projects Funded by the Agency for Healthcare Research and Quality (AHRQ), 2002

Project	Investigator
Barriers to quality improvement activities in children's health care.	Ferris, et al.
Effect of teamwork on errors in neonatal intensive care units	Thomas
Impact of electronic prescribing on medication errors in ambulatory pediatrics	Johnson
Importance of parent-doctor and child-doctor communication	Horner, et al.
Improving medication safety across clinical settings	Bates
Minimizing antibiotic resistance in Colorado	Gonzales
Reducing ER errors in treating febrile infants	Glauber, et al.
Transfer of a novel pediatric simulation program	Halamek
Using handheld technology to reduce errors in ADHD care	Lozano

provided in Table 10.6. These studies address most of the current pediatric patient safety priorities.

CONCLUSION

Communication, collaboration, and appropriate use of technology all have the potential to prevent medical errors in the vulnerable pediatric population. Development of interdisciplinary teams in all pediatric settings is the key to monitoring and addressing pediatric patient safety. Patient safety research across pediatric care settings needs to be expanded to guide future initiatives.

WEB RESOURCES

Name of Resource/URL	Description
20 Tips To Help Prevent Medical Errors in Children http://www.ahrq.gov/consumer/20tipkid.htm	AHRQ parent/consumer fact sheet

Agency for Healthcare Research and Quality
http://www.ahrq.gov/research/childbrf.htm

AHRQ statement promoting research to improve children's health

American Academy of Pediatrics
www.aap.org

Pediatric guidelines, parents' resources, position statements

Child and Adolescent Health Measurement Initiative
http://www.facct.org/facct/site/CAHMI/CAHMI/home

Assessment tools for healthy development, adolescents, prevention, and special needs

Child's Health Toolbox
http://www.ahrq.gov/news/chtoolfact.htm

AHRQ measurement tools to assess the quality of children's health care, including the many well-established measures and AHRQ quality indicators

Guidelines for preventing medical errors in pediatrics
http://www.pedsnurses.org/html/PedGuidelinesV1.doc

PDF file of article from the *Journal of Pediatric Pharmacology and Therapeutics*, published June 2001

National Association of Children's Hospitals and Related Organizations
http://www.childrenshospitals.net/

Description of health care quality related activities, including a pediatric nosocomial infection reduction and prevention of antibiotic resistance program

National Guideline Clearinghouse
www.guideline.gov

Adult and pediatric evidence-based guidelines

National Initiative for Children's Healthcare Quality
http://www.nichq.org/

Focuses on improving pediatric primary care; tool-kits available for both asthma and attention deficit hyperactivity disorder

Prevention of Infant Abduction
http://wahoo.utmb.edu/ERC/selfstud/infantab/indexinf.htm

Learning module from the University of Texas Medical Branch

Reducing Errors in Pediatric Medicine: Implications for Research and Practice
http://66.77.20.158/ahrq/childhealthwebconf/

Live Webcast of Agency for Healthcare Research and Quality conference held July 17, 2002

Summit: Setting a Research Agenda for Patient Safety

Summary statement by the American Academy of Pediatrics

http://www.aap.org/advocacy/
washing/patientsafety.htm

Vermont Oxford Network	Voluntary collaboration of health
http://www.vtoxford.org/	care providers in neonatal inten-
Vermont Oxford Network NIC/Q	sive care units focusing on the
Collaborative	care and safety of newborn infants
http://www.nicq.org/	and their families

REFERENCES

American Academy of Pediatrics (AAP). (2002). *Children's groups disappointed in FDA's decision to to appeal pediatric rule.* Retrieved March 25, 2003, from http://www.aap.org/advocacy/washing/pediatric_rule_appeal_dec17.htm

American Academy of Pediatrics (AAP). (2003). *Summit: Setting a research agenda for patient safety.* Retrieved March 29, 2003, from http://www.aap.org/advocacy/washing/patientsafety.htm

American Heritage Dictionary of the English Language, 4th ed. (2000). Retrieved May 28, 2003, from http://dictionary.reference.com/search?q=partnership

American Nurses Association (ANA). (2001). *Code of ethics for nurses with interpretive statements.* Retrieved March 31, 2003, from http://www.nursingworld.org/ethics/code/ethicscode150.htm

Byers, J. F. (2003). Components of developmental care and the evidence for their use in the NICU. *MCN: The American Journal of Maternal Child Nursing, 28(3),* 174–180.

Donald, A. (2002). Evidence based medicine: Key concepts. *Medscape General Medicine, 4(2).* Retrieved March 16, 2003, from http://www.medscape.com/viewarticle/430709

Ferris, T. G., Dougherty, D., Blumenthal, D., & Perrin, J. M. (2001). A report card on quality improvement for children's healthcare. *Pediatrics, 107(1),* 143–155.

Goldmann, D. (2003). *Serious medication errors: Evaluation of detection and prevention strategies in pediatrics.* Paper presented at the 5th Annual NPSF Patient Safety Congress, Washington, D.C.

Institute for Safe Medication Practices (ISMP). (1998). *A case riddled with latent and active failures.* Retrieved March 17, 2003, from http://www.ismp.org/msa articles/latent.html

Institute for Safe Medication Practices (ISMP). (1997). *Important error prevention advisory— cisplatin overdose.* Retrieved March 17, 2003, from http://www.ismp.org/msaarticles/cisplatin2.html

Kaushal, R. (2001). How can information technology improve patient safety and reduce medication errors in children's health care? *Archives Pediatrics & Adolescent Medicine, 155(9),* 1002–1007.

Kaushal, R. (2002). *Targeted strategies to reduce medication errors in pediatrics.* Retrieved March 30, 2003, from http://66.77.20.156/assets/AHRQ/02-265/docs/Full Transcript.doc

Kohn, L., Corrigan, J., & Donaldson, M. (Eds.). (2000). *To err is human: Building a safer health system.* Washington, DC: National Academy Press.

Lannon, C. M., Coven, B. J., France, F. L., Hickson, G., Miles, P. V., Swanson, J. T., et al. (2001). Principles of patient safety in pediatrics. *Pediatrics, 107*(6), 1473–1475.

Leape, L. L., Weissman, J. S., Schneider, E. C., Plana, R. N., Gatsonis, C., & Epstein, A. M. (2003). Adherence to practice guidelines: The role of specialty society guidelines. *American Heart Journal, 145,* 19–26.

Levine, S. R., Cohen, M. R., Blanchard, N. R., Frederico, F., Margelli, M., Lomax, C., et al. (2001). Guidelines for preventing medication errors in pediatrics. *Journal of Pediatric Pharmacology and Therapeutics, 6,* 426–442.

Miller, M. R., Elixhauser, A., & Zhan, C. (2002). *Patient safety events during pediatric hospitalizations.* Retrieved March 30, 2003, from http://www.academyhealth.org/2002/presentations/miller.pdf

National Center for Missing and Exploited Children (NCMEC). (2003). *Guidelines on prevention of and response to infant abductions.* Retrieved January 21, 2003, from http://www.missingkids.com/download/NC05_7.pdf

National Initiative for Children's Healthcare Quality (NICHQ). (2002). Retrieved April 4, 2003, from http://www.nichq.org/

Palmer, R. H., & Miller, M. R. (2001). Methodologic challenges in developing and implementing measures of quality for child health care. *Ambulatory Pediatrics, 1*(1), 39–52.

U.S. Food and Drug Administration (FDA). (1997). *Food and drug modernization act of 1997.* Retrieved March 24, 2003, from http://www.fda.gov/cder/guidance/105-115.htm

U.S. Food and Drug Administration (FDA). (1998). *FDA acts to make drugs safer for children.* Retrieved March 20, 2003, from http://www.fda.gov/bbs/topics/NEWS/NEW00666.html

U.S. Food and Drug Administration (FDA). (2002). *Best Pharmaceuticals for Children Act.* Retrieved March 25, 2003, from http://www.fda.gov/opacom/laws/pharm-kids/pharmkids.html

United States Pharmacopoeia (USP). (2003). *USP issues parent recommendations to help prevent medication errors in children,* Retrieved March 31, 2003, from http://www.onlinepressroom.net/uspharm/

Vermont Oxford Network (VON). (2003). *NIC/Q collaborative.* Retrieved March 30, 2003, from http://www.nicq.org/

Vermont Oxford Network (VON). (2002). *Welcome to the Vermont Oxford Network!* Retrieved March 30, 2003, from http://www.vtoxford.org/

Chapter 11

Patient Safety in Acute and Critical Care

Jacqueline Fowler Byers

BACKGROUND

Patients in acute care hospitals are at risk for medical errors due to common cognitive deficits, complex physiological problems, and complicated therapeutic regimens. The youngest and most elderly patients are at highest risk due to their lack of physiological and cognitive reserves. Although patients cite the presence of nurses as comforting and helping them feel secure during the critical care experience (Hupcey, 2000; Stein-Parbury & McKinley, 2000), this does not guarantee safety. Patients in the perioperative and critical care areas are at higher risk than patients in other parts of the hospital, due to the invasiveness, high complexity, and risk of interventions (Gregory-Dawes, 2002; Ridley, 2000). These areas have tight time constraints and multiple processes with tight coupling. Over 50% of hospital adverse events occur in the perioperative area (Gregory-Dawes, 2002). As a result, the American Association of PeriOperative Registered Nurses (AORN) has established a Web site and a hotline to promote perioperative patient safety (see the Web Resources section at the end of this chapter).

Ridley (2000) cites three categories related to patient safety in critical care. These include the risk of the interventions themselves, the potential for errors related to prescribed therapies (e.g., medication errors), and the dangers from outside of the critical care units (e.g., loss of electrical power, bioterrorism, etc.). Patient safety strategies need to address all of these areas. This chapter will focus on the two internal patient safety risks: the risks of interventions and the potential for errors in prescribed therapies.

Until the recent focus on patient safety, most hospitalized patients took their safety for granted. However, that is naive. The Mayo Health System (Resar, 2002) performed a chart review to determine which critical care unit (CCU) events, as identified by triggers, occurred most commonly, and the percentage that resulted in harm. These findings are listed in Table 11.1. Fifty-five percent of patients had adverse events, resulting in an increased average CCU length of stay from 4.3 days to 8.9 days with an average increase in cost of care of $2,739 (Resar, 2002). There was an average of .164 adverse events/CCU day. Eighteen percent of the adverse events were related to medication administration, which correlates with the high number of medication errors found in the Harvard Medical Practice Study described in chapter 1. Medication adverse events were related to sedatives (24%), anticoagulants (24%), narcotics (12%), antibiotics (10%), insulin (8%), electrolytes (2%), and others (17%). Four percent of all of the adverse events contributed to death, and 11.4% required a rescue intervention.

TABLE 11.1   Top 10 Critical Care Unit Adverse Event Triggers

Trigger	# Positive (out of 1450 adverse events)	# With Harm (%)
In unit procedure	629	112 (17.8%)
Hematocrit drop > 4 Grams	309	201 (65%)
Intubation or reintubation	309	166 (54%)
Need for antiemetics	233	16 (6.8%)
Radiologic tests for embolism or clot	200	35 (17.5%)
Oversedation	184	159 (86%)
Nosocomial pneumonia	158	154 (97%)
Rising blood urea nitrogen	154	104 (67%)
Positive blood culture	121	101 (83%)
Abrupt medication stoppage	112	68 (61%)

From "ICU trigger tool data," by R. Resar, 2002. Retrieved January 11, 2003, from http://www.ihi.org/conferences/natforum/handouts/L01_3.pdf

The rate of CCU adverse event triggers can be used as a measure of critical care unit safety and quality, and as a tool to prioritize patient safety intervention areas (Resar, 2002). Biddle (2003) used patient safety triggers as the themes for trigger films for staff and student sharp-end training. Three- to four-minute vignettes in a realistic medical setting show common and catastrophic themes such as grabbing the wrong syringe or giving blood to a Jehovah's Witness patient. Best and worst practices are demonstrated, including error disclosure, with pauses for participant discussion (Biddle, 2003).

Strategies to promote acute care patient safety are no different from those of any other health care area. However, the stakes are higher in acute care. Most of the global patient safety initiatives described in chapters 1 and 2 focus on acute care since that is the area in which most research has been conducted and most error data reported. Two known factors that improve patient safety in acute care are the presence of pharmacists in the critical care areas, and the availability of specialized intensive care physicians (intensivists) for daily rounds (The Leapfrog Group, 2000; Pronovost, Wu, Dorman, & Marlock, 2002). Adverse events, morbidity, and mortality are decreased when these measures are implemented. The use of intensivists and other specific acute care patient safety initiatives are discussed in the exemplars later in this chapter.

REGULATORY REQUIREMENTS

The Joint Commission for Accreditation of Healthcare Organizations (JCAHO) requires reporting of sentinel events by all accredited health care organizations as discussed in chapter 1. It is important to note that 64% of reported sentinel events occurred in inpatient units of general hospitals, and 3.9% in the emergency departments, accounting for over two-thirds of total reported sentinel events (JCAHO, 2003c).

The JCAHO has mandated six evidence-based patient safety goals and related practice change recommendations that were implemented fully into the survey process in January 2003. In 2004 a seventh goal was added and original goals were further delineated with specific unapproved abbreviations and the Universal Protocol for preventing wrong site, wrong procedure, wrong person surgery™ (JCAHO, 2003d, 2003e). The JCAHO will be expecting compliance unless a facility does not serve the patient population covered by the safety goals. Table 11.2 lists these new goals. The JCAHO believes that implementation of these recommendations will dramatically

TABLE 11.2 JCAHO Patient Safety Goals

Patient Safety Goal		Recommendations
Improve the accuracy of patient identification	a.	Use at least two patient identifiers (neither to be the patient's room number) whenever taking blood samples or administering medications or blood products.
	b.	Prior to the start of any surgical or invasive procedure, conduct a final verification process, such as a "time out," to confirm the correct patient, procedure, and site, using active—not passive—communication techniques.
Improve the effectiveness of communication among caregivers	a.	Implement a process for taking verbal or telephone orders or critical test results that requires verification "read-back" of the complete order by the person receiving the order or test result.
	b.	Standardize the abbreviations, acronyms, and symbols used throughout the organization, including a list of abbreviations, acronyms, and symbols *not* to use.
Improve the safety of using high-alert-medications	a.	Remove concentrated electrolytes (including, but not limited to, potassium chloride, potassium phosphate, sodium chloride > 0.9%) from patient care units.
	b.	Standardize and limit the number of drug concentrations available in the organization.
Eliminate wrong-site, wrong-patient, wrong-procedure surgery	a.	Create and use a preoperative verification process, such as a checklist, to confirm that appropriate documents (e.g., medical records, imaging studies) are available.
	b.	Implement a process to mark the surgical site, and involve the patient in the marking process.
Improve the safety of using infusion pumps		Ensure free-flow protection on all general-use and PCA (patient controlled analgesia) intravenous infusion pumps used in the organization.
Improve the effectiveness of clinical alarm systems	a.	Implement regular preventive maintenance and testing of alarm systems.
	b.	Assure that alarms are activated with appropriate settings and are sufficiently audible with respect to distances and competing noise within the unit.
Reduce the risk of health-care acquired infections	a.	Comply with Centers for Disease Control and Prevention (CDC) hand-hygiene guidelines.
	b.	Manage as sentinel events all identified cases of unanticipated death or permanent loss of function associated with a health-care acquired infection.

From JCAHO, 2002c; 2003.

reduce the incidence of sentinel events, since the identified areas are the highest-risk areas in acute patient care. As of February 2003, 313 surveys were performed including the patient safety goals. There were three standards with demonstrated noncompliance. These were use of prohibited abbreviations (7%), use of two patient identifiers (2.6%), and surgical site marking (2.2%) (JCAHO, 2003a). These goals will be updated on a regular basis to ensure an active, maturing patient safety program.

There are two national initiatives in place to gain insights into acute care patient safety issues and patients' experiences. In December 2002, the American Hospital Association (AHA), the Association of American Medical Colleges (AAMC), the Federation of American Hospitals (FAH), the Center for Medicare & Medicaid Services (CMS), the Agency for Healthcare Research and Quality (AHRQ), the JCAHO, the National Quality Forum (NQF), and the AFL-CIO announced a public-private collaboration for voluntary hospital reporting of ten hospital quality measures based on the JCAHO ORYX™ initiative. The ORYX reporting of outcomes and performance measures was implemented as part of the JCAHO accreditation process in 2000. The National Quality Forum has endorsed the program (Combs, 2002; JCAHO, 2002).

The selected measures for the new collaborative reporting initiative are related to best practices for high-volume clinical conditions including acute myocardial infarction, heart failure, and pneumonia. The voluntary hospital quality measures are listed in Table 11.3. This program is called The Quality Initiative: A Public Resource on Hospital Performance. The goal is the development of a public national hospital patient care quality database to drive patient safety/quality improvement initiatives. The number of measures will be expanded over time as will the number of participating hospitals. In 2003, JCAHO increased the number of required core and noncore reported performance measures in order to support this initiative. It is anticipated that measures will be expanded to include surgical infection prevention, critical care, pain management, and inpatient care of pediatric asthma (JCAHO, 2003a).

A second initiative from the Department of Health and Human Services, and the AHRQ is the development of a standardized survey of patients' hospital experiences (H-CAPS) to allow hospital-to-hospital comparisons by consumers and health care professionals. Consumer feedback will be useful for hospitals to identify areas for improvement, including areas of patient safety. This will initially be piloted in Arizona, Maryland, and New York (Combs, 2002). This is an extension of the CAPS survey used in the outpatient setting.

TABLE 11.3   Hospital Voluntary Reporting Initiative

Diagnosis	Measures
Acute myocardial infarction	• Was aspirin given to the patient when admitted to the hospital? • Was aspirin prescribed when the patient was discharged? • Was a beta blocker given to the patient when admitted to the hospital? • Was a beta blocker prescribed when the patient was discharged? • Was an ACE inhibitor given to the patient?
Heart failure	• Did the patient get an assessment of his or her heart function? • Was an ACE inhibitor given to the patient?
Pneumonia	• Was an antibiotic given to the patient in a timely manner? • Had a patient received a pneumococcal vaccination? • Was the patient's oxygen level assessed when admitted?

From "HHS, hospital groups, unveil initiative to collect, share quality information," by J. Combs, 2002. Retrieved December 12, 2003, from http://healthcenter.bna.com/pic2/hc.nsf/id/BNAP-5HBTC8?OpenDocument

FEDERAL REPORTS ON OPPORTUNITIES

In 2001, the AHRQ published the evidence report/technology assessment from the University of California at San Francisco Stanford University Evidence-Based Practice Center *Making Health Care Safer: A Critical Analysis of Patient Safety Practices* (AHRQ, 2001). This report is an extensive review of evidence-based opportunities to improve acute care patient safety and outcomes. The authors identified areas of strongest evidence for patient safety practices. The findings are listed in Table 11.4. Many of the top evidence-based practices could easily be implemented with minimal cost and complexity, yet this is not being done in most cases. The potential for decreased acute care complications is great. The top evidence-based patient safety practices can be used as a guide for implementation of patient safety initiatives.

The Institute of Medicine (IOM) also published a report of an extensive study in 2003 regarding 20 identified priority areas for national action to transform health care quality (Adams & Corrigan, 2003). These areas include both processes of care and clinical categories. Priorities across all areas of health care include care coordination and patient self-management/

TABLE 11.4   Top Acute Care Patient Safety Practice Priorities (Greatest Level of Evidence) Identified by AHRQ

Ranked from highest to lowest	Implementation cost/complexity
1. Appropriate use of venous thromboembolism prevention in patients at risk.	Low
2. Use of perioperative beta blockers in appropriate patients to prevent perioperative morbidity and mortality.	Low
3. Use of maximum sterile barriers while placing central venous catheters (CVCs) to prevent infection.	Low
4. Appropriate use of antibiotic prophylaxis in surgical patients to prevent perioperative infections.	Low
5. Asking patients to recall and restate what they have been told during the informed consent process.	Low
6. Continuous aspiration of subglottic secretions to prevent ventilator-associated pneumonia.	Medium
7. Use of pressure-relieving bedding material to prevent pressure ulcers.	Medium
8. Use of real-time ultrasound guidance during CVC insertion to prevent complications.	High
9. Patient self-management for warfarin to achieve appropriate outpatient anticoagulation and prevent complications.	High
10. Appropriate provision of nutrition, with a particular emphasis on early enteral nutrition in critically ill and surgical patients.	Medium
11. Use of antibiotic impregnated CVCs to prevent catheter related infections.	Low

From AHRQ, 2001.

health literacy. Areas specific to acute care include: end of life with advanced organ system failure; ischemic heart disease; medication management (medication errors and overuse of antibiotics); nosocomial infections; pain control in advanced cancer; pregnancy and childbirth; severe and persistent mental illness; and stroke. These areas can be used to prioritize patient safety activities or initiatives depending on the performance of the organization. A few of the areas identified by AHRQ and the IOM will be discussed in more detail in the exemplars.

PROMOTING ACUTE CARE EVIDENCE-BASED CLINICIAN PRACTICE

The vast number and varied quality of clinical research studies makes evidence-based practice a challenge (see chapter 4 for more detail on this topic). Systematic reviews assist with this process, but this information needs to be disseminated effectively to practitioners. Practice guidelines, critical pathways, and clinical decision support are examples of evidence-based knowledge dissemination. They can prevent errors in planning. Even when these practice tools are in place, compliance is relatively low (AHRQ, 2001). Having a practice protocol in place does not ensure that it will be used. Changing attitudes and behaviors is the first step.

Changing physician practice patterns is very difficult. However, it is key to ensuring acute care patient safety because physicians prescribe the majority of therapeutic activities in acute care. Strategies shown to be effective include academic detailing (one-on-one education) and using local opinion leaders to champion practice change (Landry & Sibbald, 2002; AHRQ, 2001). Computerized reminders have moderate success, which may increase as the technology improves and becomes more widespread. Least effective strategies include audit with feedback, and printed materials. The key to all change management is to have all stakeholders actively involved in the process, such as in critical pathway development (Landry & Sibbald, 2002; AHRQ, 2001).

The remainder of this chapter will provide exemplars of evidence-based patient safety activities relevant to acute care. These exemplars are intended to provide guidance to the reader for planning an acute care patient safety program.

EXEMPLARS

Intensivist Care Model

Both The Leapfrog Group and the Institute for Healthcare Improvement (IHI) endorse the use of critical care trained intensivists to manage patients in the critical care unit (The Leapfrog Group, 2000; Tibble, Pronovost, & Rainey, 2002). Intensivists may have an internal medicine, anesthesiology, or surgery background. The consistent use of intensivists reduces variation in care, ensures care by physicians with current critical care management experience, and promotes evidence-based practice and anticipation of potential complications (Tibble, Pronovost, & Rainey, 2002). This decreases errors in planning. Critical care, board certified intensivists should be available continuously to manage the care of patients throughout their critical stay using an interdisciplinary team model. The intensivist manages triage, unit admission, and discharge. Intensivists are responsible for individual patients but also for providing leadership in the critical care unit as a whole, including policies, procedures, and protocols. The intensivist leads an interdisciplinary team providing coordinated care to optimize patient outcomes (Tibble, Pronovost, & Rainey, 2002).

An open critical care unit allows any physician with medical staff privileges to admit patients to the critical care unit and to manage their care. Units with mixed care models have some patients managed by their admitting physicians and some by intensivists. In closed critical care units, care is turned over to the intensivist until critical care unit discharge. Admitting physicians are involved in the communication loop, but do not drive clinical care. Closed critical care units have the best clinical outcomes. Studies have determined that surgical mortality can be reduced by two-thirds with the use of a closed intensivist critical care unit model (The Leapfrog Group, 2000; Pronovost, Wu, Dorman, & Marlock, 2002).

Critical Care Unit Safety Checks

The Veterans Affairs Ann Arbor Healthcare System implemented a team patient safety initiative in 2000 that earned a Patient Safety Foundation Solutions Award in 2001 (Piotrowski & Hinshaw, 2002). The initiative focused on developing discipline specific standards in the areas of prevention of medication and intravenous administration errors, ventilator and restraint-related errors, and nosocomial infections. Safety standards can prevent errors in execution of care. Five core standards were developed regarding restraint use (3 standards), adherence to isolation protocols (1 standard), and assessment of sedation levels of mechanically ventilated patients (1 standard). Twenty-three additional standards were developed to promote safe medication administration. Monitoring of these additional standards was rotated weekly. Two-person teams monitored adherence to safety standards twice daily at change of shift. The safety checks take approximately a minute to complete and are done in tandem with bedside rounds. The goal was to both promote a culture of patient safety as well as to decrease medical errors. The biggest barrier to the safety checklist implementation was the staff fear of punitive action (Piotrowski & Hinshaw, 2002). Links between the patient safety checklist and other outcomes data such as nosocomial infection rates are yet to be established.

Prevention of Wrong-Site Surgery

Wrong-site surgery, an error of execution, theoretically should be totally preventable. However, from 1995 to 2003, the JCAHO received 2,034 reports of sentinel events. Of these, 11.8% (240) were wrong-site surgeries (JCAHO, 2003c). Despite sentinel event alerts, this rate has not improved over time. This number may reflect underreporting of actual events. Root cause analyses of these reported events found that 80% were caused by errors in communication, 39% lack of orientation/training, 22% lack of patient assessment, 22% unavailability of information, 19% procedural noncompliance, 16% operating room hierarchy, and 11% distraction (JCAHO, 2002b). Factors reported to contribute to wrong-site surgery include staffing issues, emergency surgery, unusual patient physical characteristics, time pressure to start or complete a procedure, unusual equipment or operating room set-up, multiple surgeons, and multiple procedures performed in the same surgical site (Chubb, 2002).

Clearly, work environment and culture have a tremendous influence on the identified root causes, including the sense of disempowerment of surgical staff vs. physicians (see chapter 7). In the operating room, every team member must be empowered to speak up when needed. Training on team communication and assertion is key. Each surgical case should start with introductions and a team briefing to ensure every one agrees with the patient and site identification. Topics to cover include case presentation, surgical procedure/plan, outcomes needed, equipment availability, special needs, and safety considerations (Calland, 2003; Leonard, 2003). Surgical briefings and debriefings have been shown to increase team efficiency, to increase team communication, and to improve situational awareness (Calland, 2003).

Several surgical professional organizations responded to the wrong-site surgery problem and its root causes by initiating campaigns to "Sign your Site" (American Academy Orthopaedic Surgeons [AAOS]) and "Sign, Mark, and X-ray (SmaX)" (North American Spine Society [NASS]). JCAHO developed recommendations for both health care practitioners and patients to prevent wrong-site surgery titled "Universal protocol for preventing wrong site, wrong procedure, wrong person surgery™" (JCAHO, 2002b; JCAHO,

2003d). The key strategies of wrong-site surgery prevention include: marking the surgical site, orally verifying the surgery (patient and all health care staff), and taking time in the operating room to double check the chart, x-rays, and patient before starting the surgical procedure (JCAHO, 2002a; JCAHO, 2003d). The professional organization guidelines place responsibility for safety on everyone caring for the patient, but places ultimate accountability on the surgeon. A concern regarding the current approaches to marking surgical site is inconsistency among hospitals. For instance, "X" may mean this is the site, or this is not the site. Use of "yes" and "no", or the surgeon's signature is preferable, because they are less open to misinterpretation (AHRQ, 2001). Surgeons need to use a consistent marking method in all of the facilities where they operate. More specific safety steps in a verification checklist that will ensure recommendation compliance are listed in Table 11.5. Each of the listed safety checks is critical to prevent wrong-site surgery. This safety checklist can be used in acute care, in freestanding surgical centers, and in office surgery. Additional prevention tools are listed in the Web Resources section of this chapter.

Promoting a High Reliability Unit

Acute care facilities are, by their very nature, high-risk organizations. The goal should be to make the organization as highly reliable as possible (see chapter 1). Dr. Preston and team at Kaiser Permanente Northern California are using human factors, assertiveness, communication training, and the principles of high-reliability organizations to address quality of care and patient safety in a high-volume labor and delivery setting (Preston, 2003).

Similar to operating rooms, labor and delivery tends to have a hierarchal structure. The first step was to establish new ground rules related to the work setting and culture. The "new" rules were: end faultfinding; team input supports the best decisions; safety first; and the goal is to improve outcomes (Preston, 2003). In high-reliability organization language, the unit had a clearly stated purpose (safety first), clear language (fetal well-being), clear operating style (guidelines and protocols), and clear policy (physicians will come to the unit when called by a registered nurse) (Preston, 2003).

Clinical practice and systems issues were identified and addressed. Evidence-based practice protocols, emergency planning, and drills were developed for high-risk clinical situations. Drill participants reviewed a video of the team's performance after the drill and debriefings examined human factors, systems, and technical issues in performance (Preston, 2003).

TABLE 11.5   Wrong-Site Surgery Patient Safety Checklist

Patient:

☐ Verbally states type of operation and surgical site (which eye, knee, etc.)
☐ Provides informed consent
☐ Active involvement in site-marking process

Surgeon:

☐ Signs surgical site prior to surgery using a permanent marker
☐ Informs the patient regarding the procedure, answers all questions, and obtains informed consent noting specific surgical site
☐ If bone or spine level is not visually identifiable, an intra-operative x-ray with nonmovable markers is obtained

Surgeon and all surgical staff:

☐ Confirms site with patient prior to surgery
☐ Have the right and duty to call a halt to the procedure if safety steps are not followed

Safety cross check:

☐ Verifies the correct identity of the patient
☐ Verifies medical records and radiology films are for the correct patient
☐ Takes a "time out" prior to initiating surgery to double check the following against the marked surgical site: medical records, informed consent, radiology films, and operating room/anesthesia records
☐ Ensure that all radiology films are marked left and right, and that they are placed on the light box correctly

Document:

☐ Sign on one form that the above steps were completed

From Chubb, 2002; North American Spine Society, 2002; American Academy of Orthopaedic Surgeons, 2002.

Communication training focused on assertiveness skills and communication clarity. The Situational Brief approach, SBAR (Situation, Background, Assessment, Recommendation) was used. The multidisciplinary team training emphasized continuing with the conversation using SBAR until the problem is solved and all parties understand the proposed action and final decision. Briefings are to occur during multidisciplinary rounds, during escalation of care, preprocedure, preoperatively, during unit transfer, and whenever needed (Preston, 2003).

Evaluation of this program includes birth outcomes data, staff attitudes (all disciplines), nurse retention, patient satisfaction, and malpractice claims. A positive impact on nurse retention has already been demonstrated (Preston, 2003).

Improving Staff Hand Washing Compliance

Another error of execution is the lack of effective hand washing in the acute care area. Prevention of nosocomial infection is a 2004 JCAHO Patient Safety Goal. The first line of defense in the prevention of nosocomial infections in acute care is hand washing. Effective hand washing reduces transmission of microorganisms and decreases morbidity and mortality (CDC, 2002; Larson, 1995). This has been known for the last 150 years, however health care provider compliance is very low (Bischoff, Reynolds, Sessler, Edmond, & Wenzel, 2000; CDC, 2002; AHRQ, 2001). Barriers to hand washing include time, skin irritation, and inconvenient locations or lack of sinks. Educational interventions demonstrate statistically significant increases in hand washing behaviors, but these gains are not maintained over time, nor does compliance reach 100% (CDC, 2002; AHRQ, 2001). A more effective strategy is to combine educational/performance improvement interventions with decreasing barriers to hand washing. Recommended strategies include: ensuring sink availability with the ability to turn off the water without using hands in unit design, providing convenient paper towels and skin lotions in the sink areas, and supplying alcohol-based waterless antiseptic in all patient areas (CDC, 2002; AHRQ, 2001; West, 2002). A recent observational study compared the frequency of hand washing in an old hospital with less sink availability, with the frequency in a new hospital where there was a sink in every patient room. The researchers found a significantly higher rate of hand washing in the old hospital (53% vs. 23%, $p = .0001$) (Lankford, et al., 2003). Therefore, physical accessibility of sinks is not enough to foster hand washing compliance. A work culture that encourages hand washing compliance in addition to administrative accountability is key (CDC, 2002; West, 2002). Lankford and colleagues (2003) found that hand washing was more likely to occur if a higher-ranking person in the room washed their hands ($p < .001$). Therefore, role modeling is critical.

Use of Perioperative Beta-Blockers to Prevent Cardiac Complications

The most common medical complication during both vascular and noncardiac surgery is myocardial ischemia and damage including infarction, with resultant high mortality. Historically, screening for patients at risk for cardiac events, with additional testing and possible preoperative revascularization interventions for high-risk patients was the standard of care. There was no perioperative intervention. In the last few years, research has demonstrated the efficacy of using perioperative beta blockade to reduce cardiac events significantly in intermediate and high-risk patients (Auerbach & Goldman, 2002a, 2002b; Poldermans, et al., 1999; AHRQ, 2001). The American College of Cardiology (ACC) and the American Heart Association (AHA) recommend perioperative use of beta-blockers in high-risk patients to reduce the risk of adverse cardiac events. High-risk patients include those with a history of angina, hypertension, or arrhythmias, or documented preoperative myocardial ischemia. Starting beta blockade therapy days before elective surgery is preferable, continuing for at least seven days postoperatively. Beta blockade doses should be titrated to achieve a heart rate of 50–70 beats per minute (American College of Cardiology & American Heart Association, 2002; AHRQ, 2001). Drs. Auerbach and Goldman provide patient management recommendations using case studies in a clinical applications article that accompanied their scientific review in the *Journal of the American Medical Association* (Auerbach & Goldman, 2002a). Consistent use of perioperative beta blockade therapy in at-risk patients (elimination of an error in planning) holds significant promise to decrease perioperative adverse events, and is very easy to implement through development of a clinical practice guideline.

Prevention of Central Venous Catheter Complications

Central Venous Catheters (CVCs) are used frequently in acute care in order to provide access to infuse both large volumes of fluid and irritating intravenous medications. The most common complication of CVCs is infection both at the catheter insertion site, in the catheter itself, and ultimately the bloodstream. The infection rate increases with duration of placement. The National Nosocomial Infections Surveillance System (NNISS) reports that CVC bloodstream infections vary from 3.3–8.8 per 1,000 CVC days in the critical care setting (NNISS, 2002). CVC bloodstream infections are associated with increased length of stay and mortality (AHRQ, 2001). Pittet and colleagues reported a 25% attributed mortality related to CVC bloodstream infections, and an average of $25,000 increase in cost/case (Pittet, Tarara, & Wenzel, 1994). Strategies that attempt to decrease the rate of CVC infection include changing out the CVC periodically by using a guide wire, removal of the old CVC and insertion of a new CVC at a new site. These procedures have been common practice for many years, but are not supported by research (AHRQ, 2001).

Two strategies found in the ARHQ report to effectively decrease the rate of CVC bloodstream infections are the use of maximum barrier precautions during CVC insertion, and the use of CVCs coated with antibacterial or antiseptic agents (AHRQ, 2001). Failure to use these precautions is an error in execution. The use of maximum barriers includes the use of sterile gloves, long-sleeved gowns, full-size sterile drapes and nonsterile masks and caps. This is compared with the routine practice of sterile gloves and a small sterile drape only. A randomized clinical trial by Raad and colleagues demonstrated a greater than 50% decrease in catheter colonization and CVC bloodstream infections using maximum barrier protection during CVC insertion (Raad, et al., 1994). Education of physicians in the use of maximum barrier techniques resulted in a 28% decrease in the rate of CVC bloodstream infections (Sherertz, et al., 2000). The cost benefit of using maximum barrier protection during CVC insertion has been demonstrated in two studies (Raad, et al., 1994; Sherertz, et al., 2000).

A meta-analysis comparing the use of CVCs coated with chlorhexidine/silver sulfadiazine to standard CVCs found a significantly decreased odds ratio of a CVC bloodstream infection in the antiseptic catheter coated group (Odds ratio .56, 96% CI: 0.37–0.84) (Veenstra, Saint, Saha, Lumley, & Sullivan, 1999). CVCs coated with minocycline/rifampin are equally effective at preventing CVC bloodstream infections for the first 10 days of CVC use. Although they are more expensive, CVCs coated with minocycline/rifampin are more effective than CVCs coated with chlorhexidine/silver sulfadiazine when CVC duration extends beyond 10 days (AHRQ, 2001). The AHRQ report recommends the use of CVCs coated with antibacterial or antiseptic agents, with the choice of coating based on the estimated duration of catheter use (AHRQ, 2001).

Promoting Patient Safety Through Unit Design

An emerging field in health care and architecture is designing units to be true healing environments. One aspect of this is to design patient care areas to promote patient safety (Henrich, 2002; IHI, 2003; Patterson, 1999). The Institute for Healthcare Improvement (IHI) and the Voluntary Hospital Association (VHA) initiated a collaborative effort in 2003 to develop idealized critical care unit design to promote patient safety and optimal patient outcomes (IHI, 2003).

A coronary care unit redesign at Clarian Health Partners, Methodist Campus was based on 1,000 hours of time-motion studies. Key aspects of the unit redesign related to patient safety included decentralization of nursing stations, maximizing information technology, and elimination of patient transfers from unit to unit by creation of a room design that could provide care from critical care through discharge. The decrease in patient transfers, consistent nurses, and nurses' improved knowledge of their patients resulted in a decrease in patient falls and medication errors. The patient fall index dropped from six to two, and the medication error index decreased from ten to three (Henrich, 2002). Even without other unit redesign, single-patient rooms decrease medication errors by decreasing the risk of delivering medication to the wrong patient (Shepley, 2003).

Similar to the Clarian project, an interdisciplinary team including experts in Failure Modes and Effects Analysis (FMEA) worked to design St. Joseph's Community Hospital of West Bend, Wisconsin based on the principles of patient-centered atmosphere, healing environment, operational efficiency, safety, quality care, technological advancements, and staff-friendly workplace (Reiling, 2002). Hospital design not only included the traditional "mock-ups" but also simultaneous major redesign of workflow and processes (Reiling, 2002; Larson, 2002). The design team created a checklist to ensure that all design principles were addressed in the new hospital blueprint. The checklist categories are listed in Table 11.6.

TABLE 11.6   Patient Safety Facility Design Principles

- Ongoing failure mode and effects analysis (FMEA)
- Staff, patients, family, vendors, architect, administrator (stakeholder) input
- Accountable leaders drive the process
- Focus on organizational processes
- Consider human factors
- Base design on specific patient populations
- Standardize wherever possible
- Provide immediate access to information
- Address known threats to patient safety
- Healing environment
- Efficient processes
- Advanced technology and automation
- Scalable, adaptive, flexible

From "Putting patient safety in the blueprint," by L. Larson, 2002. Retrieved February 26, 2003, from http://www.hospitalconnect.com/hhnmag/jsp/articledisplay.jsp?dcrpath=AHA/NewsStory_Article/data/0302HHN_Feature_Blueprints&domain=HHNMAG

AREAS FOR FUTURE RESEARCH

The authors of *Making Health Care Safer: A Critical Analysis of Patient Safety Practices* identified areas that most urgently need further research based on their review of the literature. These findings are listed in Table 11.7. The top research priorities hold the most current promise for further improving patient safety and outcomes through evidence. Additional research questions include:

- What are the best methods to promote evidence-based patient safety activities in the acute care setting?
- What will be the impact of computerized physician order entry (CPOE) on patient safety after this technology is in widespread use?
- What are the relationships among hospital patient care processes, work culture, and patient outcomes?

TABLE 11.7   Top Acute Care Patient Safety Research Priorities Identified by AHRQ

1.	Improving perioperative glucose control to decrease perioperative infections.
2.	Localizing specific surgeries and procedures to high-volume centers.
3.	Use of supplemental perioperative oxygen to decrease perioperative infections.
4.	Changes in nursing staffing to decrease overall hospital morbidity and mortality.
5.	Use of silver alloy-coated urinary catheters to prevent urinary tract infections.
6.	Computerized physician order entry with computerized decision support systems to decrease medication errors and adverse events primarily due to the drug ordering process.
7.	Limitations on antibiotic use to prevent hospital-acquired infections due to antibiotic-resistant organisms.
8.	Appropriate use of antibiotic prophylaxis in surgical patients to prevent perioperative infections.
9.	Appropriate use of venous thromboembolism prevention in patients at risk.
10.	Appropriate provision of nutrition, with a particular emphasis on early enteral nutrition in critically ill and post-surgical patients.
11.	Use of analgesics in the patient with an acutely painful abdomen without compromising diagnostic accuracy.
12.	Improved hand washing compliance (via education/behavior change, sink technology and placement, or the use of antimicrobial washing substance.

From AHRQ, 2001.

CONCLUSION

The diversity and complexity of patient care in the acute care setting makes patient safety a challenge. The use of a proactive program targeting high-priority/high-benefit areas that meets or exceeds all regulatory requirements is critical. Both errors in planning and execution must be addressed, focusing on the risks of interventions and the potential for errors in prescribing therapies. The financial and emotional cost of adverse and sentinel events can be mitigated by the use of routine patient safety practices in all acute care settings in conjunction with a culture of safety as a top priority.

WEB RESOURCES

Name of Resource/URL	Description
2003 Standards, Recommended Practices, and Guidelines http://www.aorn.org/products/standards.htm	Association of PeriOperative Registered Nurses (AORN) recommended practice standards
Patient Safety is No Accident web site http://www.patientsafety.aaos.org/	Patient safety resources from the American Academy of Orthopaedic Surgeons (AAOS)
American Hospital Association Quality and Patient Safety web page http://www.hospitalconnect.com/aha/key_issues/patient_safety/index.html	American Hospital Association Quality and Patient Safety Index
Guideline for Hand Hygiene in Healthcare Settings—2002 http://www.cdc.gov/handhygiene/	Centers for Disease Control and Prevention (CDC) hand hygiene recommendations
Guideline Update for Perioperative Cardiovascular Evaluation for Non-cardiac Surgery—Executive Summary http://www.acc.org/clinical/guidelines/perio/exec_summ/VI_medical.htm	American College of Cardiology/American Heart Association guidelines adds beta-blockade for at-risk patients

Joint Commission for the Accreditation of Healthcare Organizations 2004 national patient safety goals *http://www.jcaho.org/ accredited+organizations/ patient+safety/04+npsg/04_npsg.htm*	2004 JCAHO patient safety goals
JCAHO facts about patient safety *http://www.jcaho.org/ accredited+organizations/ patient+safety/ facts+about+patient+safety.htm*	Overview of JCAHO standards and efforts regarding patient safety
Making Health Care Safer: A Critical Analysis of Patient Safety Practices *http://www.ahrq.gov/clinic/ptsafety/ spotlight.htm*	AHRQ report on evidence-based patient safety practice opportunities
Patient Safety First from AORN *http://www.patientsafetyfirst.org/*	AORN patient safety resources
Premier Safety Institute *http://my.premierinc.com/frames/ index.jsp?pagelocation=/frames/ public/public-main.htm*	Safety information and resources for hospitals
Qualityhealthcare.org *http://www.qualityhealthcare.org*	Online authority for improving healthcare sponsored by the *British Medical Journal* and the Institute for Healthcare Improvement; sections on critical care and end of life
Sign, Mark, and X-ray (SmaX) http://www.spine.org/forms/ smaxchecklist.pdf	North American Spine Society surgical safety checklist
Universal Protocol for Preventing Wrong-Site, Wrong-Procedure, Wrong-Person Surgery www.jcaho.org/ accredited+organizations/ patient+safety/univers al+protocol/ index.htm http://www.jcaho.com/ accredited+organizations/	JCAHO consensus document regarding best practice

patient+safety/universal+protocol/
universal+protocol.pdf

Veterans Affairs National Center
for Patient Safety
http://www.patientsafety.gov/

Resources, discussions and links
from the Veterans Affairs Center
for Patient Safety, including a patient safety handbook

REFERENCES

American Academy of Orthopedic Surgeons (AAOS). (2002). *Advisory statement: Wrong site surgery.* Retrieved April 1, 2003, from http://www.aaos.org/wordhtml/papers/advistmt/wrong.htm

American College of Cardiology (ACC) and American Heart Association (AHA). (2002). *Guideline update for perioperative cardiovascular evaluation for noncardiac surgery—Executive summary.* Retrieved April 1, 2003, from http://www.acc.org/clinical/guidelines/perio/exec_summ/VI_medical.htm

Adams, K., & Corrigan, J. M. (Ed.). (2003). *Priority areas for national action: Transforming health care quality.* Washington, DC: National Academies Press.

Agency for Healthcare Research and Quality (AHRQ). (2001). *Making health care safer: A critical analysis of patient safety practices.* Rockville, MD: Author.

Auerbach, A. D., & Goldman, L. (2002a). Beta-blockers and reduction of cardiac events in noncardiac surgery: Clinical applications. *Journal of the American Medical Association, 20,* 1445–1457.

Auerbach, A. D., & Goldman, L. (2002b). Beta-blockers and reduction of cardiac events in noncardiac surgery: Scientific review. *Journal of the American Medical Association, 287,* 1435–1444.

Biddle, C. (2003, March). *Trigger films: Enhancing clinical communication and patient safety in the critical care environment.* Paper presented at the 5th Annual NPSF Patient Safety Congress, Washington, DC.

Bischoff, W. E., Reynolds, T. M., Sessler, C. N., Edmond, M. B., & Wenzel, R. P. (2000). Handwashing compliance by health care workers: The impact of introducing an accessible, alcohol-based hand antiseptic. *Archives of Internal Medicine, 160*(7), 1017–1121.

Calland, J. F. (2003, March). *Remote analysis of the surgical environment: Measuring the effects of debriefing attendings on surgical safety factors.* Paper presented at the 5th Annual NPSF Patient Safety Congress, Washington, DC.

Centers for Disease Control (CDC). (2002). *Guideline for hand-hygiene in health-care settings.* Retrieved December 12, 2003, from http://www.cdc.gov/mmwr/preview/mmwrhtml/rr5116a1.htm

Chubb (2002). *Wrong-site surgery: Focus on communication.* Retrieved December 31, 2002, from http://cber.chubb.com/publications/stat/stat_wrong_site_surgery.asp

Combs, J. (2002). *HHS, hospital groups, unveil initiative to collect, share quality information.* Retrieved December 12, 2003, from http://healthcenter.bna.com/pic2/hc.nsf/id/BNAP-5HBTC8?OpenDocument

Gregory-Dawes, B. S. (2002). Formula for success with safety—Just do it! *AORN Journal*, 75(6), 1072, 1074.

Henrich, A., Fay, J., & Sorrells, A. (2002). Courage to heal. *Healthcare Design*, 12–13.

Hupcey, J. E. (2000). Feeling safe: The psychosocial needs of ICU patients. *Journal of Nursing Scholarship*, 32(4), 361–367.

Institute for Healthcare Improvement (IHI). (2003). *Idealized design of the intensive care unit.* Retrieved February 20, 2003, from http://www.ihi.org/idealized/idicu/index.asp

Joint Commission for Accreditation of Healthcare Organizations (JCAHO). (2003). *2004 patient safety goals.* Retrieved December 12, 2003, from http://www.jcaho.org/accredited+organizations/patient+safety/04+npsg/04_npsg.htm

Joint Commission for Accreditation of Healthcare Organizations (JCAHO). (2003). *Compliance with patient safety goals.* Retrieved April 20, 2003, from http://www.jcaho.org/about+us/news+letters/jcahonline/

Joint Commission for Accreditation of Healthcare Organizations (JCAHO). (2003a). *Hospitals to gather and use additional performance data.* Retrieved August 10, 2003, from http://www.jcaho.org/news+room/news+release+archives/jcaho_072503.htm

Joint Commission for Accreditation of Healthcare Organizations (JCAHO). (2002a). *Joint commission issues alert: Simple steps by patients, health care practitioners can prevent surgical mistakes.* Retrieved December 31, 2002, from http://www.jcaho.org/news+room/press+kits/joint+commission+issues+alert+simple+steps+by+patients,++health+care+practitioners+can+prevent+surg.htm

Joint Commission for Accreditation of Healthcare Organizations (JCAHO). (2002b). *Root causes of wrong site surgery 1995–2002.* Retrieved April 18, 2003, from http://www.jcaho.org/accredited+organizations/ambulatory+care/sentinel+events/rc+wrong+site+surgery.htm3

Joint Commission for Accreditation of Healthcare Organizations (JCAHO). (2003c). *Sentinel event statistics May 7, 2003.* Retrieved May 28, 2003, from http://www.jcaho.org/accredited+organizations/ambulatory+care/sentinel+events/sentinel+event+statistics.htm.

Joint Commission for Accreditation of Healthcare Organizations (JCAHO). (2002). *Statement from the Joint Commission on Accreditation of Healthcare Organizations regarding the hospital voluntary reporting initiative.* Retrieved January 9, 2003, from http://www.jcaho.org/news+room/latest+news+release/stmnt_1212.htm

Joint Commission on Accreditation of Healthcare Organizations. (2003e). *2004 National patient safety goals—FAQs.* Retrieved December 7, 2003, from www.jcaho.org/accredited+organizations/patient+safety/universal+protocol/index.htm.

Landry, M. D., & Sibbald, W. J. (2002). Changing physician behavior: A review of patient safety in critical care medicine. *Journal of Critical Care*, 17(2), 138–145.

Lankford, M. G., Zembower, T. R., Trick, W. E., Hacek, D. M., Noskin, G. A., & Peterson, L. R. (2003). *Influence of role models and hospital design on the hand hygiene of health-care workers.* Retrieved April 10, 2003, from http://www.cdc.gov/ncidod/EID/vol9no2/02-0249.htm

Larson, E. L. (1995). APIC guidelines for hand washing and hand antisepsis in health care settings. *American Journal of Infection Control*, 23, 251–269.

Larson, L. (2002). *Putting patient safety in the blueprint.* Retrieved February 26, 2003, from http://www.hospitalconnect.com/hhnmag/jsp/articledisplay.jsp?dcrpath= AHA/NewsStory_Article/data/0302HHN_Feature_Blueprints&domain= HHNMAG

The Leapfrog Group. (2000). *ICU physician staffing.* Retrieved December 30, 2002, from http://www.leapfroggroup.org/FactSheets/ICU_FactSheet.pdf

Leonard, M. (2003, March). *Human factors skills to promote effective communication and teamwork.* Paper presented at the 5th Annual NPSF Patient Safety Congress, Washington, DC.

National Nosocomial Infections Surveillance System (NNISS). (2002). Report, data summary from January 1992–June 2002. *American Journal of Infection Control, 30,* 458–475.

North American Spine Society (NASS). (2002). *Sign your site: A checklist for safety.* Retrieved April 1, 2003, from http://www.spine.org/forms/smaxchecklist.pdf

Patterson, M. (1999). Smooth healing. *Building interiors,* 16–17.

Piotrowski, M., & Hinshaw, D. B. (2002). A team-driven approach to enhancing patient safety in the intensive care unit. *COR Clinical Excellence, 3*(5), 1–4.

Pittet, D., Tarara, D., & Wenzel, R. P. (1994). Nosocomial bloodstream infections in critically ill patients: Excess length of stay, extra costs, and attributable mortality. *Journal of the American Medical Association, 272,* 1598–1601.

Poldermans, D., Boersma, E., Bax, J. J., Thomson, I. R., van de Ven, L. L., Blankensteijn, J. D., et al. (1999). The effect of bisoprolol on perioperative mortality and myocardial infarction in high-risk patients undergoing vascular surgery. *New England Journal of Medicine, 341*(24), 1789–1794.

Preston, P. (2003, March). *Can you hear me now? Strategies to improve high risk communication.* Paper presented at the 5th Annual NPSF Patient Safety Congress, Washington, DC.

Pronovost, P., Wu, A. W., Dorman, T., & Marlock, L. (2002). Building safety into ICU care. *Journal of Critical Care, 17*(2), 78–85.

Raad, I. I., Hohn, D. C., Gilbreath, B. J., Suleiman, N., Hill, L. A., Bruso, P. A., et al. (1994). Prevention of central venous catheter-related infections by using maximal sterile barrier precautions during insertion. *Infection Control and Hospital Epidemiology, 5,* 231–238.

Reiling, J. (2002). *The impact of facility design on patient safety.* Retrieved February 26, 2003, from http://www.ihi.org/conferences/natforum/handouts/D06_E06_1.pdf

Resar, R. (2002). *ICU trigger tool data.* Retrieved January 11, 2003, from http://www.ihi.org/conferences/natforum/handouts/L01_3.pdf

Ridley, S. (2000). Safety issues in intensive care. *Care of the Critically Ill, 16*(4), 124–125.

Shepley, M. (2003). *Evidence-based research design in the NICU.* Paper presented at the physical and developmental environment of the high-risk infant conference, Clearwater Beach, FL.

Sherertz, R. J., Ely, E. W., Westbrook, D. M., Gladhill, K. S., Streed, S. A., Kiger, B., et al. (2000). Education of physicians-in-training can decrease the risk for vascular catheter infection. *Annals of Internal Medicine, 132,* 641–648.

Stein-Parbury, J., & McKinley, S. (2000). Patients' experiences of being in an intensive care unit: A select literature review. *American Journal of Critical Care, 9*(1), 20–27.

Tibble, J., Pronovost, P., & Rainey, T. G. (2002). *Rapid fire intensive care ideas.* Retrieved January 11, 2003, from http://www.ihi.org/conferences/natforum/handouts/L01_1.pdf

Veenstra, D. L., Saint, S., Saha, S., Lumley, T., & Sullivan, S. D. (1999). Efficacy of antiseptic-impregnated central venous catheters in preventing catheter-related bloodstream infection: A meta-analysis. *Journal of the American Medical Association, 281,* 261–267.

West, K. (2002). *The CDC's new hand washing guidelines.* Retrieved December 31, 2002, from http://www.merginet.com/emsnewsfiles/379_Katherine_West_20020712.shtml

Chapter 12

Patient Safety in Ambulatory Care

Susan V. White and
Jacqueline Fowler Byers

AMBULATORY CARE SETTING

The Institute of Medicine (IOM) report created widespread public attention for the problem of medical errors, citing that up to 98,000 people die each year in the United States (U.S.) as a result of preventable errors. Of particular interest is that the figures reported are only for hospitals, omitting data about other sectors of health care, while most health care is actually provided in outpatient settings (Kohn, Corrigan, & Donaldson, 2000). Data about medical errors come primarily from studies of hospital patients, with limited data about the ambulatory care sector and patient safety. In the IOM research on medical errors only one Australian study of 324 nonrandomly selected general practitioners providing self-reported data on medical errors could be considered a study of patient safety in an ambulatory setting (Kohn et al., 2000). This lack of knowledge and research limits our ability to understand the risks to patients in ambulatory settings and therefore how to design and implement safety practices for patients in ambulatory care settings

While acute care or hospital care is confined to specific facilities and is easy to describe, ambulatory care is much broader and fragmented and includes those services provided without admission to acute or long-term care facilities (Hammons, Piland, Small, Hatlie, & Burstin, 2001; Schwartz, Rudavsky, Christakis, & Conaway, 2002). The primary care physician's office is generally considered the hub of ambulatory care, but ambulatory care is provided at all of the following sites:

- Physician's office (primary care and specialty)
- Office surgery centers
- Outpatient surgery centers
- Hospital emergency departments (addressed as part of acute care)
- Dialysis clinics
- Chemotherapy and radiation therapy centers
- Diagnostic imaging centers
- Occupational health centers
- Mental health centers (addressed in chapter 14 on behavioral health) (Hammons, et al., 2001; Schwartz et al., 2002).

Ambulatory Care Characteristics

There are differences in the delivery of ambulatory care services that deserve comment since these differences provide insight into the findings about errors in this setting and the approaches to patient safety. First, ambulatory care is provided at multiple sites where there are numerous handoffs or transitions of care, which are seldom seamless. This creates a set of loosely linked components. (Refer to chapter 1 for discussion of coupling—tight or loose—and the opportunity for error). The multiple sites create complexity from a logistical perspective in terms of scheduling appointments, travel time, and travel distance. This complexity makes it difficult for patients to arrive at appointments as scheduled. Those patients who are "no shows" are a major challenge in the ambulatory setting and this hinders continuity of follow-up care. Complexity is also increased when insurer requirements force clinicians and patients to use particular services, including consultants who are unfamiliar and do not have established working relationships with the primary physician. Coordination of ambulatory care is a great challenge and a patient safety concern.

An episode of care occurs in bits and pieces over a period of time, and involves many transitions, creating loss of continuity for both the patient and the provider. There are multiple caregivers for a single patient, such as primary care practitioner and specialists, as well as multiple types of caregivers, including physicians, nurses, advanced practice nurses, physician assistants, medical assistants, and other support personnel. There is no coordinated system and no systematic infrastructure that provides support and cohesion across multiple sites, caregivers, and patients. Instead there is great diversity, breadth of services, and variation in the structure of ambulatory care.

Not only are there multiple sites for health care services, there is also a broad range of outlets providing medications to outpatients such as community pharmacies, online services, and mail-order services. Having multiple sites provide prescription medications under different requirements can create delays in approval, renewals, and coverage verification, so the patient does not always receive medication as needed. For example, many mail-order pharmacies will fill routine medications for 90 days. Often additional forms must be completed by the patient, sent to the insurer, and then forwarded to the pharmacy. However, after the 90-day period, a renewal process must be taken which can be fairly simple or complex, depending on the company. These additional steps require strict adherence by the patient. If the patient is not vigilant in watching when medications need to be refilled then gaps could arise for the patient in not having medications while following up with the physician and pharmacy. This could create serious safety issues for some patients. Each additional site adds an opportunity for an error to occur, especially when incomplete patient information is obtained.

It is particularly difficult to create and sustain a seamless continuum of care for patients due to frequent changes in job, insurance carrier, provider, pharmacy, and other health care services. This constant change forces major reliance on the patient and family to adhere or comply with medication and treatment regimens, so education and self-management are essential to success in this setting. Specific focus on the patient's role is described in chapter 5.

Ambulatory settings are also characterized by fewer regulations, which is usually evident in less developed policies and procedures, fewer checks on individuals related to adequate training and experience, greater variation in how equipment is maintained, and in the education training and experience of the personnel who use the equipment. There are fewer peer interactions such as credentialing and privileging for physicians, accompanied by greater variations in medical practice, less oversight of performance (especially procedures), and fewer protections of discussions about errors and peer performance (Schwartz et al., 2002).

While regulations for ambulatory care are generally fewer than for more acute settings, there are standards from the Joint Commission on Accreditation of Healthcare Organizations (JCAHO) on ambulatory care as well as office-based surgery. These standards were launched in 2001, with 100 practices now accredited. Standards are only applicable to those organizations that are accredited and they emphasize attention to those issues that most directly impact patients and cover essential areas such as patient care, patient safety, staffing, customer service, improving care, improving health, and responsible leadership (JCAHO, 2003). The overwhelming majority of ambulatory settings are not professionally accredited.

As the nation's leading evaluator of safety and quality in health care organizations, JCAHO now accredits more than 40 types of outpatient settings. The office-based surgery standards were established specifically for small surgical practices with up to four licensed independent practitioners. Practices eligible for accreditation include oral surgeons' offices, endoscopy suites, orthopedic surgery practices, plastic surgery practices, podiatric surgery practices, and laser eye surgery clinics (JCAHO, 2003). Similarly, the Accreditation Association for Ambulatory Health Care (AAAHC) and the American Association for Accreditation of Ambulatory Surgery Facilities (AAAASF) are organizations that also accredit ambulatory facilities.

From a financial perspective, ambulatory care settings often have fewer resources, less capital for technology, and continued pressure to see more patients, provide more services, and reduce costs. The mean duration of time spent with the physician during an ambulatory care visit at the physician's office was 19.3 minutes (Schwartz et al., 2002). There are few economic incentives for providers to implement safety practices or make changes to reduce errors. Rather the pressure to see more patients can create opportunities for errors, so strategies for scheduling, accurate and timely information, and clear communication are essential to reduce these risks.

AMBULATORY CARE ERRORS

Extrapolation from the Harvard Medical Practice Study would indicate that since more care is provided in ambulatory settings, the total number of medical errors is huge. The National Ambulatory Medical Care Survey (NAMCS) and the National Hospital Ambulatory Medical Care Survey (NHAMCS) are conducted annually by the National Center for Health Statistics and serve as tools for tracking ambulatory care utilization in the United States (Schwartz et al., 2002). In 1999, there were approximately one billion ambulatory care visits made to physicians' offices, hospital outpatient departments, and hospital emergency departments. This is a rate of 3.5 visits per person in the U.S. Visits to office-based physicians were predominant, with over 800 million visits per year compared with the 38 million times patients were hospitalized, according to Dr. Richard Roberts, board chair of the American Academy of Family Physicians (AAFP) (California Academy of Family Physicians, 2002).

Over 77% of all medical procedures are now performed in ambulatory settings (Hammons et al., 2001; Kuznets, 2002). It is estimated that 20–25% of all surgical procedures are performed in office-based settings (Schwartz et al., 2002). This volume has steadily increased over the past several decades with expectations that by 2005 an estimated ten million procedures will be performed annually in doctor's offices (Schwartz et al., 2002). Many medical and surgical procedures once provided only in hospitals are now routinely provided in ambulatory settings. Only the sickest patients receive care in the hospital, so that patients with a wide range of illness severity are receiving care in the ambulatory setting, increasing the variation in patients' conditions. Although the magnitude of the risk of medical and medication errors in the ambulatory setting is uncertain; its existence is not (Schwartz et al., 2002). Errors constitute a widespread problem in outpatient settings that cause injuries to patients and disproportionately increase expenses. That errors occur regularly is generally accepted, but the frequency, severity, preventability, cost, and impact of the events is little understood (Schwartz et al., 2002).

Types of Errors

While the data are limited, there is some information about the types of errors that occur in ambulatory settings from focused research studies, physician reports, claims data, and national utilization surveys (Hammons et al., 2001; Schwartz et al., 2002). Errors can result from single or multiple breakdowns in the system's continuum of (a) diagnosing an ailment, (b) planning a therapeutic regimen, (c) prescribing and dispensing drugs and (d) administering the drug. Errors occur in many phases of care but they can be categorized into three broad areas of care: Information, communication, and coordination.

Elder and Dovey (2002) performed a literature search of 379 articles from 1965 through March 2001 with the term medical errors, modified by adding family practice, primary health care, physicians/family, or ambulatory care and limited the search to English-language publications. Four original research studies described medical errors and adverse events in primary care, and three other studies peripherally addressed primary care medical errors. The findings led to a classification of three main categories of preventable adverse events: Diagnosis, treatment, and preventive services. Process errors were classified into four categories: Clinician, communication, administration, and blunt end. Missing from the literature on ambulatory care are studies that have patient, consumer, or health care provider perspectives.

The first step in the ambulatory care process is for the patient to be scheduled for a visit with the appropriate practitioner in a timely manner. In the office and clinic setting, patients are often "triaged" by administrative, not clinical staff. If the administrative staff does not understand the nature of the complaint or symptoms, then triaging may result in routine scheduling of a visit that is urgent. This type of problem is due to lack of education and information as well as inadequate communication of the seriousness of the condition. There have been serious consequences when triaging was not correct and there was a failure to make a timely appointment for a seriously ill person (Schwartz et al., 2002). One potential solution to scheduling issues is to "do today's work today" as suggested by Dr. Mark Murray (Murray & Tantau, 2001) in the Institute for Healthcare Improvement (IHI) collaborative on open-access scheduling. Murray and Tantau are experts on open access and changing paradigms of matching supply and demand in office practice. The *traditional* model of making office appointments is to fill the available space on a calendar with appointments and when the spaces are filled with appointments the capacity for additional patients is gone. Then, patients with serious or urgent problems are sent to a clinic or emergency room and told to "follow up with your private physician". The *advanced access* model proposed by Murray and Tantau eliminates the distinction between routine and urgent visits. The key concept in this model is to schedule the patient with his/her primary care physician when requested. When patients see their own doctor, there is less work, better continuity, and better care. The concept of open access is difficult to achieve based on traditional model scheduling. In those offices that have implemented the more advanced, open-access model for scheduling, patients are able to get appointments the same day, if necessary, unnecessary emergency room visits have been eliminated, and physicians have been reimbursed for appropriate levels of visits.

In office and clinic settings, manual records are prevalent. Another source of errors is missing patient records, missing diagnostic reports, incomplete records, and inaccurate records. Many reasons account for these problems such as sending records to consultants, especially to avoid repeating diagnostic tests, receiving diagnostic reports on multiple patients from multiple sources at irregular intervals, manually filing reports with the usual distractions and interruptions, and relying on patients for detailed, accurate information. Several studies show that in 50–70% of office visits, physicians do not have access to the information needed to answer questions that arise. These information gaps are an important issue (California Academy of Family Physicians, 2002). In one study the authors (Dovey, et al., 2002) found that misdirected laboratory paperwork is a source of many errors and that systems are needed to lessen these occurrences. Dovey and colleagues indicate further that getting results on the right patient record is a huge problem with loose paper reports coming from multiple sources.

Missing records and diagnostic reports can contribute to errors in diagnoses. Practitioners in ambulatory care are responsible for the management of multiple physiological abnormalities, coordination of the work of multiple clinicians, and the management of complex equipment and technologies. If any aspect of the information available is inaccurate or missing, then decisions are based on incomplete assessment of the patient's condition. Examples of missed diagnosis or late diagnosis of breast cancer have been noted when diagnostic reports were misplaced or not reported (Dovey, et al., 2002; Schwartz, et al., 2002). Several liability insurers have found that the largest single category of errors leading to claims and awards are delays and failures to diagnose (for example breast cancer) and the diagnostic process occurs largely in ambulatory care. Late diagnosis can also occur when appropriate screenings (such as colon cancer screening) are not performed in a timely manner. The patient has a major responsibility for following up on appointments, but responsibility for identifying screenings at various ages and providing reminders still falls to the primary practitioner.

Along with errors associated with records and diagnostic reports are issues of patient identification. These errors occur in two ways: (1) filing reports in the wrong patient's medical record, and (2) incorrectly identifying patients since most patients in ambulatory settings do not wear identification bands. The second error is more likely to occur if procedures, treatments, or medications are provided in a dialysis clinic or outpatient oncology clinic. The JCAHO's national patient safety goal for using two patient identifiers is a practice that will eventually be required in all accredited ambulatory settings (JCAHO, 2002).

A majority of patients who make a physician office visit are prescribed medication. Medication administration is less centralized and controlled in ambulatory settings, placing the responsibility on the patient, rather than the health care provider. This requires patient education, management, and compliance. Unlike the hospital setting, major data on where medication errors occur are not available for the outpatient setting. It is possible to extract some findings and consider strategies from hospital experience based on the phases of medication delivery and the primary parties who have responsibility. Strategies will be targeted to the responsible person:

Medication Phase	*Responsible Person*
Ordering	Physician or other provider
Administration	Patient and family responsibility
Dispensing	Pharmacy (community, online, mail order), some centers
Monitoring	Patient, family, and provider

Patients of all ages use ambulatory services, but certain populations are at greater risk including the elderly, children, and behavioral health patients. Persons who incur adverse drug events (ADE) in outpatient settings often fit the following profile: make more visits to their health care providers, take more drugs, take more new drugs, and have more chronic conditions (Schwartz et al., 2002).

Unfortunately, identifying adverse events, particularly adverse drug events, in ambulatory care is very difficult. The consequences of ambulatory care events may only become apparent when the patient seeks help in the emergency department or hospital. Physicians usually have less regular contact with outpatients and are less likely to be aware of drug complications experienced, unless the patient directly contacts the physician.

Many times medication histories are not accurate or do not contain a complete list of alternative therapies such as herbal supplements or over-the-counter medications. If we consider that the patient has an incomplete record, along with an abundance of available medications, then errors are likely to occur with inappropriate medications or dosing. The lack of information creates significant communication and coordination problems when patients visit several different specialists who may each prescribe medication. If the patient has not accurately communicated with each specialist then several medications of the same type or medications that cause adverse interactions may be prescribed.

Barriers to Advancing Patient Safety in Ambulatory Care

There has been a lack of sustained public and provider awareness of the issue of medical error, with most attention concentrated on acute care.

Most research on medical errors has been conducted on inpatients with funding supporting these efforts. As of this writing no national legislation has been passed on patient safety and reducing medical errors for the ambulatory care setting. Most physicians believe they provide good care even though the adoption of evidence-based medicine is slow, and the general public believes it is protected from errors (Schwartz et al., 2002). There is such fragmentation in the delivery system with diffuse responsibility that advancing safety initiatives in the ambulatory setting is difficult.

Similar to acute care, there is a lack of standardized definitions and calculations of medical errors for ambulatory care, so identifying and documenting types of errors varies. Comparative data that is available covers a broad range. There is a lack of sophisticated management and clinical information systems for tracking and no universal electronic prescribing or documentation standards. Finally, ambulatory care settings are less likely to have the tools, expertise, or capability to analyze data, evaluate processes, and redesign systems.

Reporting Errors in the Ambulatory Setting

Mandatory reporting has been focused on the acute care setting with less attention on ambulatory care. As specific events have raised public attention, such as deaths in physician offices, then attention from the regulatory sector has increased. Reporting of adverse events in ambulatory settings is mandatory in at least ten states (Kohn, Corrigan, & Donaldson, 2000) with most of the focus on ambulatory surgery centers and physicians' offices in which surgery is performed. In the JCAHO database of sentinel events, 2,034 have been reported to date from all settings with a total of 39 (1.9%) sentinel events from ambulatory settings (JCAHO, 2003). Since most ambulatory settings are not accredited by the JCAHO, this number grossly underrepresents the incidence of sentinel events.

Just as the characteristics of ambulatory care, such as multiple sites and practitioners, illustrate the difficulties in identifying medical errors, these characteristics also make reporting difficult. For example, if a patient suffers an adverse drug reaction and seeks care in an urgent care clinic or emergency department, then the prescribing physician may never know about the problem. If the adverse event is the result of an error from the pharmacy, or a consulting physician, or the patient following directions incorrectly, then the investigation now crosses multiple settings and caregivers who may not be willing to share information, especially if it poses a liability for them. Most of the reporting bills proposed at the federal level focus on hospitals since there is still no national reporting system, rather than attempting to design an ambulatory reporting system. Lack of infrastructure and inability to track, categorize, and quantify ambulatory medical errors make it difficult to design any kind of reporting system in this setting. There is also risk of being able to identify the patient in a small or solo practice in a limited geographical area, which is less likely with hospital reporting (Kuznets, 2002). Refer to chapter 9 for a detailed discussion of reporting issues.

MEDICATION ERRORS

Medication mismanagement constitutes the largest quality concern in ambulatory care. Medication therapy is widely prescribed and was provided at 631 million ambulatory visits or 66.8% of visits. At least one or more drugs were provided or prescribed at 500.6 million physician office visits and there were about 1.1 billion drug mentions at visits to office-based physicians (Schwartz et al., 2002). There is evidence that office-based physicians frequently prescribe inappropriate medications for the elderly, and adverse drug events appear to be common in older outpatients who are taking multiple medications (Hammons et al., 2001; Donnell & Jacobs, 2002). Over three billion prescriptions are dispensed annually from ambulatory care pharmacies, and by 2004 the number of retail prescriptions is estimated to reach four billion per year (Schwartz et al., 2002).

A study using 1992 National Ambulatory Medical Care Survey data found that 7.75 million office visits by the elderly resulted in the prescribing of at least one medication from a list of 20 drugs judged highly inappropriate for the elderly, and about 720,000 visits resulted in the prescribing of two inappropriate medications. Overall about 7.8% of elderly patients who received prescriptions were given inappropriate medication. Adverse drug events appear to be more common in older outpatients who are taking multiple medications. The elderly make twice as many visits to medical providers as those less than 65 years (Hammons, Piland, Small, Hatlie, & Burstin, 2003). See chapter 13 for further discussion about the elderly population.

Based on the 1998 NAMCS and NHAMCS data, about 6.2 million ambulatory visits to physician offices, outpatient departments, and emergency departments were the result of medical misadventure, including adverse drug events and complications from medical and surgical procedures. Errors are difficult to document because different criteria have been used to detect adverse drug events (ADE), and rates vary by definition. The incidence of outpatient ADEs has been reported to range from 2.6–50.6% depending on data collection methods and definitions used. Studies of ADEs in ambulatory settings using patient surveys rather than records report higher rates of 30–50% while studies based on chart reviews in small clinics, in which ADEs are narrowly defined, report a lower incidence of 1–3%. Many ADEs may not even be noted in the medical record, so any estimates may represent a low figure. Lack of information at the time of prescribing appears to be an important component of preventable ADE rates in the ambulatory setting (Hammons et al., 2003).

Gandhi (2000) studied 2,248 patients from 11 Boston ambulatory clinics, of which 18% reported a drug complication. Drug complications were common and resulted in increased use of medical care to manage adverse events. Communication to patients of medication instructions and potential side effects was often inadequate, particularly when the primary language was not English. Strategies that have been identified for patient education that address both language and literacy issues are extremely important for self-management. One study of primary care ambulatory settings found over a period of 5.5 years that adverse events occurred at a rate of 3.7 per 100,000 clinic visits. Of the adverse events, 83% were deemed preventable medical errors, 14% resulted in permanent disability, and 3% resulted in death. The authors concluded that serious adverse events occur infrequently but the consequences can be significant (Fischer, Fetters, Munro, & Goldman, 1997).

Brigham and Women's Hospital in Boston (Gandhi, et al., 2003; Schwartz, et al., 2002) used a computerized search of patient records to identify ADEs and found that they are frequent with an ADE rate of 5.5/ 100 outpatients presenting for care. Among the ADEs, 23% were life-threatening or serious and 38% were preventable. Of the ADEs reviewed:

- 9.1% resulted in hospitalization
- 15.7% required multiple ambulatory or emergency department visits
- 12.4% had a laboratory abnormality requiring a change in therapy
- 62.4% required at least one additional clinic visit for prescription changes

A recent study illustrates that there is still a gap in our knowledge about errors in the ambulatory setting (Gandhi, et al., 2003). The authors concluded that adverse events related to medications are common in primary care, and many are preventable. The study goal was to determine the rates, types, severity, and preventability of such events among outpatients and to identify preventive strategies. This prospective study included a survey of patients and a chart review, at four adult primary care practices in Boston (two hospital-based and two community-based), for a total of 1,202 outpatients who received at least one prescription during a four-week period. At two of the practices prescriptions were computerized; they were handwritten at the other two. Of the 661 patients who responded, 162 had adverse drug events (25%), with a total of 181 events (27 per 100 patients). Twenty-four of the events (13%) were serious, 51 (28%) were able to be ameliorated, and 20 (11%) were preventable. Of the 51 events that could be ameliorated, 32 (63%) were attributed to the physician's failure to respond to medication-related symptoms and 19 (37%) to the patient's failure to inform the physician of the symptoms. The medication classes most frequently involved in adverse drug events were selective serotonin reuptake inhibitors (10%), beta blockers (9%), angiotensin-converting enzyme inhibitors (8%), and nonsteroidal anti-inflammatory agents (8%) (Gandhi, et al., 2003).

Monitoring for and acting on symptoms are important, and improving communication between outpatients and providers may help prevent adverse events related to medications (Gandhi, et al., 2003). Results from a 2001 study in an integrated health care network found 3.2% of hospital admissions were caused by ADEs with 76% of these ADEs classified as preventable (Schwartz et al., 2002). An earlier study (Beard, 1992) suggested that between 3–11% of hospital admissions were due to ADEs.

A recent analysis suggested that more than one million outpatients in the United States experienced an ADE that required admission to the hospital in a year and that 4.7% of all admissions were caused by drugs. Another study found that drug-related problems, including ADRs, account for nearly 10% of all hospital admissions and up to 140,000 deaths annually in the U.S. It is easy to see that while reported admission rates due to drug events have ranged widely from 2.3–28.2%, it is definitely a problem. In a 2001 review of unplanned admissions in the elderly, 30.4% were the result of an ADE with 53.4% considered preventable. A meta-analysis estimated that 5.3% of hospitalizations are due to patient noncompliance with medication administration instructions (Schwartz et al., 2002).

Outpatient deaths attributed to medication error rose 848% between 1983 and 1993 (Kozak, Hall, & Owings, 2001). By 1993 the risk of death was 6.5 times greater for outpatients than inpatients, with one out of 131 outpatient deaths from medication error compared with one out of 854 inpatient deaths (Schwartz et al., 2002). A study of ambulatory care patients drawn from a community office-based medical practice found medication side effects in 4.2% of patients with 54% of these preventable (Quality Interagency Coordinating Task Force [QuIC], 2000).

In a recent review of pharmacists, the Massachusetts State Board of Registration in Pharmacy estimated that 2.4 million prescriptions are filled improperly each year in that state, with 90% of the prescriptions filled improperly being related to wrong drug or dosage. These errors are usually the result of inadequate point-of-care access to current clinical knowledge or unavailable patient data. Drugs used for long-term therapies seemed to have more ADEs. Of the ADEs, 56% were associated with drugs from four classes: Antihypertensives, angiotensin converting enzyme (ACE) inhibitors, antibiotics, and diuretics. Nonsteroidal anti-inflammatory gastropathy was identified as the most common cause of ADE hospitalization of the elderly with up to 90% of the admissions considered preventable (Schwartz et al., 2002).

Medication errors are costly as well as harmful. Johnson and Bootman developed an economic model to estimate the cost of medication-related problems in ambulatory care. The cost of medication-related illness and death in 1995 was estimated at $76.6 billion annually. The total amount of money spent on medications for ambulatory patients is about $80 billion per year. For every dollar spent on medications, another dollar is spent to treat new health problems caused by medications (Alliance for Aging Research, 1998). Updated data for 2000 now reveal that the cost of medication-related problems has increased to $177.4 billion with hospital admissions and long-term care admissions accounting for the majority (Schwartz et al., 2002).

There is great overlap on medication safety practices between acute care and ambulatory care. Applying consistent standard approaches for medication administration in both settings will ensure the best patient outcomes. Major differences in ambulatory care are noted in the increased role of patients/families in the ambulatory setting as well as in multiple sites. Table 12.1 summarizes recommended patient safety practices for medication safety in ambulatory care.

SURGERY AND PROCEDURE ERRORS

In ambulatory settings where procedures, treatments, or surgery are performed, many strategies for safety identified from the inpatient setting can be applied to ensure that the correct patient, correct procedure, and correct

TABLE 12.1   Medication Safety Practices in Ambulatory Care Settings

Ordering	Adopt prescription writing standards for manual systems: specify abbreviations; use leading zeroes but not trailing zeroes; spell out units; write the reason for the medication
	Standardize and limit formularies to avoid drug mix-ups and dosing issues
	Leverage with technology and consider electronic ordering with handheld PDA, or implement information systems of CPOE or EMR
	Reduce reliance on memory with standardized protocols and standing orders based on best practice
	Train staff on protocols and prescribing standards and orient new staff on procedures
	Use drug-drug interaction alert programs
	Post prescribing guidelines for the elderly with list of inappropriate meds for the elderly
	Post weight-based guidelines for children
	Use decision algorithms for warfarin (especially in the elderly); consider anticoagulation dosing services or clinic, including flow sheets with doses and coagulation studies
Administration	Patient education/return demonstration
	Patient identification system if administered in office/clinic
	Standardize flow sheets and checklists
	If clinic/office staff administer medications then refer to general practices for safe administration of medications
Monitoring	Tele-management of chronic conditions (e.g., heart failure)
	Pharmacy reminders when medications are due for reorder (e.g., long-term meds for asthma)
	Develop standardized patient education materials including patient self-management programs (e.g., diabetes, asthma)

From JCAHO, 2002b; IHI, n.d.; California Academy of Family Physicians, 2002; Dovey, Meyers, Phillips Jr., Green, Fryer, Galliher, Kappus, & Grob, 2000.

site are selected. The Joint Commission's Universal Protocol for preventing wrong site, wrong procedure, wrong person surgery™ was developed for all settings including ambulatory (JCAHO, 2003a).

Ambulatory settings often have complex equipment, but may have fewer trained personnel due to fewer regulations. The availability of rescue drugs and equipment as well as regular training in emergency procedures is often limited as well. The concern about outpatient or office surgery is being addressed by several states and medical associations to propose a consistent standard for safe surgery (Green, 2001; Iverson & the ASPS Task Force, 2002; Prager, 2000). At least six states have passed regulations on office surgery including Florida, Illinois, and New York (Green, 2001).

Invasive procedures in the inpatient and outpatient setting present some degree of risk to the patient. Characteristics of ambulatory care settings described earlier present those risks. One area of safety concern for outpatient and office-based surgery is the administration of anesthesia. At least one state, New York, has developed guidelines for patient safety, sedation, monitoring, emergency care, equipment maintenance, and infection control for practitioners (Committee on Quality Assurance in Office-Based Surgery, 1999). In another state, Florida, the Board of Medicine responded to five reported patient deaths and more than 20 adverse events in 1999, and first imposed a 90-day moratorium on office-based surgeries. Later it developed new rules. Most of the problems reported in Florida involved elective, cosmetic procedures, so several rules were developed regarding abdominoplasty and liposuction performed during the same procedure, as well as improved monitoring and screening of patients. The Accreditation Association for Ambulatory Health Care (AAAHC) is also conducting two studies on liposuction since it is frequently performed in the ambulatory setting (Kuznets, 2002).

The issue of wrong-site surgery can be compounded by a number of events in which "we see what we expect to see." In Florida, an orthopedic surgeon faces a lawsuit after he operated on the incorrect leg during tendon surgery at an ambulatory center (Liberto, 2003). The surgeon saw the patient while she was being anesthetized for surgery on a ruptured Achilles tendon in her left leg. When the surgeon left the room to scrub, the patient was turned over onto her abdomen. When the surgeon returned to the room and approached the left side of the table, he expected to see the left leg but did not realize the patient's legs were now on opposite sides.

Another area being addressed is the risk of nosocomial infections. With short stays in ambulatory surgery centers, it is very difficult to identify infection problems. The Centers for Disease Control and Prevention (CDC) has identified that nosocomial infections are a problem in multiple settings and proposed expanding the National Nosocomial Infections System to ambulatory settings (Kuznets, 2002).

Best practices for surgery safety in the ambulatory setting match most practices for acute care. The major differences in ambulatory surgery are the severity of the patient's condition, the length of stay, the availability of staff and resuscitative equipment, and regulations. Table 12.2 summarizes recommended patient safety practices for ambulatory care surgery.

TABLE 12.2   Surgery Safety Practices in Ambulatory Care Settings

Preparation	Patient verification
	Site verification
	Checklist preoperatively
	Stop procedure for any variance
	Staff education of process
	Standardize forms for surgery, anesthesia, recovery
	Ensure rescue and resuscitative equipment are available and staff are trained in use on a regular basis
	Have preventive maintenance/checks on all equipment
Procedure	Site Verification
	Standardize room setup
	Standardize equipment

From JCAHO, 2002; IHI, n.d.; California Academy of Family Physicians, 2002; Dovey, Meyers, Phillips Jr., Green, Fryer, Galliher, Kappus, & Grob, 2000.

OTHER ERRORS IN AMBULATORY CARE

The Robert Graham Policy Center supported a study by The National Network for Family Practice and Primary Care Research. A qualitative analysis was performed to identify categories of errors reported during a randomized controlled trial of computer and paper reporting methods. The study categorized 344 errors reported by 42 primary care physicians between May and September 2000 (Dovey, et al., 2000). For the study, "error" was defined as "something that should not have happened, was not anticipated, and made physicians say, "That should not happen in my practice, and I don't want it to happen again". According to analyst Dr. Sharon Dovey errors fell into the following seven categories:

- 24%—Communication problems
- 20%—Discontinuity of care
- 19%—Lab results
- 13%—Missing values/charting
- 8%—Clinical mistake
- 8%—Prescribing errors
- 8%—Other

This study provides information that identifies problem areas so potential strategies can be implemented. In this study, errors associated with prescribing were small, but the volume of medications prescribed, the risks associated with high-risk medications, and the monitoring required for certain medications emphasize the importance of medication safety. Ten errors, made by the 50 physicians in the study resulted in patients being admitted to the hospital, and one patient died.

In additional analysis of the errors:

- 284 (82.6%) were considered system malfunctions such as administrative mistakes, investigation failures, communication lapses, and payment problems
- 46 (13.4%) were considered errors made due to gaps in knowledge or skills, such as wrong or missed diagnosis, and wrong treatment decisions arising from a lack of knowledge or skills
- 14 reports (4.1%) were reclassified as "adverse events" instead of errors (Dovey, et al., 2000).

Further categorization of these errors from family physicians demonstrated other systems problems that are special to ambulatory settings: administrative failures (102; 30.9% of errors), investigation failures (82; 24.8%), treatment delivery lapses (76; 23.0%), miscommunication (19; 5.8%), payment systems problems (4; 1.2%), error in the execution of a clinical task (19; 5.8%), wrong treatment decision (14; 4.2%), and wrong diagnosis (13; 3.9%) (Dovey, et al., 2000).

In other aspects of care, research shows that for a wide variety of conditions, about half of Americans did not receive recommended preventive care, including 40% who did not receive recommended chronic care (Becher & Chassin, 2001; Centers for Disease Control and Prevention, 2001). This lack of care is evident among the elderly, in whom avoidable hospitalizations have increased. Avoidable conditions are those for which timely and effective ambulatory care should prevent the illnesses, control acute episodes, or manage the chronic condition to prevent deterioration so that hospitalization is not necessary. Chronic conditions such as diabetes, heart failure, and asthma can be managed in the ambulatory setting, but are dependent on self-management, compliance, and regular monitoring to prevent adverse events. The avoidance of hospitalization in these patients is difficult when it has been estimated that 50% of prescriptions are used incorrectly (Schwartz et al., 2002).

The Agency for Healthcare Research and Quality (AHRQ) has developed a set of quality indicators that are based on inpatient administrative data. The prevention quality indicators identify hospital admissions for 16 conditions that suggest failure of ambulatory management. These indicators can be used to assess primary care access or outpatient services. "With high-quality, community-based primary care, hospitalization for these illnesses can be avoided" (AHRQ, 2001). The specific indicators are listed in Table 12.3.

The Center for Medicare and Medicaid Services (CMS) has supported ambulatory care quality of Medicare beneficiaries in several of these conditions through its scopes of work. Practices in the ambulatory setting, based on the best practices in the literature to reduce morbidity and mortality, are found in Table 12.4. Preventive care for conditions of pneumonia, influenza, breast cancer, diabetes, and heart disease are included in the CMS quality program for Medicare beneficiaries. These conditions have been monitored under the sixth and seventh scopes of work with projects in each state. There is now a physician office project being piloted in New York, California, and Iowa to study performance in this ambulatory setting (CMS, 2003).

For example, one condition under the CMS 6th and 7th scope of work includes influenza, which poses significant risks for the elderly. Yet only 60% of elderly Caucasians were immunized in 1995, and rates were even lower for minority groups—50% for Hispanics and 40% for Blacks. The

Table 12.3   AHRQ Prevention Quality Indicators for Ambulatory Care Sensitive Conditions

---

Bacterial pneumonia
Dehydration
Pediatric gastroenteritis
Urinary infections
Perforated appendicitis
Low birth weight
Angina without an in-hospital procedure
Congestive heart failure
Hypertension
Adult asthma
Pediatric asthma
Chronic obstructive pulmonary disease
Uncontrolled diabetes
Diabetes (short-term complications and long-term complications)
Lower extremity amputations among patients with diabetes.

From AHRQ, 2001.

TABLE 12.4   Practices Supported by CMS for Ambulatory Care Quality

Disease	Practice Recommendation
Diabetes	Monitoring Hgb A1C
Asthma	Use of metered dose inhalers
Flu/pneumonia	Vaccination for both conditions
Heart disease	Continuation of beta blockers and Angiotensin Converting Enzyme (ACE) inhibitors after discharge from hospital with acute myocardial infarction
Stroke	Monitoring hypertension; administration of aspirin at onset

From CMS, n.d.

Quality Improvement Organizations (QIO) have worked on projects to increase influenza and pneumonia immunization. For other conditions such as cardiac care, from 1996–1999, projects focused on increasing warfarin use in patients with atrial fibrillation with appropriate clinical indications. These projects also looked at whether patients discharged on warfarin received proper education about their condition and medication. Some projects also evaluated atrial fibrillation patients taking warfarin who maintain an international normalized ratio (INR) between 2 and 3, indicating that warfarin therapy is properly managed.

Practices for the ambulatory care setting include areas that are common such as scheduling issues, diagnostics performed and reported by agencies other than the primary care provider, and multiple handoffs. Tables 12.5, 12.6, and 12.7 summarize recommended patient safety practices for ambulatory care in the areas of access to care and services, diagnostics, process management, and communication flow. Incorporation of these practices into daily ambulatory health care can decrease medical errors, decrease adverse events, and minimize complications.

STUDIES AND INITIATIVES

The IOM report To Err is Human: Building a Safer Health System (Kohn, Corrigan, & Donaldson, 2000) prompted numerous studies and initiatives on patient safety. The AHRQ has been the primary funding agency for research including studies on ambulatory care. Many of the studies have been developed in collaboration with professional organizations representing ambulatory sectors, specific health care organizations, and other agen-

TABLE 12.5   Access to Care Safety Practices in Ambulatory Care Settings

Scheduling Appointments	Clinical triage system (not just clerical)
	Standardize information obtained by support staff
	Email with patients when visits not needed
	Consider group visits/education
	Open access system for same day appointments; recategorize patient types
	Extend hours for seeing patients to reduce emergency department visits
	Follow up system for missed appointments
	Nurses to manage certain at risk subpopulations
	Daily "huddles" to assess work day
Preventive activities and screening	Tracking system for preventive activities (screenings) and disease specific interventions
	Utilize stickers on medical record to alert staff to follow up activities
	Create registries to track certain subpopulations
Referrals	Patient information to be sent to consultant/referral (Copies not originals)
	Tracking system for ensuring referral is completed and information posted to record for follow up
	Use geriatric and other specialists as needed
Office/Clinic Visit	Review medical record before patient arrives including any diagnostics
	Standardize exam rooms with minimum inventory list posted per room
	Standardize stocking procedures
	Provide small notepads for patients to write questions and instructions

From JCAHO, 2002b; IHI, n.d.; California Academy of Family Physicians, 2002; Dovey, Meyers, Phillips Jr., Green, Fryer, Galliher, Kappus, & Grob, 2000.

cies. Much of the research is in progress, so findings and application for practice are not yet available. As data on ambulatory care errors and patient safety are presented, an evidence-based approach with new strategies can be introduced to improve patient safety. AHRQ has funded at least 13 studies targeted to ambulatory care that are listed in Table 12.8.

The AAFP is leading research in office settings with The Robert Graham Center and is coordinating phase one of an international study of primary care in six countries. Their support of an earlier study (Dovey, et al., 2000)

TABLE 12.6   Clinical Diagnostics Safety Practices in Ambulatory Care Settings

Ordering	Provide diagnosis/reason for test
	Patient education/instructions prior to test to ensure adequate preparation
Follow-up	Tracking and reminder system to follow up on results; ensure available staff to batch and manage paper reports; ensure clinical staff reviews each message and contacts patient with normal results with physician reporting abnormal results
	Develop protocol for notification of results; ensure primary provider sees/initials reports before filing
	Instruct patient to call for results or "Office will contact you with results. If you do not hear from us in ___ time, call us"
	Secure system for reports (not loose paper or sticky notes)
	System to clearly flag abnormal results

From JCAHO, 2002b; IHI, n.d.; California Academy of Family Physicians, 2002; Dovey, Meyers, Phillips Jr., Green, Fryer, Galliher, Kappus, & Grob, 2000.

TABLE 12.7   Process Management Practices in Ambulatory Care Settings

Process Management	Use decision support aids for tracking and managing processes of care
	Use risk management applications software for tracking adverse events and potential events to make improvements
	Use trigger tools to identify complications (such as HgA1C and INR values)
	Create a culture of safety (policies and procedures; reporting errors)
Communication	Standardize messaging process for all providers
	Utilize a priority process for messages and reports (such as "bins")
	Create reminder systems and tracking systems for follow-up appointments and reports
	E-mail communication with patients
	Spread accountability for checks and balances to team for follow up items
	Document in standard format so omissions of care do not occur

From JCAHO, 2002b; IHI,n.d.; California Academy of Family Physicians, 2002; Dovey, Meyers, Phillips Jr., Green, Fryer, Galliher, Kappus, & Grob, 2000.

TABLE 12.8   AHRQ Funded Studies Related to Ambulatory Care

Title/Institution	Project Summary
Project Title: Impact of Personal Digital Assistant Devices on Medication Errors Institution: Creighton University	The objective of this research is to determine the impact of the use of personal digital assistants (PDAs) by prescribers on medication errors in primary care, office-based practices.
Project Title: Improving Primary Care Patient Safety with Handheld DSS Institution: University of Alabama	The objective of this research is to develop, implement, and evaluate computer-based decision support systems (DSS) in ambulatory care settings. The researchers will look at what keeps clinicians from using the stand-alone, handheld devices, and they will assess the impact of DSS on patient safety, targeting prevention of the risks of inappropriate prescribing of medications.
Project Title: PDA-CT: Informatics for Community Treatment Teams Institution: Simulation Technologies, Inc.	The purpose of the contract is to develop an integrated informatics system using handheld wireless devices to enhance the quality of care provided by assertive community treatment (ACT) teams serving mentally ill patients living in the community.
Project Title: Web-Enabled Asthma Application for Personalized Medical Communication Institution: Pharmacon International, Inc.	The purpose of the contract is to develop an integrated medical system that facilitates communication between physicians and asthma patients. It will facilitate compliance with therapeutic regimens and enable self-management through peak-flow monitoring.
Project Title: Applied Strategies for Interventions for Patient Safety Institution: University of Colorado Health Center	The purpose of this demonstration project is to analyze the causes and effects of medical errors in primary care settings and to reduce the incidence of those errors. The project will be carried out by the University of Colorado Department of Family Medicine in collaboration with a number of primary care, practice-based research networks, including ones that serve rural, urban, minority, and other underserved populations.

TABLE 12.8 *(continued)*

Title/Institution	Project Summary
Project Title: The Effect of Using Rules Technology with Provider Order Entry in Medication Error Reduction Institution: Denver Health	This project examines the effectiveness of utilizing computerized provider order entry (CPOE) systems on the potential reduction in medication errors. The CPOE system in Denver Health is capable of incorporating rules that will trigger a warning for a potential adverse drug event, not only in the inpatient setting but also in outpatient clinics. As part of the implementation at a large clinic in the Denver Health System later this year, rules will be implemented in the CPOE that will assist the provider in preventing adverse drug events when they are ordering medications.
Project Title: Improved Patient Safety With Information Technology Institution: Indiana University	The purpose of this demonstration project is to use an established clinical information system to identify indicators of medical errors within the ambulatory settings of a primary care, practice-based research network. Based on these indicators, the project will test two strategies (academic detailing and computerized decision support) for using this information to improve patient safety. The project will focus on two prevalent and costly conditions: congestive heart failure and asthma.
Project Title: Increasing Patient Safety by Improving Compliance to Clinical Practice Guidelines for Diabetes Management through Electronically Generated Reminders Institution: Marshfield Medical Research Foundation	This proposal will conduct a randomized control trial of physicians in Marshfield Clinics who treat diabetes patients to determine if low-cost alerts/prompts can increase compliance for testing in the treatment of diabetic patients.
Project Title: The CERTs Prescribing Safety Program Institution: Harvard Pilgrim Healthcare	The purpose of this demonstration project is to improve the detection of medication prescribing errors in outpatient settings and to develop new uses of this information to improve care. The project will be carried out by seven AHRQ-funded Centers for Education and Research on Therapeutics (CERTs) and will involve a network of HMOs with 16,000 primary care providers serving 7 million people.

(continued)

TABLE 12.8 (*continued*)

Title/Institution	Project Summary
Project Title: Improving Medication Safety Across Clinical Settings Institution: Brigham and Women's Hospital	This program establishes a Center of Excellence for Patient Safety at the Brigham and Women's Hospital in Boston. The center's focus is on improving drug safety across the continuum of care in diverse patient groups. Projects include the evaluation of tools to report and analyze medical errors, adverse events, medication errors, and adverse drug events in pediatric ambulatory patients, along with epidemiology and prevention of medication errors in psychiatric inpatients, safe intravenous infusion systems, improving anticoagulation therapy in nursing homes, and the role of organizational culture in promoting patient safety.
Project Title: The American Academy of Family Physicians DCERPS-PC Institution: The American Academy of Family Physicians	This developmental center will address patient safety improvements in primary care offices by focusing on family practice offices and residency training clinics. Family physicians and their staffs will collaborate with patients to identify opportunities for error reduction and safety improvement.
Project Title: Patient Safety for Vulnerable Populations Institution: Boston University	The aim of this developmental center is to focus on understanding and reducing medical errors, particularly those that commonly occur in ambulatory care, for low-income and culturally disadvantaged patients.
Project Title: Addressing Preventable Medication Use Variance in Mississippi Institution: University of Mississippi Medical Center	The purpose of this demonstration project is to collect data on medication use in nine ambulatory care sites in Mississippi that already use the same mandatory system for reporting medical errors. The goals of the project are to identify the causes of preventable errors and injury; develop, demonstrate, and evaluate strategies for reducing errors; and to share the results with others in the health care field.

From AHRQ, n.d.c.

illustrated categories of errors to guide improvement efforts. The American College of Physicians-American Society of Internal Medicine also launched a three-year initiative to raise awareness to reduce medical errors in doctor's offices and nonhospital settings. AAFP is doing research through the Developmental Centers for Evaluation and Research in Patient Safety (DCERPS) funded by the AHRQ (Kuznets, 2002).

The Medical Group Management Association (MGMA) is the nation's oldest and largest medical group practice organization representing over 7,100 physician group practices in which over 185,000 physicians practice medicine. In October 1999, MGMA launched its patient safety initiative to maximize patient safety in medical group practice and ambulatory care settings. They cosponsored a patient safety symposium that examined challenges, obstacles, and solutions regarding patient safety. Other conference partners included The University of Minnesota's Carlson School of Management, the Partnership for Patient Safety, Premier, Inc., Voluntary Hospitals of America (VHA), Inc., The Harvard Risk Management Foundation, The National Business Coalition on Health, and the JCAHO (MGMA, 2002).

The MGMA Center for Research is also conducting a project aimed at improving office-based practice systems for early diagnosis and treatment of breast cancer. The Breast Management Outcomes Assessment Study is designed to assess the effects of the use of specifically designed guidelines for the diagnosis of breast lumps and lesions in clinical practice. The project has a unique program intervention, the Breast Evaluation System (B.R.E.S.T.), to substantially increase guideline use and improve the process of care and patient outcomes and reduce rates of diagnostic delay and treatment discontinuity for breast care.

MGMA has also entered into a partnership with the American Hospital Association (AHA) to focus attention on medication safety issues in ambulatory care settings. A survey of MGMA members showed that 30% consider drug interactions to be the greatest patient safety risk faced in their practices. Through AHA's partnership with the Institute for Safe Medication Practices (ISMP), MGMA is working on tools to be used by physicians in their medical groups and in hospitals.

The American Medical Group Association (AMGA), the National Committee for Quality Assurance (NCQA), and Pharmacia have created a demonstration project to support patient safety in ambulatory settings called the Safety Collaborative for the Outpatient Environment (SCOPE). The goals of SCOPE are to "promote patient safety improvement innovations in the ambulatory setting through grants and to establish a collaborative of physician-led organizations to standardize patient safety definitions and evaluation criteria, share information on best practices, and recognize outstanding performance" (Schwartz et al., 2002). The partnership of the AMGA, NCQA, and Pharmacia are funding several studies that are described in Table 12.9.

EXEMPLARS

Idealized Design of Clinical Office Practice

The Idealized Design of Clinical Office Practice (IDCOP) initiative was developed by the Institute of Healthcare Improvement (IHI) to improve the performance of clinical office practices. IDCOP designs, tests, and

TABLE 12.9 AMGA, NCQA and Pharmacia Safety Collaborative for the Outpatient Environment (SCOPE) Demonstration Projects

Site	Project
Deaconess Billings Clinic	Pharmacy Intervention to Prevent Outpatient Medication Errors in Elderly Patients after Acute Hospital Stay
Gunderson Clinic	Improving Patient Safety for Rural Ambulatory Clinics
Henry Ford Medical Group	Improving Medication Safety Through the Reduction of Polypharmacy
Lahey Clinic	Enhanced Coordination of Time-Sensitive Consultations
Midwest Heart Specialists	Improving Patient Safety in the Outpatient Medication Refill Process by Providing Enhanced Digital Decision Support
Partners in Health Clinics	Evaluating the Effect of Enhanced Medication Oversight During the Hospital Discharge Process
Scott and White Clinic	Miscommunication and Medication Errors in Elderly Ambulatory Patients
The Everett Clinic	Use of Electronic Prescribing Technology to Impact Medication Errors in the Multispecialty Setting

From "Collaborative leadership for patient safety for ambulatory surgery in the office setting: Phase I Report of the National Patient Safety Consensus for the Community of Stakeholders for Ambulatory Surgery in the Office Setting," by P. Schwartz, S. Rudavsky, A. N. Christakis, & D. S. Conaway, 2002. Retrieved March 27, 2003, from www.npsf.org/download/ASOSFinalReport.pdf

deploys new models of office-based practices capable of fundamentally improved performance levels, better clinical outcomes, lower costs, higher satisfaction, and improved efficiency. Key components of this model include access to care, individualized interaction, reliability based on best practice, vitality with a sustainable and continually innovating practice, and other criteria such as alternatives to 1:1 visits and optimized care teams that match patient needs to the team (IHI, n.d.). Prototype site participants include 44 organizations.

Technologies

The use of technologies such as handheld devices for ordering and prescribing medications are being implemented. It is estimated that doctors receive 100 million calls annually from pharmacists about illegible prescriptions, potential medication errors, and substitutions with only about 5% of physicians prescribing electronically (Chin, 2001). In specific organizations, Brigham and Women's Hospital has launched a computerized provider order entry (CPOE) system in its outpatient clinics; Kaiser Permanente is investing in a computer-based clinical information system capable of delivering guidelines at the point of care. See chapter 8 on the use of technology for patient safety.

Additional technology for medication prescribing is used with an Internet online communication system. Three of the largest pharmacy benefit managers (PBM) in the country (AdvancePCS, Express Scripts, Inc. and Merck-Medco Managed Care LLC) are planning to develop an online exchange that will electronically connect physicians offices to the PBMs and pharmacies. The online exchange, RxHub LLC, will allow doctors to transmit electronic prescriptions to pharmacies while patients are still in their office. This tool allows physicians to know immediately if prescriptions are covered, provides alerts to potential adverse drug events, and asks if insurer's preferred meds can be substituted. RxHub would spare physicians from either making or receiving phone calls and additional paperwork because prescription-related problems would be caught at the blunt end rather than the sharp end when the patient obtains medications at the pharmacy (see chapter 1 for discussion of sharp- vs. blunt-end errors).

Massachusetts Coalition for the Prevention of Medical Errors

The Massachusetts Coalition for the Prevention of Medical Errors is leading state initiatives in ambulatory care. This leadership role is based on the coalition membership, which includes 24 members representing a variety of consumers, physicians, pharmacists, nurses, researchers, regulators, and managed-care plans. An ambulatory medication coalition has been created to identify the common contributing factors to medication errors in the ambulatory setting. This coalition will then identify best practices to reduce those errors, develop tools and educational programs to promote their adoption, and support consumer education. Members of the Ambulatory Medication Workgroup are currently undertaking a review of the root causes of ambulatory medication errors reported in the literature and from their own experience to help guide the focus of this initiative. One of the areas of interest is anticoagulation monitoring, which is discussed in the next section (Massachusetts Coalition for the Prevention of Medical Errors, n.d.).

Anticoagulation Clinic for Outpatient Monitoring

Chronic oral anticoagulation is widely prescribed in the ambulatory setting, especially for atrial fibrillation, peripheral vascular disease, deep vein thrombosis, and for other heart conditions (Gibbons, 2003). Lack of adherence to therapy prompts a variety of complications (bleeding or stroke) that increase morbidity and mortality. The most common causes of nonadherence include lack of prescribing standards, lack of patient education, and lack of follow-up. The use of anticoagulation clinics provides standardized monitoring, early warning of complications, notice of nonadherence, and maintenance of therapeutic dosing by monitoring international normalized ratio (INR). The Virginia Mason Medical Center provides an example in which an anticoagulation clinic reduced adverse events of bleeding, stroke, intracranial bleed, and other complications at a much greater rate than treatment of patients not at the clinic. The clinic has been able to achieve a reduction in complications in a population at great risk for problems, and thereby create safer care (Gibbons, 2003).

Telephonic Interventions for Heart Failure Patients

Providing educational materials is not sufficient for behavior change and self-management compliance in certain chronic diseases, notably heart failure. Telemanagement is used as daily reinforcement of education and early symptom management for those persons at high risk for rehospitalization, including those (1) having myriad comorbidities, (2) receiving medications with noncompliance or adverse reactions, (3) exhibiting dietary noncompliance, (4) having psychosocial concerns such as depression, (5) having financial constraints, and (6) experiencing cognitive dysfunction (Moser & Riegel, 2001). Telemanagement can include a variety of methods such as simply phoning in weight and symptoms or using video technology. "Telephonic weight monitoring and daily reporting of symptoms have been shown to have a compliance rate of 90% to decrease heart failure rehospitalization rates and to reduce health care costs" (Moser & Riegel, 2001, p. 187). Providers can react quickly to symptom changes and take action to prevent further deterioration in clinical status while the patient begins to correlate their behaviors to symptom changes.

AREAS FOR FUTURE RESEARCH

Research in the ambulatory care setting is challenging due to the variability and fragmentation of care. There is a lack of integrated data sources for searching for medical errors and greater fear of liability and litigation. The multiple sites and caregivers presents a methodological challenge in study design, which explains why focused studies in specific settings have been primarily conducted in ambulatory surgery, endoscopy, and a few office practices. Due to the volume of care provided in the ambulatory care setting, more research in broader settings is critical for patient safety.

Research in ambulatory care is just beginning to address the problems related to clear identification of the problem of medical errors, including types and numbers. This is a needed first step. A number of practices that are being implemented are also being tested to provide the evidence about those practices that are most beneficial in reducing errors and harm. The AHRQ and other agencies are funding research in the ambulatory care setting to increase knowledge and understanding about the use of technologies that may reduce errors, specifically medication errors. Technologies are also being implemented and tested to simplify scheduling and documentation of critical patient information.

CONCLUSION

Strategies for safe practices in the ambulatory setting are challenging as ambulatory care is fragmented and includes multiple sites of care delivery and providers. Implementation of known best practices and the pursuit of safety in this care setting are paramount. This chapter described problems and safety practices known to decrease medical errors and harm to patients.

WEB RESOURCES

Name of Resource/URL	Description
AAFP Family Practice Management www.aafp.org/fpm	Process improvement issues in family practice
Accreditation Association for Ambulatory Health Care www.aaahc.org	Describes accreditation services for ambulatory care
American Association for Accreditation of Ambulatory Surgery Facilities www.aaaasf.org	Describes accreditation services for ambulatory surgery
American Medical Group Association (AMGA), the National Committee for Quality Assurance (NCQA), and Pharmacia www.amga.org/QMR/SCOPE/scope_omc.asp	Safety Collaborative for the Outpatient Environment SCOPE
Agency for Healthcare Research and Quality www.ahrq.gov/about/cpcr/ptsafety/index.html	Conference synthesis of research agenda in ambulatory care for patient safety
Agency for Healthcare Research and Quality Prevention Quality Indicators www.ahrq.gov/data/hcup/prevqi.htm	List of prevention indicators that can be used to assess ambulatory care
Agency for Healthcare Research and Quality www.ahrq.gov	Critical analysis of patient safety practices

Assessing Care of Vulnerable Elders (ACOVE) www.amda.com	Comprehensive set of evidence-based indicators to assess quality of healthcare received by community dwelling elders
American Association of Family Practice (AAFP) www.aafp.org/x20104.xml	AAFP initiatives on patient safety
Center for Medicare and Medicaid Services www.cms.hhs.gov/qio/2b.pdf	CMS quality program
How's Your Health? www.howsyourhealth.com	Sample health assessment survey
Institute for Clinical Systems Improvement www.icsi.org	Resources on guidelines
Institute for Healthcare Improvement www.ihi.org/idealized/idcop/index.asp	Idealized design of clinical office practices
Joint Commission on the Accreditation of Healthcare Organizations www.jcaho.org	Multiple resources on six national patient safety goals, sentinel event alerts, and safety standards
Massachusetts Coalition for the Prevention of Medical Errors www.macoalition.org	Statewide coalition on medical error prevention; includes an initiative on ambulatory care
Medical Group Management Association www.mgma.com	Office practice resources
Medication Safety Self Assessment for Community/Ambulatory Pharmacy www.ismp.org/pdf/book.pdf	Self assessment tool online for community pharmacies
National Patient Safety Foundation www.npsf.org	Contains numerous resources on ambulatory care safety, including special report on ambulatory surgery
National Quality Forum www.qualityforum.org/safe_practices_report.pdf	List of 26 safety practices
Physician Practice www.physicianspractice.com	Downloadable forms for office practice

Practice Management   Sample pre-employment tests
www.practicemgmt.com/
test_book_details.html

REFERENCES

Agency for Healthcare Research and Quality (AHRQ). (2001). *AHRQ quality indicators. Prevention quality indicators.* Retrieved May 18, 2003, from www.ahrq.gov

Alliance for Aging Research. (1998). *When medicine hurts instead of helps.* Washington, DC: Author. Retrieved May 20, 2003, from www.agingresearch.org/brochures/medicinehurts/wmh_text.html

Beard, K. (1992). Adverse reactions as a cause of hospital admissions in the aged. *Drug Aging, 2,* 356–361.

Becher, E. C., & Chassin, M. R. (2001). Improving the quality of health care: Who will lead? *Health Affairs, 20*(5), 164–179.

California Academy of Family Physicians. (2002). *Diagnosing and treating medical errors in family practice.* San Francisco, CA: Author. Retrieved March 27, 2003, from www.familydocs.org/PDFs/MonographMedErrors.pdf

Centers for Disease Control and Prevention (CDC). (2001). CDC Study ranks prevention practices, finds that preventive medicine 'not always' covered or delivered. *Kaiser Daily Health Policy Report,* June 22.

Center for Medicare and Medicaid Services (CMS). (2003). *Doctors office quality project.* Retrieved March 31, 2003, from www.cms.hhs.gov/quality.doq

Chin, T. (2001, March 26). PBMs make their way into electronic prescriptions. *AMNews.*

Committee on Quality Assurance in Office-Based Surgery. (1999). A report to New York State Public Health Council and New York State Department of Health.

Donnell, P., & Jacobs, M. (2002). Hospital admissions resulting from preventable adverse drug reactions. *Annals of Pharmacotherapy, 36*(9), 1331–1336.

Dovey, S. M., Meyers, D. S., Phillips, Jr., R. L., Green, L. A., Fryer, G. E., Galliher, J. M., et al. (2000). *A preliminary taxonomy of medical errors in family practice.* Washington, DC: The Robert Graham Center.

Elder, N. C., & Dovey, S. M. (2002). Classification of medical errors and preventable adverse events in primary care: A synthesis of the literature. *Journal of Family Practice, 51,* 927–932.

Fischer, G., Fetters, M. D., Munro, A. P., & Goldman, E. B. (1997). Adverse events in primary care identified from a risk management database. *Journal of Family Practice, 45*(1), 40–46.

Gandhi, T. K. (2000). Drug complications in outpatients. *Journal of General Internal Medicine, 15,* 149–154.

Gandhi, T. K., Weingart, S. N., Borus, J., Seger, A. C., Peterson, J., Burdick, E., et al. (2003). Adverse outpatient drug events:A problem and an opportunity. *New England Journal of Medicine, 348*(16), 1587–1589.

Gibbons, E. F. (2003, March 12–15). *A comprehensive anticoagulation clinic program.* Presentation at the 5th Annual Patient Safety Congress, Washington, DC.

Green, J. (2001, January 1/8). AMA weighs national guidelines for office-based surgery. *AMNews*.

Hammons, T., Piland, N. F., Small, S. D., Hatlie, M. J., & Burstin, H. R. (2001). *Agenda for research in ambulatory patient safety: Synthesis of a multidisciplinary conference.* Rockville, MD: Agency for Healthcare Research and Quality. Retrieved March 27, 2003, from www.ahrq.gov/about/cpcr/ptsafety/index.html

Hammons, T., Piland, N. F., Small, S. D., Hatlie, M. J., & Burstin, H. R. (2003). Ambulatory patient safety: What we know and need to know. *Journal of Ambulatory Care Management, 26*(1), 63–82.

Institute for Healthcare Improvement (IHI). (n.d.). *Idealized design of clinical office practices.* Retrieved April 1, 2003, from www.ihi.org/idealized/idcop/index.asp

Iverson, R. E., & ASPS Task Force on Patient Safety in Office-Based Surgery Facilities (2002). Patient safety in office-based surgery facilities, I: Procedures in the office-based setting. *Plastic and Reconstructive Surgery, 110,* 1337–1342.

Joint Commission on Accreditation of Healthcare Organizations (JCAHO). (2002). *2003 national patient safety goals.* Retrieved January 12, 2003, from *www.jcaho.org/accredited+organizations/patient+safety/npsg/index.htm*

Joint Commission on Accreditation of Healthcare Organizations (JCAHO). (2003). *Sentinel event statistics—May 7, 2003.* Retrieved May 20, 2003, from *www.jcaho.org/accredited+organizations/hospitals/sentinel+events/sentinel+event+statistics.htm*

Joint Commission on Accreditation of Healthcare Organizations. (2003a). *Universal protocol for preventing wrong site, wrong procedure, wrong person surgery*™ Retrieved December 7, 2003, from www.jcaho.org/accredited+organizations/patient+safety/universal+protocol/index.htm.

Kohn, L. T., Corrigan, J. M., & Donaldson, M. S. (Eds.). (2000). *To err is human. Building a safer health system.* Washington, DC: National Academy Press.

Kozak, L. J., Hall, M. J., & Owings, M. F. (2001). Trends in avoidable hospitalizations, 1980–1998. *Health Affairs, 20*(2), 225–242.

Kuznets, M. (2002). Spotlight on ambulatory care patient safety. *Focus on Patient Safety. A newsletter from the National Patient Safety Foundation, 5*(4), 1–2.

Liberto, J. (2003, April 21). Suit says doctor botched surgery. *St. Petersburg Times*, St. Petersburg, FL.

Massachusetts Coalition for the Prevention of Medical Errors. (n.d.). *Reducing ambulatory medication errors.* Retrieved May 18, 2003, from www.macoalition.org

Medical Group Management Association. (2002). *Additional Statement. National summit on medical errors and patient safety research.* Retrieved March 31, 2003, from http://www.quic.gov/summit/amgma.htm

Moser, D. K., & Riegel, B. (Eds.). (2001). *Improving outcomes in heart failure: An interdisciplinary approach.* Gaithersburg, MD: Aspen Publishers, Inc.

Murray, M., & Tantau, C. (2001, December 9–12). *Exploding the myth of open access: How to create sustainable improvement.* Presentation at the 2001 IHI Conference in Orlando, Florida.

Prager, L. (2000, November 13). Regulators look at ways to control office-based surgery. *AMNews*.

Quality Interagency Coordinating Task Force (QuIC). (2000). Doing what counts for patient safety: Federal actions to reduce medical errors and their impact. Report of the QuIC Task Force to the President.

Schwartz, P., Rudavsky, S., Christakis, A. N., & Conaway, D. S. (2002). *Collaborative leadership for patient safety for ambulatory surgery in the office setting: Phase I Report of the National Patient Safety Consensus for the Community of Stakeholders for Ambulatory Surgery in the Office Setting*. Chicago, IL: National Patient Safety Foundation. Retrieved March 27, 2003, from www.npsf.org/download/ASOSFinalReport.pdf

Chapter 13

Safety Issues With the Elderly and Chronically Ill

Janice Z. Peterson

OVERVIEW

The physical and psychosocial changes of aging predispose the elderly to a variety of safety problems. The chronically ill, who may also be elderly, are vulnerable to similar safety problems. This chapter will focus on the most common safety problems related to the elderly and the chronically ill, including falls, restraints, medication errors, and pressure ulcers. Nosocomial infections, dehydration, and fluid imbalance will be considered briefly, as well as risk assessment and best practices for the prevention and management of these safety problems.

In general, as people age there is physiologic decline in function, structure, and functional reserve. These changes vary greatly from one individual to another, with chronological age not being a strong predictor of the extent of change (Alcee, 2000; Arking, 1998; Luekenotte, 2000a). For instance, one 70-year-old person may have little physical change while another has a great deal of change. The problem of loss of functional reserve may not be apparent until the individual is stressed, as with an acute illness. These changes predispose the elderly to a multitude of safety risks. Similarly, chronic illness may also predispose individuals to safety problems. While not all people who suffer chronic illness are elderly, the incidence of chronic disease increases with age. Often, there is overlap between the effects of aging and the effects of chronic illness. Risk factors for safety problems related to age and chronic illness are listed in Table 13.1 (Arking, 1998; Luekenotte, 2000b). Environment interacts with these physical changes to play an important role in the risk to the safety of the elderly and chronically ill across the continuum of care, including acute care, long-term care, home health care, and the community (Meiner & Miceli, 2000). See also Table 13.1.

FALLS

Falls are among the most frequent and potentially serious safety problem for elderly and chronically ill in all settings—acute care, long-term care, and the home. Annually, it is estimated that nearly one-third of community dwelling older adults and one-half of those in acute or long-term care institutions will fall (National Center for Injury Prevention and Control [NCIP], 2000b). The elderly tend to suffer more serious consequences of falling than younger persons. The National Center for Injury Prevention (NCIP) used visits to the emergency department to estimate the annual rate of non-fatal injuries due to falls. In 2000, the rate of nonfatal injuries due to falls was 2,377 per 100,000 for those aged 65 to 69. The rate increased with each 5 years of age, with the sharpest increase for those older than 85. Deaths due to falls per 100,000 population was less than 1% of the rate for non-fatal injuries, but followed a similar pattern of sharp increase after age 85 (NCIP, 2000a). The rates of nonfatal injuries and deaths due to falls are illustrated in Figures 13.1 and 13.2. Falls among persons under age 65 accounted for only 16% of all traumatic brain injuries while among those over age 65, falls accounted for 64% of traumatic brain injuries (NCIP, 2000b). Another serious consequence of falling is hip fracture. According to Medicare statistics, older adults suffer 270,000 hip fractures per year. When older adults suffer hip fracture, they tend to require longer hospitalization and rehabilitation, and those over 75 are more likely to die within one year of fracture (NCIP, 2000b).

In addition to the morbidity and mortality associated with falls in the elderly, falling has serious meaning for the older person. For some, developing a fear of falling has a serious impact on quality of life and may be one factor in the decision to enter a long-term care facility (Donald & Bulpitt, 1999). Further, a series of falls may be a sign of impending physical and mental decline, although it is unclear which comes first (Laird, Studenski, Perera, & Wallace, 2001).

TABLE 13.1 Potential Safety Problems in the Elderly and Chronically Ill: Intrinsic and Extrinsic Risks

Potential problems	Intrinsic risk factors due to changes of aging	Intrinsic risk factors from chronic illness	Extrinsic or environmental factors
Falls	Orthostatic hypotension Nocturia Sleep pattern changes Posture and gait changes Slowing reflexes Decreased muscle tone and strength Decline in vision changes—depth perception, clarity, dark adaptation, visual fields, color sensitivity Changes in inner ear Acute or chronic confusion	Hypertension—medication induced orthostatic hypotension Chronic neurological problems such as Parkinson's disease Cardiac—dysrhythmias Arthritis Stroke Dementia	Poor lighting Slick or irregular floor surfaces Bathroom fixtures that are too high or too low Unsafe stairways
Medication errors/adverse drug events	Reduced liver and renal function with age may limit ability to metabolize medications. Cognitive deficits may have overlay of multiple chronic health problems	May be taking a large number of medications to treat the chronic illness, including self medication (polypharmacy) The chronic disease may limit ability to metabolize medications Dementia or other memory problems may limit reliability of self-administration of medications	Availability of over-the-counter (OTC) medications Current health care system promotes multiple specialties with lack of communication among prescribers Inadequate income to purchase medications

(continued)

TABLE 13.1   *(continued)*

Pressure ulcers/skin breakdown	Skin thinning Reduced circulation Reduced tactile sense	Diabetes Circulatory problems	Immobility imposed by treatment (bed rest, lengthy surgery, restraints) Shearing forces Pressure
Potential problems	Intrinsic risk factors due to changes of aging	Intrinsic risk factors from chronic illness	Extrinsic or environmental factors
Nosocomial infections	Aging immune system	Immune suppression through treatment of chronic health problem	Invasive treatment Communal living such as nursing homes Neglect of immunizations
Fluid imbalance • Over-hydration • Dehydration	Kidneys less able to regulate fluid Reduced thirst sensation	Renal disease Congestive heart failure Dementia or other illness that may inhibit ability to get fluids	Medications Intravenous fluid therapy Staff neglecting to offer or assist with oral fluids

From Arking, 1998; Luekenotte, 2000b.

Assessing the Risk for Falls

The first step in preventing falls is to identify who is at risk. As listed in Table 13.1, multiple intrinsic factors related to normal aging as well as chronic disease can play a role in the risk for falling. Research has helped to identify pertinent risks for falling, which include: a history of falling, chronic health conditions, cognitive impairment, depression, perceptual dysfunction (including depth perception, visual impairment, balance, and gait deficits), and multiple medications (Buri, Picton, & Dawson, 2000; Fuller, 2000; Hausdorff, Rios, & Edelberg, 2001; Laird et al., 2001).

Parkinson's disease and type 2 diabetes are among several chronic illnesses that have been shown to increase the risk of falling. A community-based study confirmed the high risk of falling in Parkinson's disease and identified factors that compounded the risk. When those with Parkinson's disease who had fallen were compared with those who had not fallen, the

Non-fatal Fall Injuries by Age - 2000

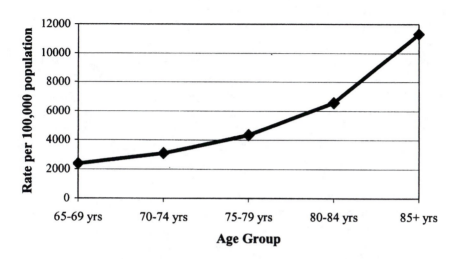

FIGURE 13.1   Non-fatal fall injuries by age for year 2000.

From National Center for Injury Prevention and Control, 2000.

Fall Deaths for Year 2000

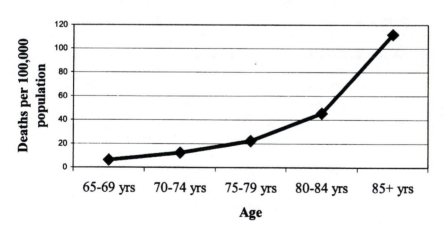

FIGURE 13.2   Fall deaths for year 2000.

From National Center for Injury Prevention and Control, 2000.

following factors were ascertained: multiple medications, greater physical disability, depression, anxiety, more steps to complete a mobility test, and greater postural sway (Ashburn, Stack, Pickering, & Ward, 2001). Elderly individuals with type 2 diabetes in an urban day care center and those in a rural community center were evaluated for fall risk. In both groups, more than half reported falling. Loss of lower extremity protective sensation was found in all individuals with type 2 diabetes in the urban center and two-thirds of those in the rural center; and the majority of those with sensory impairment had impaired balance (Conner-Kerr & Templeton, 2002).

Many tools have been developed to assess risk for falling. After evaluating 20 fall assessment tools, the authors of an integrated review recommended that the choice of assessment tool would depend on the setting (Perell, et al., 2001). For acute care settings, a tool is needed that is sensitive to the risk for falling while not requiring so much time to complete that the patient and nurse are overtaxed. For community settings, where independent walking is often the case, gait and balance take on greater importance and should be emphasized in the screening. In long-term care, so many patients are at risk for falling that universal fall precautions may be more appropriate (Perell, et al., 2001). A sampling of the many tools and methods for assessment of risk for falling is listed in Table 13.2 (Conley, 1999; Duncan, Studenski, Chandler, & Prescott, 1992; Eagle, et al., 1999; Morse, Morse, & Tylko, 1989; O'Connell & Myers, 2002; Simpson, Worsfold, Reilly, & Nye, 2002). A discussion of selected examples of these tools follows.

A short, but sensitive tool for predicting patients at risk for falling was developed and tested by Conley (1999). The original scale consisted of ten items based on a review of research literature. An eleven-month prospective study was conducted, testing the instrument on all admissions over age 50. Of the 1168 patients who had the fall risk assessment scale administered, 59 subsequently fell. More than half the patients fell within the first three days of admission. Based on the statistical analysis of the most sensitive items, the scale was condensed to six weighted items. The final version of the tool includes questions about recent falls, dizziness, and problems with urinary urgency or incontinence. In addition, the nurse makes observations about three other items: impaired judgment or lack of safety awareness, agitation, and impaired gait. See Table 13.3 (Conley, 1999).

Multiple factors should be considered in assessing the risk for falls. However, tools that assess gait and balance are particularly useful for community residing elderly and chronically ill. The TURN 180 is a quick and simple assessment of postural stability. The person is asked to take a few step, turn 180 degrees, and return. People who take more than four steps to complete a 180-degree turn are at increased risk for falling (Simp-

TABLE 13.2   Assessing Risk for Falling: A Sampling of Tools and Methods

Tool/Reference	Comment	Setting
Conley Scale (Conley, 1999)	6-item, weighted scale, found to be sensitive in an acute care setting	Acute care
Functional Ambulation Performance (FAP) Score (Nelson, et al., 1999)	A compilation of several ambulation skills, showed a similar ability to discriminate between fallers and nonfallers.	Community
Functional Reach Test (Duncan, Studenski, Chandler, & Prescott, 1992)	Balance test: the minimal distance a person can reach beyond arm's length in the horizontal plane while standing in a fixed base of support. If reach is 7.4 inches or less, considered high risk for falls.	Community
Morse Fall Scale (Morse, Morse, & Tylko, 1989) (O'Connell & Myers, 2002)	Includes history of falling, secondary diagnosis, ambulatory aid, intravenous therapy, gait, and mental status. Primarily designed and tested in acute care settings.	Acute care. Has also been tested in long-term care.
Primary Nurse's Clinical Judgment (Eagle et al., 1999)	Found by Eagle and colleagues to be as sensitive as the Morse Fall Scale and Functional Reach Test in predicting risk of falls.	Acute care
TURN 180 Simpson, Worsfold, Reilly, & Nye, 2002)	Gait and posture evaluation. People who require more than 4 steps to complete a 180-degree turn have an increased risk for falls.	Community

son, Worsfold, Reilly, & Nye, 2002). The Functional Ambulation Performance (FAP) score, a compilation of several ambulation skills, showed a similar ability to discriminate between fallers and nonfallers. Generally these two assessments are done by physical therapists, indicating the need for a multidisciplinary approach to assessing for risk of falls among the elderly (Nelson, et al., 1999).

Interventions to Prevent Falls

Findings of fall prevention programs were summarized using a meta-analysis of 12 studies. Overall, a 4% decrease in rate of falls was found

TABLE 13.3   Conley Scale

History

- On admission, history of falling in last 3 months (2)

Observation

- Impaired judgment/lack of safety awareness (3)
- Agitation (2)
- Impaired gait, shuffle/wide base, unsteady walk (1)

Direct Questions

- Do you ever experience dizziness or vertigo? (1)
- Do you ever wet or soil yourself on way to bathroom? (1)

Scoring: Score of 2 or greater or a fall during hospitalization should initiate fall prevention strategies.

From Conley, 1999. Reprinted with permission.

with fall prevention programs. The largest mean weighted effect size was reported with interventions that used a comprehensive risk assessment to individualize the intervention. A smaller effect size was reported with interventions that included exercise and risk modification; and the smallest effect was with exercise alone. In addition, only studies that followed the participants for at least 12 months demonstrated any effect on outcome (Hill-Westmoreland, Soeken, & Spellbring, 2002). Several evidence-based guidelines have been developed for prevention of falls in the elderly. The American Geriatrics Society, the British Geriatrics Society, and the American Academy of Orthopaedic Surgeons Panel on Falls Prevention (2001) developed one of the most comprehensive evidence-based guidelines for falls. An algorithm summarizing the assessment and management of falls begins with periodically asking all patients about falls in the past year (see Figure 13.3). No further intervention is required if there is no history of falls. If there has been a single fall, balance and gait should be evaluated. If there have been multiple falls or if the patient presents to a medical facility after a fall, a full fall evaluation is recommended with multifactoral interventions as indicated according to level and place of care: home, long-term care, or acute care (American Geriatrics Society, British Geriatrics

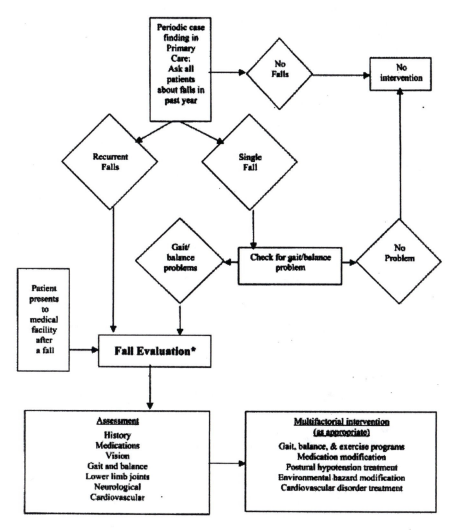

*See text for details

FIGURE 13.3 Algorithm summarizing the assessment and management of falls.

From American Geriatrics Society, et al., 2001. Reprinted with permission of Blackwell Publishing, Ltd.

Society, & American Academy of Orthopedic Surgeons, 2001). The following sections summarize the key points in preventing falls in each setting.

Key Points in Fall Prevention Intervention—in Community-Dwelling Elderly

Multifactoral assessment and interventions are more effective than any one individual intervention and should include, if indicated:

- Exercise, individually tailored, and combined with balance training such as T'ai Chi (Rubenstein, et al., 2000)
- Home assessment with safety improvements
- Group teaching on prevention of falls
- Use of assistive devices and proper shoes
- Assessment and management of medications, polypharmacy, and alcohol use
- Assessment and management of chronic health problems, especially cardiovascular and neuromuscular (Close, et al., 1999; Feder, Cryer, Donovan, & Carter, 2000; Gillespie, et al., 2001; Lightbody, Watkins, Leathley, Anil, & Lye, 2002; American Geriatrics Society, British Geriatrics Society, & American Academy of Orthopedic Surgeons, 2001; Steinweg, 1997).

Key Points in Fall Prevention Intervention—in Long-Term Care Settings

Multifactoral intervention should include:

- Staff education programs
- Gait training and advice on appropriate assistive devices such as canes and walkers. External hip protectors can be effective in reducing hip fractures, but compliance may be difficult (Parker, Gillespie, & Gillespie, 2001). Elders may reject assistive devices such as canes and walkers due to the social stigma, saying there is no need or that the cost is prohibitive (Aminzadeh & Edwards, 2001).
- Review and management of medications, especially psychotropic medications
- Toileting interventions
- Use of signage and/or name bands to identify high-risk patients (Jensen, Lundin-Olsson, Nyberg, & Gustafson, 2002; Lightbody, Watkins,

Leathley, Anil, & Lye, 2002; Mills, Waldron, Quigley, Stalhandske, & Weeks, 2003; American Medical Directors Association, 1998; Rubenstein, Powers, & MacLean, 2001; Society, et al., 2001).

Key Points in Fall Prevention Intervention—in Acute Care

Limited research and no evidence-based guidelines were found specific to reducing patient falls in acute care settings. The limited research mainly focused on identifying those at risk rather than on intervention. One researcher reported an extensive evaluation of factors related to falls in an acute care setting and described the interventions that were being instituted in response to the findings. However, outcomes had not been measured at the time of publication (Alcee, 2000). An attempt at a meta-analysis of outcomes of fall prevention programs in hospitals was inconclusive. Only three studies were found that met criteria for meta-analysis, and those were inconclusive (Oliver, Hopper, & Seed, 2000). Based on suggestions made by experts and risk factors in acute care, possible interventions to reduce falls in the acute care setting may include:

- Staff education and reorientation on fall risk assessment and intervention
- Attention to call bell, bed, and chair height
- Hourly rounds strictly enforced
- Visible signage in patient rooms and bright orange arm bands when patients are at risk for falls
- Develop and implement a fall investigation report form
- Regular toileting, or commode near bed
- Staff, patient, and family education and awareness program.

Quality Indicators for Management and Prevention of Falls

These quality indicators were based on research evidence, similar to the process for developing evidence-based guidelines. While they could be applied to any setting, they are based mainly on research in community-dwelling elderly and those in long-term care.

- Ask all vulnerable elders about falls at least once a year.
- Examine vulnerable elders at least once for gait and balance disturbances.

- If a vulnerable elder has reported two or more falls in the past year, complete a basic fall evaluation.
- If a vulnerable elder reports new or worsening difficulty with ambulation, balance, or mobility, there should be an evaluation with appropriate referral.
- An appropriate exercise program should be prescribed and the vulnerable elder should be evaluated for assistive devices if there is decreased balance or proprioception, or increased postural sway.
- If the vulnerable elder is found to have gait, strength, or endurance problems, an exercise program should be prescribed. (Rubenstein, et al., 2001)

RESTRAINTS

In the United States, restraints were once thought to be a way to prevent falls. However, the work of Strumpf and Evans (1998) has reversed that thinking. Strumpf and Evans examined long-term care institutions in Europe and found that restraints were practically never used. Moreover, there were actually fewer falls than were occurring in long-term care in the United States (Strumpf & Evans, 1998). Subsequent research in the United States has revealed that restraints actually cause more injuries than they prevent (Evans & Strumpf, 1990). In a matched case-control study, patients with orders for restraints were more likely to fall than patients without orders. However, having orders for restraints did not necessarily mean the restraints were being used at the time of the fall, and it was hypothesized that orders for restraints may have been written more frequently for those who were at greater risk of falling (Shorr, et al., 2002).

While restraints have not been shown to reduce the incidence of falls, there are multiple potentially harmful physical and psychological consequences of using restraints (Capezuti, Strumpf, Evans, Grisso, & Maislin, 1998; Evans & Strumpf, 1990; Strumpf & Evans, 1998). By restricting mobility, restraints may create for many elders the hazards of immobility, as well as confusion, agitation, incontinence, and emotional distress (Watson, 2002). Restraints can cause physical injury, even death. ("JCAHO warns of bedrail-related entrapment," 2002; "Restrained victim dies," 2002).

Since the Omnibus Budget Reconciliation Act (OBRA) of 1987, there has been a significant decrease in the use of restraints to prevent falls (U.S. Congress, 1987). OBRA emphasized patients' rights not to be restrained. The Joint Commission on Accreditation of Healthcare Organizations

(JCAHO) and the Health Care Financing Administration (HCFA) recently issued new guidelines that emphasize safety (Abrahamsen, 2001). The newer guidelines limit the use of restraints but more clearly define the situations in which restraints can be used temporarily. Both organizations recognize that restraints may be needed at certain times; however they recommend that restraints be used only in an emergency and with careful monitoring. The American Physical Therapy Association and the American Geriatrics Association have also issued position statements strongly advocating reduction and elimination of the use of restraints (American Geriatrics Society, 2002; Ciolek, 2000).

Reduction of Restraints

Restraints are typically applied because the individual exhibits challenging behavior such as trying to get out of bed unassisted when there is potential for falling or pulling at therapeutic tubes or lines. The first step is assessing the challenging behavior for the meaning and cause of the problem behavior. Identify possible solutions based on the assessment and select the least restrictive alternative. Possible solutions include treating the underlying physical disease, alleviating depression, alleviating pain and discomfort, modifying the environment, providing space and security, and reviewing medications for possible adjustment. Restraints should only be used as a last resort, only when potential benefits outweigh the potential harm, and only at the minimum level that ensures safety. If restraints must be used, apply them safely, limit the time in restraints, and recheck frequently for continued need of the restraints ("Physical restraint," 2002; Watson, 2002).

Key Points in Guidelines for the Reduction of Restraints

While restraints may not be eliminated totally, there are creative strategies to reduce their use. One evidence-based guideline for restraints was developed with the University of Iowa Gerontological Nursing Interventions Research Center (Ledford & Mentes, 1999). Another guide for restraint reduction, while not fully research-based, is very comprehensive. It includes several flow charts to aid in decision making about how to reduce the use of restraints (Colorado Foundation for Medical Care, 1998). Key points include:

- Restrain only if necessary for safety.
- Consider alternatives, for instance, dress the patient in mitts or sweat pants to reduce the possibility of pulling out a urinary catheter.

- If the patient is restless, evaluate the need for toileting.
- If restraints must be applied, be sure they are applied correctly so that the patient does not become entangled or suffer injury from the restraint chafing.
- Reassess frequently for possible injury from the restraint such as circulatory problems, possible change in patient status, and possible discontinuance of the restraint.

EXEMPLAR: "RESTRAINTS ARE EXTINCT"

Promoting a restraint-free environment in a not-for-profit tertiary care center was accomplished through a six-year continuous quality improvement initiative (Baggett & Powell, 2001). Gathering data was the first step. A chart review clearly demonstrated that restraint usage was higher than required by accreditation. Restraints were primarily being used to prevent falls and disruption of tubes and lines in patients with altered mental status. The results of a survey of the staff were plotted on a root cause analysis of reasons for restraints being used (see Figure 13.4). Some of the reasons for using restraints were: alternatives to restraints not available, outdated attitudes, outdated knowledge, fear of legal action, and bed alarms not in good repair. Based on this analysis, a plan was devised to provide the staff with adequate equipment and teach them how to use alternatives to restraints effectively. A 45-bed unit with a large geriatric population and a history of the largest number of restraints was selected for a trial implementation of the plan (Baggett & Powell, 2001).

The trial began with the development of protocols for fall prevention and for patients at risk of pulling out tubes and lines (Baggett & Powell, 2001). The Restraint Reduction Team considered well-known techniques as well as creative alternatives to restraints. One of the creative approaches for fall prevention was using deep cushions to make getting out of chairs difficult. A more basic approach to fall prevention was toileting every two hours to reduce the number of patients getting out of bed unaided. For patients who had trouble walking to the bathroom, bedside commodes were used. When the hospital did not own enough commodes, arrangements were made to rent them. The staff learned that by simply covering a site where there was a tube or line, the patient was less likely to disrupt the treatment. Staff attitude and knowledge about restraint reduction were addressed through education and involvement of the staff in developing and testing the strategies. At the completion of the 4-month trial, restraint

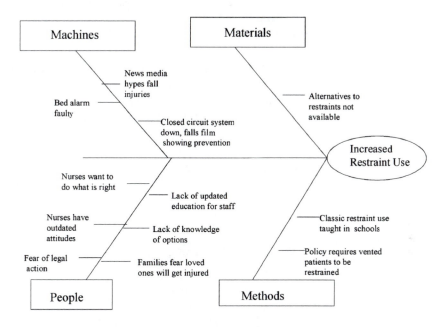

FIGURE 13.4   Restraint use root cause analysis.
From Baggett & Powell, 2001. Reprinted with permission of The Kendall™ Corporation.

usage had dropped by 80% on the trial unit. When the program was instituted hospital-wide, there was an overall reduction in restraint usage of 27%. The educational program has since become a permanent part of the hospital orientation and required annual competency skills. The name of the Restraint Release Committee was changed to RELEASE, for "Restraints Are Extinct Letting Each Achieve Safety for Everyone" (Baggett & Powell, 2001).

MEDICATION ERRORS AND ADVERSE DRUG EVENTS

The problems of medication errors and adverse drug events are especially salient for the elderly, in terms of incidence, preventability, and severity of outcomes. The incidence and preventability of adverse drug events was studied among noninstitutionalized older persons by examining Medicare enrollees in a multi-specialty group practice during a one-year period. Of the 1523 adverse drug events that were identified, 27% were considered preventable. The overall rate of adverse drug events was 50 per 1000 person/years, with a rate of 13.8 preventable events per 1000 person/years (Gurwitz, et al., 2003). A six-year, retrospective analysis of mortalities associated with medication errors reported to the Food and Drug Administration (FDA) revealed that nearly half of the deaths occurred in patients over 60 years of age, demonstrating that the consequences of medication errors are more severe in the elderly (Phillips, et al., 2001).

Risk for Medication Errors and Adverse Drug Events

As mentioned in the beginning of this chapter, multiple physiological and situational factors contribute to the risk of medication errors and adverse drug effects in the elderly and chronically ill. The major risks include: physical changes of aging and chronic disease that reduce the ability to break down and eliminate drugs, complex medical regimes related to the treatment of chronic illness, and polypharmacy. An expert panel reviewed the medications of a national sample of noninstitutionalized people over age 65 (N = 2455). The panel determined that up to 23% of the community-dwelling elderly were receiving potentially inappropriate medications, and 2.6% were receiving medications that the panel agreed should never be used. Risks for inappropriate medication use were poor health and taking more prescription medications (Zhan, et al., 2001). In another study, the most common factors in preventable adverse drug events were related to prescribing, monitoring, and patient adherence (Gurwitz, et al., 2003). In a study of 20 long-term care facilities, 40% of the residents were prescribed at least one inappropriate medication, and 10% were prescribed two inappropriate medications (Lombardi & Kennicutt, 2001). Adverse drug events were also found to be preventable among nursing home residents in a prospective study of adverse drug events among residents in 18 nursing homes. Being newly admitted to the nursing home, having multiple medical conditions, and taking multiple medications were identified in the study as risk factors for adverse drug events. High-risk medications were psychoactives, opioids, and anti-infectives (Field, et al., 2001).

In a study of home health care patients, two sets of criteria were used to evaluate the frequency of possible medication errors: Beers' Criteria that identify medications that experts have deemed generally inappropriate for older adults and Home Health Criteria that identify patterns of medication use and symptoms that indicate need for reevaluation of the medical regimen (see Table 13.4). Of the patients surveyed, nearly one-third had evidence of potential medication problems based on both sets of criteria. Patterns of potential medication problems that were identified by the Home Health Criteria included therapeutic duplication, over or undertreatment of hypertension, use of psychotropic medications despite a recent fall or development of confusion, and use of NSAIDS concurrently with anticoagulants (Meredith, et al., 2001).

Guidelines/Suggestions for Prevention of Medication Errors and Adverse Drug Events

Three main areas for addressing medication errors and adverse drug events are appropriate prescribing, monitoring for drug response, and appropriate administration, which includes both patient adherence and administration by staff. The elderly and those who suffer chronic disease are more sensitive to medication, and some medications are more likely to cause adverse reactions in these groups (Johnson, 2000). A panel of nationally recognized experts developed what are frequently referred to as Beers' Criteria for appropriate medication use by the elderly (Beers, 1997; Beers, Baran, & Frenia, 2000, 2001; Beers, Fink, & Beck, 1991; Beers, et al., 1992; Stuck, et al., 1994). These criteria, along with the Home Healthcare Criteria can be used as starting points for evaluating and making recommendations for adjustments of elderly clients' medication regimens (Brown, et al., 1998; Meredith, et al., 2001).

While no specific, evidence-based guidelines were found for the prevention of medication errors and adverse drug events in the elderly and chronically ill, several recommendations were found. For example, the American Medical Directors Association has published a "Multidisciplinary Medication Management Tool Kit," a multimedia approach to avoiding medication errors and adverse drug events in long-term care, available for order on the Internet (American Medical Directors Association, 2003). The existing criteria for appropriate medication use could be more widely implemented in consultation with pharmacists or geriatric nurse specialists to evaluate potential problems; however these criteria are based primarily on expert panels rather than extensive research. More pharmaceutical research is needed to establish a better knowledge base about what is appropriate medication prescribing for the elderly (Gurwitz & Rochon, 2002; Lombardi & Kennicutt, 2001). Technology could be used to apply the various criteria to medication prescription and to monitor outcomes

TABLE 13.4   Potential Medication Problems in Rank Order

Problem	Drug(s) Considered
1. Unnecessary therapeutic duplication	Top 100 drugs[1]
2. SBP/DBP ≥ 180/110 mm Hg	Antihypertensives[2]
3. Symptoms of confusion	Benzodiazepines, antidepressants, antipsychotics
4. Fall in past 3 months	Benzodiazepines, tricyclic antidepressants, antipsychotics
5. SBP ≤ 100 mm Hg	Antihypertensives[2], loop diuretics, nitrates
6. Symptoms of *orthostasis*	Antihypertensives[2], loop diuretics
7. Symptoms of *orthostasis*	Tricyclic antidepressants, antipsychotics
8. Pulse < 55 bpm	β-blockers, verapamil/diltiazem, thyroid replacement, digoxin
9. NSAID use with age ≥ 80 years	NSAIDs
10. NSAIDs with drugs increasing risk of gastrointestinal bleeding complications	NSAIDs with anticoagulants or oral corticosteroids
11. Warfarin and a newly started potentially interacting drug	Warfarin
12. Dose outside geriatric range	Top 100 drugs[1]
13. SBP/DBP ≥ 180/110 mm Hg	Antihypertensives with NSAIDs or oral corticosteroids
14. SBP/DBP ≤ 180/110 mm Hg	No treatment
15. NSAIDs with antiulcer drugs	NSAIDs with antiulcer drugs
16. Symptoms of digoxin toxicity	Digoxin
17. Symptom of poorly controlled heart failure	Diuretics, ACEIs, diltiazem, verapamil, beta-blockers, digoxin, nitrates
18. ACEI and angioedema or cough	ACEIs
19. Beta-blockers and obstructive lung disease	Beta-blockers
20. Pulse > 100	Tricyclic antidepressants, theophylline, Beta-agonists, thyroid replacement
21. Extrapyramidal symptoms	Antipsychotics, metoclopramide
22. Symptoms of anticholinergic toxicity	Multiple anticholinergic drugs
23. Poorly controlled angina	CCBs, beta-blockers, nitrates
24. Edema	Diuretics, ACEIs, diltiazem, verapamil, nifedipine, beta-blockers, nitrates, other antihypertensives[2]

TABLE 13.4   (continued)

Problem	Drug(s) Considered
25. Constipation	Verapamil, opioids
26. Dipyridamole absent artificial valve	Dipyridamole
27. Chlorpropamide and hypoglycemia symptoms	Chlorpropamide
28. Propoxyphene	Propoxyphene and propoxyphene-containing drugs

[1]Most commonly used medication in 1994 from the medication database of a large home health agency in Los Angeles (includes over-the-counter and prescribed drugs).
[2]Antihypertensives include diuretics, beta-blockers, ACEIs, CCBs, and others.
ACEI = angiotensin-converting enzyme inhibitor; bpm = beats per minute; CCB = calcium channel blocker; DBP = diastolic blood pressure; NSAID = nonsteroidal anti-inflammatory drug; SBP = systolic blood pressure.
Note: Rankings were tied for problems 1–5, 6–11, 12–13, 14–15, 16–22, and 24–27.
From Brown, et al., 1998. Copyright © 1998 by the American Pharmacy Association. Reprinted with permission.

(Eastman, 2002; Gurwitz & Rochon, 2002). Ensuring that medications are administered correctly is important. In acute and long-term care, proper identification of patients is imperative. If cognitive dysfunction is present, proper identification requires even more careful verification. For community-dwelling elderly and chronically ill, health education becomes one mechanism for promoting safe administration and management of medications. The FDA Consumer Magazine has published guidelines for the elderly lay public to manage medications (Williams, 1997).

Key Points in Medication Errors and Adverse Drug Events

- Monitor all medications, including over-the-counter and herbal supplements to eliminate duplications, monitor drug interactions and medications that are not recommended for elderly using guides or checklists such as Beers' Criteria or the Home Healthcare Criteria.
- Start with the lowest recommended dose and increase dosages slowly. Monitor for signs and symptoms of untoward effects of treatment.
- Use technology as described in Chapter 8. The Beers' Criteria or the Home Healthcare Criteria might be computerized and linked to the medication dispensing system.

- Locate relevant patient information at point of patient care—wristbands for identification and allergies.
- Community-dwelling elderly need sufficient education about safe management of medications, how to communicate with physicians about medications, and memory aids.

PRESSURE ULCERS

Pressure ulcers are significant across settings in rate of occurrence, influence on morbidity and mortality, and impact on health care costs. The occurrence of pressure ulcers varies greatly depending on the setting, case mix, and definition. In hospitals, pressure ulcers are reported to occur in 3.5% to 29.5% of acute care patients and 2.4% to 23% of long-term care residents (Agostini, Baker, & Bogardus, 2001b; Horn, et al., 2002). The identification of pressure ulcers in home health care is not as clear; estimates have been as low as 4% and as high as 25% (Bliss, 1998; Horn, et al., 2002). In addition to the pain and disfigurement caused by pressure ulcers, infection such as cellulites, osteomyelitis, and sepsis may result (Agostini, Baker, & Bogardus, 2001a, 2001b). Hospital-acquired pressure ulcers have been associated with a greater risk of death. However, in a recent study, after adjusting for predisposing factors such as nutritional and functional status, comorbidity, and other hospital complications, pressure ulcers were not associated with increased morbidity (Thomas, Goode, Tarquine, & Allman, 1996). The development of a pressure ulcer is associated with substantial increase in length of stay, hospital cost, and postdischarge resource use (Allman, Damiano, & Strauss, 1996; Allman, Goode, Burst, Bartolucci, & Thomas, 1999). Furthermore, lawsuits over the development of pressure ulcers add to the potentially avoidable financial burden of pressure ulcer development. For example, in a review of forty cases of litigation over pressure ulcers that occurred in residents of nursing homes, about half might have been prevented if standard guidelines had been followed for risk identification and prevention, a potential saving of over eleven million dollars (Goebel & Goebel, 1999). Thus, prevention of pressure ulcers could save money in addition to reducing morbidity and mortality.

Risks for Pressure Ulcers

Pressure ulcers develop when skin and supporting tissue break down, usually due to pressure being exerted over bony prominences or other hard surfaces for prolonged periods. The most commonly involved bony prominences are the sacrum, ischial tuberosity, grater trochanter, lateral malleolus, and heels. Often the largest area of tissue damage is nearest the bone. Generally pressure ulcers are rated or staged on a scale from 1 to 4, with 1 being nonblanchable, redness, induration, warmth or hardness of the skin, and 4 being full thickness skin loss and extensive tissue destruction to muscle, bone, and supporting structures (Agostini, et al., 2001b; Wiersema-Bryant, 2000).

In addition to prolonged pressure, mechanical risks for pressure ulcers include friction and shearing. Increased exposure to pressure may be due to immobility, reduced activity, or reduced sensitivity to pressure or pain. Friction damages skin by mechanical action and may be caused by skin rubbing on sheets or other surfaces. Shearing is the sliding of the parallel structures of skin and deeper tissue in opposite directions. Shearing occurs most commonly when the head of the bed is elevated and the individual slides downward. The skin stays in place due to resistance while the deeper tissue is pulled down with the body, stretching and occluding the blood vessels (Graff, Bryant, & Beinlich, 2000; Jay, 1995; Wiersema-Bryant, 2000).

There are multiple intrinsic factors that increase tissue vulnerability, explaining why some individuals risk skin breakdown after half an hour in one position while others can lie in the same position for several hours without tissue damage. Increased age, poor nutrition, limited mobility, and multiple chronic health problems are among the intrinsic factors that increase tissue vulnerability (Agostini, et al., 2001b; Bliss, 1998; Wiersema-Bryant, 2000).

Identifying Risk

The first step in implementing a program to prevent pressure ulcers is risk assessment in order to target preventive strategies most effectively. Several tools have been developed for identifying people who are at risk for developing pressure ulcers, the Norton Scale and the Braden Scale being the most widely recognized (Gooderidge, et al., 1998). The more recently developed Braden Scale (see Table 13.5) has been widely tested. The Braden Scale guides the assessment of six variables commonly associated with the development of pressure ulcers—sensory perception, moisture, activity, mobility, nutrition, friction, and shear. The variables are rated on a scale of 0 to 3 or 4, with higher scores denoting lower risk. A total score of 18

TABLE 13.5   Braden Scale

SENSORY PERCEPTION Ability to respond meaningfully to pressure-related discomfort	1. Completely Limited: Unresponsive (does not moan, flinch, or grasp) at painful stimuli, owing to diminished level of consciousness or sedation OR Limited ability to feel pain over most of body	2. Very Limited: Responds only to painful stimuli. Cannot communicate discomfort except by moaning or restlessness OR Has sensory impairment that limits the ability to feel pain or discomfort over half of body	3. Slightly Limited: Responds to verbal commands but cannot always communicate discomfort or the need to be turned OR Has some sensory impairment, which limits ability to feel pain or discomfort in 1 or 2 extremities.	4. No Impairment: Responds to verbal commands. Has no sensory deficit that would limit ability to feel or voice pain or discomfort
MOISTURE Degree to which skin is exposed to moisture	1. Constantly Moist: Skin is kept moist almost constantly by perspiration, urine, etc. Dampness is detected every time patient is moved or turned	2. Very Moist: Skin is often, but not always, moist. Linen must be changed at least once a shift	3. Occasionally Moist: Skin is occasionally moist, requiring an extra linen change approximately once a day	4. Rarely Moist: Skin is usually dry. Linen only requires changing at routine intervals
ACTIVITY Degree of physical activity	1. Bedfast: Confined to bed	2. Chairfast: Ability to walk severely limited or nonexistent. Cannot bear own weight and/or must be assisted into chair or wheelchair	3. Walks Occasionally: Walks occasionally during day, but for very short distances, with or without assistance. Spends majority of each shift in bed or chair	4. Walks Frequently: Walks outside the room at least twice a day and inside room at least once every 2 hours during waking hours

TABLE 13.5 *(continued)*

MOBILITY Ability to change and control body position	1. Completely Immobile: Does not make even slight changes in body or extremity position without assistance	2. Very Limited: Makes occasional slight changes in body or extremity position, but unable to make frequent or significant changes independently	3. Slightly Limited: Makes frequent though slight changes in body or extremity position independently	4. No Limitation: Makes major and frequent changes in position without assistance
NUTRITION Usual food intake pattern	1. Very Poor: Never eats a complete meal. Rarely eats more than 1/3 of any food offered. Eats 2 servings or less of protein (meat, or dairy products) per day. Takes fluids poorly. Does not take a liquid dietary supplement OR Is NPO and/or maintained on clear liquids or IVs for more than 5 days	2. Probably Inadequate: Rarely eats a complete meal and generally eats only about 1/2 of any food offered. Protein intake includes only 3 servings of meat or dairy products per day. Occasionally will take a dietary supplement. OR Receives less than optimum amount of liquid diet or tube feeding	3. Adequate: Eats over half of most meals. Eats a total of 4 servings of protein (meat, dairy products) each day. Occasionally will refuse a meal, but will usually take a supplement if offered. OR Is on a tube feeding or TPN regimen, which probably meets most of nutritional needs	4. Excellent: Eats most of every meal. Never refuses a meal. Usually eats a total of 4 or more serving of meat and dairy products. Occasionally eats between meals. Does not require supplementation.

(continued)

TABLE 13.5   *(continued)*

FRICTION AND SHEAR	1. Problem: Requires moderate to maximum assistance in moving. Complete lifting without sliding against sheets is impossible. Frequently slides down in bed or chair, requiring frequent repositioning with maximum assistance. Spasticity, contractures or agitation leads to almost constant friction.	2. Potential Problem: Moves feebly or requires minimum assistance. During a move, skin probably slides to some extent against sheets, chair, restraints, or other devices. Maintains relatively good position in chair or bed most of the time but occasionally slides down	3. No Apparent Problem: Moves in bed and in chair independently and has sufficient muscle strength to lift up completely during move. Maintains good position in bed or chair at all times

From Braden & Bergstrom, 1994. Copyright © 1994 John Wiley & Sons, Inc. Reprinted with permission.

or less indicates high risk for development of pressure ulcers (Bergquist, 2001; Bergstrom & Braden, 2002; Bergstrom, Braden, Kemp, Champagne, & Ruby, 1998; Braden & Bergstrom, 1994).

Rosenberg (2002) constructed a checklist for pressure ulcers that adds the dimensions of preventive strategies and client and caregiver knowledge and ability to participate in pressure ulcer prevention (see Figure 13.5). While this checklist has not been tested for predictive value and the items are not weighted, it appears to have particular value in community settings to guide the professional caregiver in assessing risk and need for teaching prevention strategies to patients and caregivers (Rosenberg, 2002).

Prevention of Pressure Ulcers

Numerous evidence-based guidelines have been developed for the prevention and treatment of pressure ulcers; however they have not been univer-

CHECKLIST FOR PRESSURE ULCER PREVENTION

Please put a check mark next to each item that applies. Check marks may indicate possible risk for skin disruption

PATIENT PHYSIOLOGICAL ASSESSMENT

—— Patient is bedridden
—— Patient is immobile
—— Patient has impaired mobility
—— Patient is dependent in transfer or mobility
—— Patient has diminished mentation or neurological impairment
—— Patient has undergone prolonged operation under general aesthesia
—— Patient has urinary incontinence
—— Patient has fecal incontinence
—— Patient has diabetes mellitus
—— Patient has peripheral vascular disease
—— Patient has spinal cord injury
—— Patient has metasatic carcinoma
—— Patient is advanced in age
—— Patient has history of smoking
—— Patient has had a recent weight loss.
—— Patient has had pressure ulcer in the past.
—— Patient has low diastolic pressure.
—— Patient is of male gender.

PREVENTION STRATEGIES

—— Patient not turned every hour or as needed.
—— Patient not on pressure support system.
—— Patient not ingesting dietary protein of 1.2 to 1.5 grams per kilogram of body weight per day.
—— Patient not exposed to complementary therapies like therapeutic touch
—— Caregiver/patient needs copy of risk scales, such as Braden.

AHCPR Web site: http.//www.ahcpr.gov/

CAREGIVER KNOWLEDGE ASSESSMENT

—— Caregiver not educated on complexity of pressure ulcers
—— Caregiver not educated regarding pressure ulcer prevention
—— Caregiver does not have knowledge of skin care
—— Caregiver feels skin care detection not a top priority
—— Caregiver not educated on who to call for help in assessing skin.
—— Caregiver not educated on where to obtain support system like foam overlay
—— Caregiver not educated on repositioning and how often (hourly?)
—— Caregiver does not have a copy of the AHCPR guidelines for pressure ulcer prevention and care
—— Caregiver has a copy of AHCPR guidelines but no knowledge of contents.
—— Caregiver has difficulty understanding AHCPR guidelines.

PATIENT KNOWLEDGE ASSESSMENT

—— Patient not able to assess own skin.
—— Patient not interested in preventing pressure ulcers.
—— Patient feels pressure ulcer occurrence inevitable
—— Patient feels skin detection not a top priority.
—— Patient feels caregiver not knowledgeable about pressure ulcers.
—— Caregiver or patient needs AHCPR guidelines.

AHCPR Clearinghouse: 1-800-358-9295

FIGURE 13.5   Checklist for pressure ulcer prevention.

From Rosenberg, 2002. Reprinted with permission of Slack, Inc.

sally implemented (Rutledge, Donaldson, & Pravikoff, 2000). (See chapter 4 for more on this topic). For instance, in a sample of 35 geographically diverse Veterans Affairs nursing homes, overall adherence to pressure ulcer prevention guidelines ranged from 29% to 51% (Saliba, et al., 2003). Guidelines have been developed under the auspices of several organizations, including the Agency for Health Care Policy and Research, the American Medical Directors Association, the Royal College of Nursing, and the University of Iowa Gerontological Nursing Interventions Center (Agency for Health Care Policy and Research, 1992; Folkdahl & Frantz, 2002; MacLean, 2003; Royal College of Nursing, 2001). In general, the guidelines focus on assessing for those at risk and implementing strategies aimed at the identified risk factors, particularly alleviation of pressure, shearing, nutritional and hydration deficits, and incontinence. One guideline was aimed at prevention of pressure ulcers specifically on heels. In justifying the need for specific attention to heels, the authors cited the increasing incidence of heel breakdown, the potential loss of the affected limb if a heel ulcer develops, and the uniqueness of the problem (Graff et al., 2000).

Relief of pressure and shearing was the focus of several studies and integrated reviews of pressure-alleviating devices. After reviewing 10 years of research on pressure reduction support surfaces, Whittemore (1998) concluded that the choice of support surface is complex, with level of patient risk being a major determinant. Foam overlays were found to be convenient and inexpensive, but efficacy depended on thickness and construction. Thus foam overlays were recommended for moderate risk. Replacement mattresses, relatively new at the time of Whittemore's review, were mattresses that appear similar to regular mattresses on the outside but are designed with internal construction to reduce pressure and provide support. Specific brands appeared to be comparable to foam overlays in preventing pressure ulcers in low- to moderate-risk clients. However several brands were no better than regular mattresses. Static air overlay devices reduced tissue-interface pressures sufficiently for most moderate to high-risk situations. Whittemore found conflicting results in the research concerning alternating air overlays, insufficient evidence to recommend the higher cost of alternating air over static air overlays. Specialty beds were recommended for extremely high-risk situations. Since there was some variability among brands of all types of devices, a trial program was suggested before an agency makes a major purchase (Whittemore, 1998).

Other support surface considerations include heat and moisture control, redistribution of pressure, reduction of friction, flammability, infection control, and service requirements. For example, foam is good for pressure redistribution, but may hold in heat and is not resistant to moisture, posing a possible infection control problem. Air overlays are good for reducing pressure if properly inflated and are resistant to moisture damage, but may hold in heat and cause sweating (Sprigle, 2000). Because the heel is so small in comparison to the pressure exerted, i.e., high pressure in pounds per square inch, preventing heel breakdown depends on dispersing the pressure over a larger area. There are multiple devices available to protect heels, but the least expensive is to suspend the heels off the bed with pillows. However, care must be taken to position the limb correctly to avoid contractures and undue pressure on the knee (Graff et al., 2000).

Key Points in Prevention of Pressure Ulcers

- A valid tool such as the Braden Scale should be used in the initial assessment to identify those who may be at risk. Reevaluation should be on a regular basis, depending on the level of risk and changes in health status.
- Skin should be inspected on a daily basis at minimum, more frequently in acute care settings, for those who are identified as being at risk.
- All bed-bound, wheelchair-bound persons and those who are unable to reposition themselves should be considered at risk.
- In addition to reducing and dispersing pressure, design the pressure ulcer prevention plan according to the specific risks identified.
- Specific strategies may include: keeping the skin clean, dry, and moisturized, and managing incontinence and nutritional supplements.
- Patients, families, caregivers, and staff should receive education about preventing pressure ulcers (Agency for Health Care Policy and Research, 1992; Agostini, et al., 2001b; Bates-Jensen, 2001; Mayo Foundation of Medical Education and Research, 2001; Royal College of Nursing, 2001; Wiersema-Bryant, 2000).

OTHER SAFETY PROBLEMS

Based on changes related to the aging process and chronic illness, other potential safety problems that should be considered in the elderly and chronically ill are nosocomial infections and fluid imbalance. The general principles in addressing these problems are similar to those discussed for the previous safety problems.

Nosocomial Infections

The elderly may be at greater risk for nosocomial infections due to loss of immune function with aging (Garrison, 2000). Similarly, immune function may be suppressed by some treatments for certain chronic illness. Scrupulous infection control measures such as handwashing are particularly important when providing care for the elderly and chronically ill in any setting. In acute care, nosocomial infections of all types have been found to occur more frequently in the elderly than in younger persons (Bochicchio, Joshi, Knorr, & Scalea, 2001; Stephan, Cheffi, & Bonnet, 2001). In long-term care, indwelling urinary catheters are a major culprit for infections (Garrison, 2000). Compared with other age groups, identified tuberculosis case rates are highest among the elderly. Frequently additional cases are only discovered at autopsy. The possible reactivation of childhood cases of tuberculosis must also be considered in the elderly. In settings such as long-term care where patients are in close contact, some form of screening for tuberculosis is highly recommended (Zevallos & Justman, 2003; Rajagopalan & Yoshikawa, 2000).

Another consideration for the prevention of infections in the elderly and chronically ill is immunizations. Guidelines for immunization of adults are available through the Centers for Disease Control (CDC) and other organizations. For the elderly and those who have chronic illnesses that put them at risk, pneumococcal and influenza vaccines are recommended in addition to updating the usual childhood immunizations. Health care providers that work with these vulnerable populations should also receive influenza immunization annually to avoid exposing this vulnerable population to potentially fatal influenza infection (Gardner, Pickering, Orenstein, Gershon, & Nichol, 2002).

Fluid Imbalance

The elderly and chronically ill are prone to both dehydration and overhydration. They are prone to dehydration in part due to not drinking enough fluid. As people age, they may not feel thirsty when dehydrated as a younger person would. Confusion, depression, delirium, and lack of independence in functional status may also cause a person to neglect taking in sufficient fluids. Medications such as diuretics, laxatives, and steroids that may be administered for certain chronic health problems can add to the potential for dehydration (Orr, 2000). In addition infection, vomiting, and diarrhea can precipitate dehydration. The elderly and chronically ill are often dependent on others for fluids, and the care providers may not understand the importance of providing fluids, or they may even mistakenly believe that withholding fluids is a treatment for incontinence.

Overhydration is another problem of fluid balance in the elderly and chronically ill. The aging process affects the ability to handle fluids, and chronic diseases such as congestive heart failure and renal disease are among the chronic illnesses that increase risk of overhydration. Thus, intravenous therapy must be managed carefully in the elderly and chronically ill (Gerontological Nursing Interventions Research Center, 1998).

The Gerontological Nursing Interventions Research Center and the American Medical Directors Association have each developed guidelines for fluid management for the elderly. Recommendations include attention to fluid intake in those who are at risk, offering fluids frequently if not at risk for overhydration, and monitoring for signs and symptoms of fluid imbalance (Gerontological Nursing Interventions Research Center, 1998; American Medical Directors Association, 2001).

AREAS FOR FURTHER RESEARCH

There are gaps in the research related to preventing and managing safety problems in the elderly and chronically ill. While preventing falls and pressure ulcers has been well studied in some settings, there is a smaller body of research related to preventing medication errors, adverse drug events, nosocomial infections, and fluid imbalances. The research on prevention of falls in acute care settings is weak. Evidence-based guidelines have been developed for most of these problems, but they have not been universally implemented. Further research is needed to focus on these gaps and to test best practices for implementing the guidelines.

CONCLUSION

The elderly and chronically ill are vulnerable to a variety of safety problems that may be preventable, or their incidence reduced in many cases. When those who are at risk are identified, preventive interventions can be targeted. As described in this chapter, there are many well-developed risk assessment tools for falls and pressure ulcers, and a number of criteria for potentially risky medications have been compiled. These tools can be used to identify who is at risk as well as to identify the most important strategies for prevention. Further, increasing staff sensitivity to the potential vulnerability of the elderly and chronically ill can add to the early identification of risk and the institution of preventive strategies.

WEB RESOURCES

Name of Resource/URL	*Description*
American Family Physicians http://www.aafp.org/x19449.xml	Index of algorithms, including evaluation of falls and treatment of osteoporosis
American Family Physicians Patient Information http://www.aafp.org/afp/20000401/2173ph.html	Patient information sheet—"What Can I Do To Prevent Falls?"
American Geriatrics Society http://www.americangeriatrics.org	See "Guidelines and Positions Statement" for • Use of restraints • Prevention of falls in the elderly • Adult immunization schedule
American Medical Directors Association http://www.amda.com/	Publishes selected articles from *Caring for the Aged,* a journal for long-term care practitioners. Several safety tool kits for long-term care are available: Multidisciplinary Medication Management, Pressure Ulcers, Immunizations, and Infection Control
Colorado Foundation for Medical Care with the Colorado Department of Public Health and Environment, Health Facilities Division http://www.cms.hhs.gov/cop/2e.pdf	Restraint reduction: Assessment and alternative help guide; includes several flow charts

National Center for Injury Prevention and Control, Centers for Disease Control and Prevention
http://www.cdc.gov/ncipc/factsheets/fallcost.htm

The cost of fall injuries among older adults

Oklahoma State Department of Health
http://www.health.state.ok.us/program/injury/updates/tbifalls.pdf

Fall-related traumatic brain injuries among adults 65 years of age and older: Oklahoma, 1992–1998

Omnibus Budget Reconciliation Act. Subtitle C: Nursing Home Reform Act. Public Law #100-203
http://www.ssa.gov/OP_Home/ssact/title19/1919.htm#c1

Residents' rights related to freedom from restraints

Safety Without Restraints
http://www.health.state.mn.us/divs/fpc/safety.htm

A new practice standard for safe care related to elimination of restraints

Veterans Administration Midwest Patient Safety Center of Inquiry
http://www.gapscenter.org/

VA GAPS Center: Getting at patient safety

Veterans Administration National Center for Patient Safety
http://www.patientsafety.gov/

Multiple safety resources including "Fall Prevention and Management," found under "NCPS Spotlight"

REFERENCES

Abrahamsen, C. (2001). Patient restraints: JCAHO and HCFA issue new restraint guidelines. *Nursing Management, 32*(12), 69–70, 72.

Agency for Health Care Policy and Research (AHCPR). (1992). *Pressure ulcers in adults: Prediction and prevention.* Rockville, MD: U.S. Department of Health and Human Services.

Agostini, J. V., Baker, D. I., & Bogardus, S. T. (2001a). Geriatric evaluation and management units for hospitalized patients. In K. G. Sojania, B. W. Duncan, K. M. McDonald, & R. M. Wachter (Eds.), *Making health care safer: A critical analysis of patient safety practices* (Vol. AHRQ Publication No. 01-E058, pp. 323–330). Rockville, MD: Agency for Healthcare Research and Quality.

Agostini, J. V., Baker, D. I., & Bogardus, S. T. (2001b). Prevention of pressure ulcers in older patients. In K. G. Sojania, B. W. Duncan, K. M. McDonald, & R. M. Wachter (Eds.), *Making health care safer: A critical analysis of patient safety practices*

(Vol. AHRQ Publication No. 01-E058, pp. 301–306). Rockville, MD: Agency for Healthcare Research and Quality.

Alcee, D. (2000). The experience of a community hospital in quantifying and reducing patient falls. *Journal of Nursing Care Quality, 14*(3), 43–53.

Allman, R. M., Damiano, A. M., & Strauss, M. J. (1996). Pressure ulcer status and post-discharge health care resource utilization among older adults with activity limitations. *Advances in Wound Care: Journal for Prevention and Healing, 9*(2), 38–44.

Allman, R. M., Goode, P. S., Burst, N., Bartolucci, A. A., & Thomas, D. R. (1999). Pressure ulcers, hospital complications, and disease severity: Impact on hospital costs and length of stay. *Advances in Wound Care: Journal for Prevention and Healing, 12*(1), 22–30.

American Geriatrics Society. (2002). *American Geriatrics Society position statement on restraint use.* Retrieved April 22, 2003, from http://www.americangeriatrics.org/products/positionpapers/restraintsupdate.shtml

American Geriatrics Society, British Geriatrics Society, & American Academy of Orthopedic Surgeons. (2001). Guideline for the prevention of falls in older persons. *Journal of the American Geriatrics Society, 49*(5), 664–672.

American Medical Directors Association. (1998). *Falls and fall risk.* Columbia, MD: American Medical Directors Association.

American Medical Directors Association. (2001). *Dehydration and fluid maintenance.* Columbia, MD: American Medical Directors Association.

American Medical Directors Association. (2003). *Multidisciplinary medication management tool kit.* Retrieved March 15, 2003, from http://www.amda.com/info/ltc/m3toolkit.htm

Aminzadeh, F., & Edwards, N. (2001). Exploring seniors' views on the use of assistive devices in fall prevention. *Public Health Nursing, 15*(4), 297–304.

Arking, R. (1998). *Biology of aging* (2nd ed.). Sunderland, MA: Sinauer Associates.

Ashburn, A., Stack, E., Pickering, R. M., & Ward, C. D. (2001). A community-dwelling sample of people with Parkinson's disease: Characteristics of fallers and non-fallers. *Age and Ageing, 30*(1), 47–52.

Baggett, D., & Powell, R. (2001). Moving toward a restraint-free environment in the acute care setting. *Untie the elderly, 13*(2), 1–5.

Bates-Jensen, B. M. (2001). Quality indicators for prevention and management of pressure ulcers in vulnerable elders. *Annals of Internal Medicine, 135*, 744–751.

Beers, M. H. (1997). Explicit criteria for determining potentially inappropriate medication use by the elderly: An update. *Archives of Internal Medicine, 157*, 1531–1536.

Beers, M. H., Baran, R. W., & Frenia, K. (2000). Drugs and the elderly, part 1: The problems facing managed care. *American Journal of Managed Care, 6*, 1313–1320.

Beers, M. H., Baran, R. W., & Frenia, K. (2001). Drugs and the elderly, part 2: Strategies for improving prescribing in a managed care environment. *American Journal of Managed Care, 7*(1), 69–72.

Beers, M. H., Fink, A., & Beck, J. C. (1991). Screening recommendations for the elderly. *American Journal of Public Health, 81*, 1131–1140.

Beers, M. H., Ouslander, J. G., Fingold, S. F., Morgenstern, H., Ruben, D. B., Rogers, W., et al. (1992). Inappropriate medication prescribing in skilled-nursing facilities. *Annals of Internal Medicine, 117*, 684–689.

Bergquist, S. (2001). Subscales, subscores, or summative score: Evaluating the contribution of Braden Scale items for predicting pressure ulcer risk in older adults receiving home health care. *Journal of WOCN, 28,* 279–289.

Bergstrom, N., & Braden, B. J. (2002). Predictive value of the Braden Scale among black and white subjects. *Nursing Research, 51,* 398–403.

Bergstrom, N., Braden, B. J., Kemp, M., Champagne, M., & Ruby, E. (1998). Predicting pressure ulcer risk: A multisite study of the predictive value of the Braden Scale. *Nursing Research, 47,* 261–269.

Bliss, M. R. (1998). Prevalence, etiology, and prevention of pressure sores. Part I: Prevalence and etiology. *Clinical Geriatrics, 1,* 16, 18, 21–22.

Bochicchio, G. V., Joshi, M., Knorr, K. M., & Scalea, T. M. (2001). Impact of nosocomial infections in trauma: Does age make a difference? *Journal of Trauma: Injury, Infection, and Critical Care, 50,* 612–619.

Braden, B. J., & Bergstrom, N. (1994). Predictive validity of the Braden Scale for pressure sore risk in a nursing home population. *Research in Nursing and Health, 17,* 459–470.

Brown, N. J., Griffin, M. R., Ray, W. A., Meredith, S., Beers, M. H., Marren, J., et al. (1998). A model for improving medication use in home health care patients. *Journal of American Pharmacy Association, 38,* 696–702.

Buri, H., Picton, J., & Dawson, P. (2000). Perceptual dysfunction in elderly people with cognitive impairment: A risk factor for falls? *British Journal of Occupational Therapy, 63,* 248–253.

Capezuti, E., Strumpf, N. E., Evans, L. K., Grisso, J. A., & Maislin, G. (1998). The relationship between physical restraint removal and falls and injuries among nursing home residents. *Journals of Gerontology, 53A*(1), M47–M52.

Ciolek, C. H. (2000). American Physical Therapy Association's recent initiatives in restraint reduction. *Untie the elderly, 12*(1), 1–5.

Close, J., Ellis, M., Hooper, R., Glucksman, E., Jackson, S., & Swift, C. (1999). Prevention of falls in the elderly trial (PROFET): A randomized controlled trial. *The Lancet, 353,* 93–97.

Colorado Foundation for Medical Care. (1998). *Restraint reduction: Assessment and alternative help guide.* Retrieved April 22, 2003, from http://www.cms.hhs.gov/cop/2e.pdf

Conley, D. (1999). The challenge of predicting patients at risk for falling: Development of the Conley Scale. *Medsurg Nursing, 8,* 348–355.

Conner-Kerr, T., & Templeton, M. S. (2002). Chronic fall risk among aged individuals with type 2 diabetes. *Ostomy/Wound Management, 48*(3), 28–32.

Donald, I. P., & Bulpitt, C. J. (1999). The prognosis of falls in elderly people living at home. *Age and Ageing, 28,* 121–125.

Duncan, B. W., Studenski, S., Chandler, J., & Prescott, B. (1992). Functional reach: A new clinical measure of balance. *Journals of Gerontology, 45,* M192–M197.

Eagle, D. J., Salama, S., Whitman, D., Evans, L. A., Ho, W., & Olde, J. (1999). Comparison of three instruments in predicting accidental falls in selected inpatients in a general teaching hospital. *Journal of Gerontological Nursing, 25,* 40–45.

Eastman, P. (2002). Call to action: Reduce inappropriate drug use in elderly. *Caring for the Ages, 3*(3), 1, 28–30.

Evans, L. K., & Strumpf, N. E. (1990). Myths about elder restraint. *Image Journal of Nursing Scholarship, 22,* 124–128.

Feder, G., Cryer, C., Donovan, S., & Carter, Y. (2000). Guidelines for the prevention of falls in people over 65. *British Medical Journal, 321,* 1007–1011.

Field, T. S., Gurwitz, J. H., Avorn, J., McCormick, D., Jain, S., Eckler, M., et al. (2001). Risk factors for adverse drug events among nursing home residents. *Archives of Internal Medicine, 161,* 1629–1634.

Folkdahl, B. A., & Frantz, R. A. (2002). *Prevention of pressure ulcers.* Iowa City, IA: University of Iowa.

Fuller, G. F. (2000). Falls in the elderly. *American Family Physician, 61,* 2159–2168, 2173–2174.

Gardner, P., Pickering, L. K., Orenstein, W. A., Gershol, A. A., & Nichol, K. L. (2002). Guidelines for quality standards for immunization. *Clinical Infectious Diseases, 35,* 503–511.

Garrison, T. M. (2000). Infection. In A. G. Leuckenotte (Ed.), *Gerontologic nursing.* St. Louis: Mosby.

Gerontological Nursing Interventions Research Center. (1998). *Hydration management* (Guideline). Iowa City, IA: University of Iowa.

Gillespie, L. D., Gillespie, W. J., Robertson, M. C., Lamb, S. E., Cumming, R. G., & Rowe, B. H. (2001). Interventions for preventing falls in elderly people. *Cochrane Database for Systematic Reviews.* Retrieved August 19, 2003, from http://www.cochrane.org/

Goebel, R. H., & Goebel, M. R. (1999). Clinical practice guidelines for pressure ulcer prevention can prevent malpractice lawsuits in older patients. *Journal of Wound, Ostomy, and Continence Nursing, 26,* 175–184.

Gooderidge, D. M., Sloan, J. A., LeDoyen, Y. M., McKenzie, J., Knight, W. E., & Gayari, M. (1998). Risk-assessment scores, prevention strategies, and the incidence of pressure ulcers among the elderly in four Canadian health-care facilities. *Canadian Journal of Nursing Research, 30*(2), 23–44.

Graff, M. K., Bryant, J., & Beinlich, N. (2000). Preventing heel breakdown. *Orthopaedic Nursing, 19*(5), 63–70.

Gurwitz, J. H., Field, T. S., Harrold, L. R., Rothschild, J., Debellis, K., Seger, A. C., et al. (2003). Incidence and preventability of adverse drug events among older persons in the ambulatory setting. *Journal of the American Medical Association, 289,* 1154–1156.

Gurwitz, J. H., & Rochon, P. (2002). Improving the quality of medication use in elderly patients: A not so simple prescription. *Archives of Internal Medicine, 162,* 1670–1672.

Hausdorff, J. M., Rios, D. A., & Edelberg, H. K. (2001). Gait variability and fall risk in community-living older adults: A 1-year prospective study. *Archives of Physical Medicine and Rehabilitation, 82,* 1051–1056.

Hill-Westmoreland, E. E., Soeken, K., & Spellbring, A. M. (2002). A meta-analysis of fall prevention programs for the elderly: How effective are they? *Nursing Research, 51,* 1–8.

Horn, S. D., Bender, S. A., Bergstrom, N., Cook, A. S., Ferguson, M. L., Rimmasch, H. L., et al. (2002). Description of the National Pressure Ulcer Long-Term Care Study. *Journal of the American Geriatrics Society, 50,* 1816–1825.

Jay, R. (1995). Pressure and shear: Their effects on support surface choice. *Ostomy/ Wound Management, 41*(8), 36–38.

JCAHO warns of bedrail-related entrapment. (2002). *Healthcare Risk Management, 24,* 130–131.

Jensen, J., Lundin-Olsson, L., Nyberg, L., & Gustafson, Y. (2002). Fall and injury prevention in older people living in residential care facilities: A cluster randomized trial. *Annals of Internal Medicine, 136,* 733–741.

Johnson, J. F. (2000). Pharmacologic management. In A. Luekenotte (Ed.), *Gerontologic nursing* (2nd ed., pp. 435–447). St. Louis: Mosby.

Laird, R. D., Studenski, S., Perera, S., & Wallace, D. (2001). Fall history is an independent predictor of adverse health outcomes and utilization in the elderly. *American Journal of Managed Care, 7,* 1133–1138.

Ledford, L., & Mentes, J. (1999). *Restraints.* Iowa City, IA: University of.

Lightbody, E., Watkins, C., Leathley, M., Anil, S., & Lye, M. (2002). Evaluation of a nurse-led falls prevention programme versus usual care: A randomized controlled trial. *Age and Ageing, 31,* 203–211.

Lombardi, T. P., & Kennicutt, J. D. (2001). Promotion of a safe medication environment: Focus on the elderly and residents of long-term care facilities. *Medscape Pharmacists, 2*(1).

Luekenotte, A. (2000a). Overview of gerontologic nursing. In A. Luekenotte (Ed.), *Gerontologic nursing* (2nd ed., pp. 1–33). St. Louis: Mosby.

Luekenotte, A. (Ed.) (2000b). *Gerontologic nursing* (2nd ed.). St. Louis: Mosby.

MacLean, D. S. (2003). Preventing and managing pressure sores. *Caring for the Aged, 4*(3), 34–37.

Mayo Foundation of Medical Education and Research. (2001). *Pressure ulcers: Prevention and management.* Retrieved April 10, 2003, from http://www.mayo.edu/geriatrics-rst/PU.html

Meiner, S. E., & Miceli, D. G. (2000). Safety. In A. Luekenotte (Ed.), *Gerontologic nursing* (2nd ed., pp. 232–255). St. Louis: Mosby.

Meredith, S., Feldman, P. H., Frey, D., Hall, K., Arnold, K., Brown, N. J., et al. (2001). Possible medication errors in home healthcare patients. *Journal of the American Geriatrics Society, 49,* 719–724.

Mills, P. D., Waldron, J., Quigley, P. A., Stalhandske, E., & Weeks, W. B. (2003). *Reducing falls and injuries due to falls in the VA system.* Paper presented at Department of Veterans Affairs, Veterans Health Administration National Center for Patient Safety.

Morse, J. M., Morse, R. M., & Tylko, S. J. (1989). Development of a scale to identify the fall-prone patient. *Canadian Journal on Aging, 8,* 866–876.

National Center for Injury Prevention and Control (NCIP). (2000a). *The cost of fall injuries among older adults.* Retrieved February 28, 2003, from http://www.cdc.gov/ncipc/factsheets/fallcost.htm

National Center for Injury Prevention and Control (NCIP). (2000b). *Falls and hip fractures among older adults.* Retrieved April 22, 2003, from http://www.cdc.gov/ncipc/factsheets/falls.htm

Nelson, A. J., Certo, L. J., Lembo, L. S., Lopez, D. A., Manfredonia, E. F., Vanichpong, S. K., et al. (1999). The functional ambulation performance of elderly fallers and non-fallers walking at their preferred velocity. *NeuroRehabilitation, 13,* 141–146.

O'Connell, B., & Myers, H. (2002). The sensitivity and specificity of the Morse Fall Scale in an acute care setting. *Journal of Clinical Nursing, 11*(1), 134–136.

Oliver, D., Hopper, A., & Seed, P. (2000). Do hospital fall prevention programs work? A systematic review. *Journal of the American Geriatrics Society, 48*, 1679–1689.

Orr, M. E. (2000). Nutrition. In A. Luekenotte (Ed.), *Gerontologic nursing* (2nd ed., pp. 181–198). St. Louis: Mosby.

Parker, M. J., Gillespie, L. D., & Gillespie, W. J. (2003). Hip protectors for preventing hip fractures in the elderly. *Cochrane Library*. Retrieved August 18, 2003, from http://www.cochrane.org/cochrane/revabstr/AB001255.htm

Perell, K. L., Nelson, A., Goldman, R. L., Luther, S. L., Prieto-Lewis, N., & Rubenstein, L. Z. (2001). Fall risk assessment measures: An analytic review. *Journals of Gerontology, 56A*, M761–M766.

Phillips, J., Beam, S., Brinker, A., Holquist, C., Honig, P., Lee, L. Y., et al. (2001). Analysis of mortalities associated with medication errors. *American Journal of Health-System Pharmacy, 58*, 1824–1829.

Physical restraint—Part 1: Use in acute and residential care facilities. (2002). *Best Practice, 6*(3), 1–6.

Restrained victim dies: Confidential settlements. (2002). *Healthcare Risk Management, 24*(4), 3–4.

Rajagopalan, S., & Yoshikawa, T. T. (2000). Topics in long-term care: Tuberculosis in long-term-care facilities. *Infection Control and Hospital Epidemiology, 21*, 611–615.

Rosenberg, C. J. (2002). Assessment: New checklist for pressure ulcer prevention. *Journal of Gerontological Nursing, 28*(8), 7–12.

Royal College of Nursing. (2001). *Pressure ulcer risk assessment and prevention*. London: Royal College of Nursing.

Rubenstein, L. Z., Josephson, K. R., Trueblood, P. R., Loy, S., Harker, J. O., Pietruszka, F. M., et al. (2000). Effects of a group exercise program on strength, mobility, and falls among fall-prone elderly men. *Journals of Gerontology, 55A*, M317–M321.

Rubenstein, L. Z., Powers, C. M., & MacLean, C. H. (2001). Quality indicators for the management and prevention of falls and mobility problems in vulnerable elders. *Annals of Internal Medicine, 135*, 686–693.

Rutledge, D. N., Donaldson, N. E., & Pravikoff, D. S. (2000). Protection of skin integrity: Progress in pressure ulcer prevention since the AHCPR 1992 guidelines. *Online Journal of Clinical Innovations, 15*(3), 1–67.

Saliba, D., Rubenstein, L. V., Simon, B., Hickey, E., Ferrell, B., Czarnowski, E., et al. (2003). Adherence to pressure ulcer prevention guidelines: Implications for nursing home quality. *Journal of the American Geriatrics Society, 51*, 56–62.

Shorr, R. I., Guillen, M. K., Rosenblatt, L. C., Walker, K., Caudle, C. E., & Kritchevsky, S. B. (2002). Restraint use, restraint orders, and the risk of falls in hospitalized patients. *Journal of the American Geriatrics Society, 50*, 526–529.

Simpson, J. M., Worsfold, C., Reilly, E., & Nye, N. (2002). A standard procedure for using TURN180: Testing dynamic postural stability among elderly people. *Physiotherapy, 88*, 342–353.

Sprigle, S. (2000). Effects of forces and the selection of support surfaces. *Topics in Geriatric Rehabilitation, 16*(2), 47–62.

Steinweg, K. K. (1997). The changing approach to falls in the elderly. *American Academy of Family Physicians, 56,* 1815–1822.

Stephan, F., Cheffi, A., & Bonnet, F. (2001). Nosocomial infections and outcome of critically ill elderly patients after surgery. *Anesthesiology, 94,* 407–414.

Strumpf, N. E., & Evans, L. K. (1998). Achieving restraint-free care. In N. E. Strumpf (Ed.), *Restraint-free care: Individualized approaches for frail elders* (pp. 1–19). New York: Springer Publishing.

Stuck, A. E., Beers, M. H., Steiner, A., Aronow, H. U., Rubenstein, L. Z., & Beck, J. C. (1994). Inappropriate medication use in community-residing older persons. *Archives of Internal Medicine, 154,* 2195–2200.

Thomas, D. R., Goode, P. S., Tarquine, P. H., & Allman, R. M. (1996). Hospital-acquired pressure ulcers and risk of death. *Journal of the American Geriatrics Society, 44,* 1435–1440.

U.S. Congress. (1987). Omnibus Budget Reconciliation Act. Subtitle C: Nursing home reform act. Public Law #100-203. Retrieved April 22, 2003, from http://www.ssa.gov/OP_Home/ssact/title19/1919.htm#c1

Watson, R. (2002). Assessing the need for restraint in older people. *Nursing Older People, 14*(4), 31–32.

Whittemore, R. (1998). Pressure-reduction support surfaces: A review of the literature. *Journal of WOCN, 25*(1), 6–25.

Wiersema-Bryant, L. (2000). Integumentary system. In A. Luekenotte (Ed.), *Gerontologic nursing* (2nd ed., pp. 655–694). St. Louis: Mosby.

Williams, R. D. (1997). Medications and older adults. *U.S. Food and Drug Administration, FDA Consumer Magazine.* Retrieved March 5, 2003, from http://www.fda.gov/fdac/features/1997/697_old.html

Zevallos, M., & Justman, J. E. (2003). Tuberculosis in the elderly. *Clinics in Geriatric Medicine, 19,* 121–138.

Zhan, C., Sangl, J., Bierman, A. S., Miller, M. R., Friedman, B., Wickizer, S. W., et al. (2001). Potentially inappropriate medication use in community-dwelling elderly: Findings from the 1996 Medical Expenditure Panel survey. *Journal of the American Medical Association, 286,* 2823–2829, 2883–2884.

Chapter 14

Patient Safety in Behavioral Health

Christy L. Beaudin

INTRODUCTION

In 1998, there were nearly 11 million episodes of treatment in mental health organizations—24% were in 24-hour hospital services and 76% were in less than 24-hour hospital services (Mandescheid, et al., 2001). The volume of services underscores the need for effective strategies to reduce errors and ensure patient safety in mental health and substance abuse services. This requires an integrated and coordinated approach to synthesize knowledge and experience. Behavioral health care organizations and providers can encourage learning about what constitutes a potential or actual error, promote internal reporting of what has been found, take actions to reduce risk, and focus on process and system improvement to minimize individual blame. Even though research is scarce, there is information available to inform the development of initiatives targeting the reduction of errors, regardless of treatment setting. Much has been written on risk management, especially regarding the assessment of a person's level of suicide risk. The failure to detect suicide risk and take appropriate action is one of the most prevalent and preventable clinical errors in behavioral health care.

While there are effective treatments for mental health and substance use disorders, the diagnosis and treatment of persons at risk for depression or suicide may be untimely or unavailable. According to the Agency for Healthcare Research and Quality (AHRQ) (2002), the following are current mental health concerns impacting the safety and welfare of Americans:

- Suicide is the third leading cause of death among adolescents in the United States (U.S.)
- About 22% of Americans age 18 and older suffer from mental disorders that interfere with the productivity and enjoyment of life, with sequelae of disability and death
- About 6–10% of persons treated in primary care settings have depression, but it is often undetected
- More than 50% of patients suffering from schizophrenia do not receive proper doses of antipsychotic medications or appropriate psychosocial interventions.

While movement has occurred in general health services, priorities have yet to be established at a national level for reducing medical errors and improving patient safety in behavioral health care. Information is difficult to locate about patient safety practices or effective interventions across the health care continuum. This is confounded by the deficiencies in integration between the public sector programs (Medicaid, Medicare, Veterans Benefits, Federal Mental Health Services Funding, Institutions for the Mentally Diseased (IMDs), Community Reinvestment, Dual-Diagnosis Funding, and Developmental Disabilities) and private sector providers (primarily employer-sponsored programs with fee-for-service and managed care arrangements). Behavioral health care organizations and providers need to foster a culture of safety, but the absence of information makes it difficult to identify appropriate interventions and anticipate outcomes when systemic change is desired. What evidence-based patient safety behavioral health information is available to health care practitioners and organizations?

Quality improvement (QI) offers the opportunity to apply known mechanisms for promoting patient safety. Any behavioral health provider, organization, or delivery system can strive to be *highly reliable* with an exemplary track record for patient safety (see chapter 1). This can be accomplished through analyses of errors, which reveal organizational failures and technical failures related to system performance, as well as human limitations related to human behavior (Pizzi, Goldfarb, & Nash, 2001).

This chapter addresses strategies, tactics, and opportunities for establishing, maintaining, and/or improving patient safety in behavioral health. The current state of behavioral health is discussed and approaches to addressing safety needs in everyday behavioral health practice are described. Exemplars are provided.

CURRENT STATE OF BEHAVIORAL HEALTH SAFETY PRACTICES

The treatment of mental health and substance use disorders frequently involves different types of agencies and professionals, not just those from the behavioral health delivery system. The array can include traditional medical settings, schools, agencies for the developmentally disabled, correctional facilities, and a multitude of professionals such as psychiatrists, psychologists, masters prepared therapists, primary care and specialty providers, teachers, occupational and speech therapists, judges, and court advocates. An additional layer is the third-party payer. And because a mental health or substance use disorder may not be as discrete as a coronary artery bypass graft surgical procedure, the boundaries for errors and root cause analysis are fluid. Finding the root cause(s) of an error in behavioral health treatment then becomes relative to:

- Setting: community or institutional
- Intent: the provider (clinician, facility, or agency) rendering treatment, support or intervention
- Time: current versus past; unfolding of error over time
- Person: age, gender, race/ethnicity, culture, and underlying condition
- Circumstance: precipitating factors to current episode; chronic or acute mental health disorder

Successful root cause analysis (RCA) cannot occur without acknowledging assumptions that underlie the treatment of behavioral health disorders—assumptions that have been influenced by the history of medicine and human factors, such as biological, psychological, social, and cultural (Paget, 1988; Institute of Medicine [IOM], 2002b). These assumptions envelope clinical practice and include:

- Illness is the basis for the relationship between the patient/person and the entities responsible for treatment (e.g., payers and providers)
- Clinicians work with knowledge-based probabilities and it is probability of a certain outcome that drives action (e.g., use of the *Diagnostic Statistical Manual IV-R* [*DSM-IV-TR*™] APA, 2000)

- Mistakes and errors have potential to unfold over time (e.g., persons with serious and persistent mental disorders, misdiagnosis of conditions associated with aging)
- Remedies for errors are often sought through jurisprudence (e.g., negligence, breach of confidentiality, involuntary hospitalizations)
- The language of disorders (i.e., *DSM-IV-TR*™) and the information/evidence collected (assessment) and interpreted to determine actions (treatment plan) occurs in a routine and similar manner, regardless of setting or type of treating clinician
- Clinical diagnosis and treatment errors are inevitable

Acknowledging these assumptions is important when using RCA in different treatment settings. One source of information about errors in settings can be found in the Joint Commission for Accreditation of Healthcare Organizations (JCAHO) sentinel event trend analysis. Behavioral health treatment settings are most at risk for sentinel events after general hospitals, in the following order: psychiatric hospitals, psychiatric units, and outpatient behavioral health (JCAHO, 2003).

Safety in behavioral health is confounded by the fact that unlike infectious diseases or surgical procedures, there are no laboratory tests to be performed resulting in a definitive diagnosis and treatment approach found in biomedicine. Discovering pathology and acting on it does not neatly fit a classification system. While the *DSM-IV-TR*™ serves as the professional guide for determining a diagnosis, it serves more as clinical reassurance and reimbursement tool than a framework for driving treatment decisions. For example, absent are parameters to promote safe treatment such as an appropriate length of stay in an inpatient facility for mania, the number of outpatient sessions optimal for treating depression, or the most effective medication/combination of medications to treat schizophrenia.

CURRENT SAFETY AND ERROR REDUCTION ACTIVITIES

In behavioral health, crisis looms when errors are made—health care costs increase, loss of life and/or litigation ensue, and an *individual's* freedom may be lost (i.e., jail detention, involuntary hospitalization, or unnecessary use of physical restraints). The deconstruction of an error surely influences any subsequent action taken by a clinician, facility, or health plan. Learning opportunities may be lost when the approach is blame versus RCA or failure mode and effects analysis (FMEA). See Table 14.1 for a summary of error types by treatment setting and possible strategies to minimize risk of occurrence.

Safety Through Regulation and Accreditation

Regulation and accreditation have probably been the most influential in establishing practice standards for patient safety in behavioral health. Regulation related to mental health commenced in the late 1950s and continues today. Starting with the Community Mental Health Services Act of 1963, attention to public policy in mental health services began to shift. With a focus on deinstitutionalization, Congress moved to address major problems of persons with mental illness. While the Community Mental Health Centers proliferated, "the interests of persons with severe and long-term mental illnesses—clearly the group with the most formidable problems—slowly receded into the background" (Gerald, 2001). Through the 1970s, deinstitutionalization created safety concerns as many persons with mental illness were being discharged to community settings without adequate support. In 1980, Congress passed the Mental Health Systems Act that provided an outline for a national system to ensure the availability of both care and treatment in community settings, but its provisions became moot with the Omnibus Reconciliation Act (Grob, 1994).

The Americans with Disabilities Act (ADA) (42 U.S.C. §§ 12101–12213) was signed into law on July 26, 1990. The ADA is designed to protect people with disabilities and integrate them fully into the mainstream of American life. It protects people with a history of current disability, people deemed by others to be disabled, and those who encounter discrimination on the basis of an association with a person who has a disability. The ADA explicitly includes people with mental disabilities, including individuals with psychiatric impairments. It prohibits discrimination in employment (Title I), in the provision of state and local government programs, services, and benefits (Title II), and by private businesses and other entities that operate places of "public accommodation" (Title III) (Bazelon Center, 2003). All of these protections are important to health care, social services, and employment. On March 28, 1997, the Equal Employment Opportunity Commission (EEOC) released policy guidance concerning persons with psychiatric disabilities and the ADA.

In 1996, Congress passed the Mental Health Parity Act (42 USCS § 300 gg–5), which took effect January 1, 1998. The law provides for mandated

TABLE 14.1 Errors and Risk Management Strategies in the Behavioral Health Treatment Setting

Treatment Setting*	Error	Strategy for risk management
Acute inpatient Partial hospital Outpatient Residential treatment	Environmental • Contraband • Elopement • Security of facilities (e.g., elopement) • Cooking and exercise equipment	• Environmental safety checks • Unit design
Acute inpatient Partial hospital Outpatient Residential treatment	• Suicide attempt • Successful suicide	• Environmental considerations such as break-away bars and location of nurse's station • Staffing levels • Policies and procedures • Workforce education and training • Root Cause Analysis (RCA) • Debriefings
Acute inpatient Emergency Partial hospital Outpatient Residential treatment	Psychiatric Assaults (physical and sexual) • Patient-Patient • Patient-Staff • Staff-Patient	• Policies and procedures • Program structure (e.g., Assaulted Staff Action Program, coping skills) • Workforce training • Credentialing/peer review
Emergency Acute inpatient Partial hospital Residential treatment	Seclusion and restraint (physical and chemical) • Deaths due to asphyxiation, strangulation, cardiac arrest, and blunt trauma • Injuries due to broken bones and coma • Additional psychiatric trauma affecting current and future therapeutic relationships	• Policies and procedures • Staffing levels • Workforce education and training • Root Cause Analysis (RCA) • Debriefings • Trauma-informed tools

(continued)

TABLE 14.1 *(continued)*

Treatment Setting*	Error	Strategy for risk management
Clinician and/or treatment team • Acute inpatient • Partial hospital • Outpatient • Residential treatment	Boundary violation/therapeutic relationship • Trust, dignity respect • Sexual • Symbiotic	• Training and education • Credentialing/state board licensing • Consumer education • Complaint management system • Quality of care reviews • Root Cause Analysis (RCA)
Emergency room Acute inpatient Partial hospital Outpatient	Detoxification • Overmedication to prevent withdrawal • Undetected detoxification leading to nutritional repletion, withdrawal and seizures • Oversedation leading to aspiration	• Policies and procedures • Workforce education and training • Root Cause Analysis (RCA)
Acute inpatient Partial hospital Outpatient	Electroconvulsive therapy (ECT) • Anesthesia problems (e.g., local at IV site and very rare adverse reaction and death) • Retrograde amnesia	• Policies and procedures • Workforce education and training • Root Cause Analysis (RCA)
Emergency room	Unnecessary jail detention	• Policies and procedures • Workforce training and education • Protocols for accurate assessment and diagnosis of mental disorders, particularly serious mental illness • Root Cause Analysis (RCA)

TABLE 14.1 *(continued)*

Treatment Setting*	Error	Strategy for risk management
Any psychiatric setting Emergency Pharmacy	Medication • Type: prescribing, transcribing, dispensing, and administration (Hritz, et al., 2002) • High-risk medications • Side effects (e.g., risk for postural hypotension and falls) • Dosage • Monitoring (e.g., lithium with bipolar disorder) • Polypharmacy • Adherence and premature discontinuance • Instructions	• Policies and procedures • Information technology (e.g., computerized physician order entry systems) • Workforce education and training • Root Cause Analysis (RCA)
Any psychiatric setting Medical treatment setting Schools Foster care Legal system	Uncoordinated care across or between delivery systems: • Primary care practitioner or facility fails to communicate with behavioral health providers • Behavioral health providers, in particular prescribing practitioners, fail to communicate with medical delivery system	• Policies and procedures • Workforce education and training • Tools to promote communication between and within delivery system(s) • Root Cause Analysis (RCA)
Any psychiatric setting Any medical setting	Misdiagnosis and treatment planning • Psychiatric diagnosis • Comorbidities • Psychiatric, when medical (i.e., delirium and dementia) • Differential • Individual characteristics (i.e., gender, age, race/ethnicity, cultural)	• Clinical practice guidelines • Policies and procedures • Workforce education and training • Root Cause Analysis (RCA)

(continued)

TABLE 14.1   *(continued)*

Treatment Setting*	Error	Strategy for risk management
Any psychiatric setting	Clinician or treatment setting does not meet community standards	• Policies and procedures • Credentialing/ recredentialing • Peer review • Accreditation • Licensure (facility or provider) • Root Cause Analysis (RCA)
Any psychiatric setting	Ineffective and/or inappropriate treatment modality/ approach: • Cognitive when other indicated • Regression • Prognosis (near and/or long-term)	• Clinical practice guidelines • Root Cause Analysis (RCA)

*Based on setting where problems are most likely to occur

coverage for employer health plans to cover mental illness at the same annual and lifetime coverage limits that they would set for coverage of physical ailments. Although thirty-four states and the federal government have enacted full or partial mental health parity, definitive findings on this issue remain elusive. Published studies on the effects of parity suggest that managed care techniques can be highly effective in ensuring against overutilization of mental health services. Both equitable benefits coverage and assurance of appropriate levels of care advance the safety needs of the individual.

With its roots in structure, accreditation standards provide behavioral health care organizations and providers with parameters for practice. With compliance and monitoring activities implemented by the organization, evidence of health care quality and continuous quality improvement in organizational management, leadership, service delivery, and clinical outcomes will follow. Accreditation is also intended to demonstrate value in that purchasers and consumers receive treatment consistent with industry practices. The four most dominant agencies in behavioral health are the

JCAHO, the National Committee for Quality Assurance (NCQA), the Utilization Review Assessment Commission (URAC), and the Commission on Accreditation of Rehabilitation Facilities (CARF).

The Joint Commission on Accreditation of Healthcare Organizations (JCAHO) is the oldest agency for accreditation and is a leader in patient safety. Most recently it established that voluntarily reportable sentinel events under the JCAHO's Sentinel Event Policy would include "any suicide of a patient in a setting where the patient is housed around the clock, including suicides following elopement from such a setting" (JCAHO, 2003). Patient safety approaches in URAC standards include implicit standards (i.e., quality management and improvement, credentialing, complaints/grievances. and appeals) and explicit standards (required response to urgent situations posing immediate threat). See Table 14.2 for a summary of accreditation standards related to patient safety.

Behavioral Health Clinical Practice Guidelines

Practice guidelines provide evidence-based guidance for clinical practice, thus aiding assessment, diagnosis, and treatment planning for certain mental health disorders. Publicly available guidelines are based on reasonable scientific knowledge and best practices for the treatment of disorders. Challenges of guideline implementation include:

- Selection of a guideline when there is more than one guideline for the same condition. Using Attention Deficit Hyperactivity Disorder (ADHD) as an example, there are currently guidelines available from the National Institutes of Health (NIH) Consensus Development Panel, the American Academy of Pediatrics, the American Academy of Child and Adolescent Psychiatry, the Scottish Intercollegiate Guideline Network, and the Institute for Clinical Systems Improvement (ICSI).
- Dissemination, training, and maintaining or updating guidelines so they are current with community standards and advances in science.

Commonly used strategies for implementing evidence-based practice or using clinical practice guidelines are adopting existing guidelines or adapting/creating new ones (see chapter 4). Guidelines that are adopted are those from recognized sources, including professional behavioral health care and medical associations, such as the American Psychiatric Association

TABLE 14.2   Patient Safety Accreditation Standards in Behavioral Health

Agency	Standards	Compliance Activities
NCQA	QI 1: Program Structure The organization clearly defines its quality improvement (QI) structures and processes and assigns responsibility to appropriate individuals. There is an annual written evaluation of the QI program that includes: • a description of completed and ongoing QI activities that address quality and safety of clinical care and quality of service • trending of measures to assess performance in the quality and safety of clinical care and quality of service • analysis of the results of QI initiatives, including barrier analysis • Evaluation of the overall effectiveness of the QI program, including progress toward influencing network-wide safe clinical practices.	Examines organization's documentation to include: • Policies and procedures • Quality Improvement (QI)/ Utilization Management (UM) Program documents • Meeting minutes • UM and credentialing files • Quality improvement activity summaries Examples of activities that demonstrate a commitment to improving safe clinical practice include: • Distributing information to enrollees that improves their knowledge about clinical safety in their own care such as: –Questions to ask about drug-to-drug interactions –Research findings that facilitate decision making. • Collaborating with network providers and practitioners to: –Conduct in-service training focused on improving knowledge of safe practices. Examples include improving treatment record legibility and establishing systems for timely follow-up of lab results –Combine data on adverse outcomes or polypharmacy issues –Distribute research on proven safe clinical practice –Develop incentives for achieving safer clinical practices.

TABLE 14.2 *(continued)*

Agency Standards	Compliance Activities
	• Focusing existing quality improvement activities on improving patient safety such as: –Analyzing and taking actions on complaint and satisfaction data that relates to clinical safety –Evaluating clinical practice against aspects of practice guidelines that improve safe practices –Improving continuity and coordination of care between practitioners to avoid miscommunication that leads to poor outcomes –Improving continuity and coordination between sites of care, such as hospitals and partial hospitalization programs or ambulatory follow-up care to assure timely and accurate communication –Implementing pharmaceutical practices that require safeguards to enhance patient safety –Using site visit results from initial practitioner credentialing and organizational –Credentialing to improve safe practices –Tracking and trending adverse event reporting to identify systems issues that contribute to poor safety. • Distributing information to enrollees that facilitates informed decisions based on safety. For example, disseminating the following information:

(continued)

TABLE 14.2   *(continued)*

Agency	Standards	Compliance Activities
		–Facilities with computerized pharmacy order entry systems –Organizations that have best practices or outcomes often based on volume –Pharmacies that provide patient counseling and research on proven safe clinical practices.
JCAHO	Almost 50% of JCAHO standards are directly related to safety, addressing such issues as: • Medication use • Infection control • Surgery and anesthesia • Transfusions • Restraint and seclusion • Staffing and staff competence • Fire safety • Medical equipment • Emergency management • Security In January 2003, standards were effective for behavioral health care, which originated in the January 2001 hospital standards. These standards address a number of significant patient safety issues including: the responsibility of organization leadership to create a culture of safety; the implementation of patient safety programs; the response to adverse events when they occur; the prevention of accidental harm through the prospective analysis and redesign of vulnerable patient systems (e.g., the ordering, preparation and dispensing of medications); and the hospital's	

TABLE 14.2 *(continued)*

Agency	Standards	Compliance Activities
	responsibility to tell a patient about the outcomes of the care provided to the patient—whether good or bad. Implemented in 1996, the Sentinel Event Policy is a patient safety cornerstone.	Evidence for compliance include: • Policies and procedures • Governance documents • Minutes Sentinel events require an appropriate response, which includes timely, thorough, and credible root cause analysis, action plan, implementation of improvements to reduce risk, and monitoring of effectiveness.
CARF	Behavioral health criterion related to Health and Safety, "CARF-accredited organizations maintain accessible, safe, and clean environments through both external and internal safety reviews and personnel commitment to this philosophy." General program standards address: • Rights and responsibilities • Assessment • Individual plan • Transition/recovery support services • Pharmacotherapy • Seclusion and restraints • Emergency intervention procedures Treatment settings include behavioral health and opioid treatment programs.	• Policies and procedures • QI program • Performance outcomes

(continued)

TABLE 14.2 *(continued)*

Agency	Standards	Compliance Activities
URAC	URAC patient safety related standards are quite numerous. Indirectly, credentialing and quality management standards address patient safety. Directly, URAC's core standard speaks to patient safety and is required of all applicants.	Compliance documentation relates to: • Policies and procedures • QI/UM program documents • Staff structure and qualifications • Staff management and development • Clinical oversight For example URAC Standard Core 25 (The organization has a mechanism to respond on an urgent basis to situations that pose an immediate threat to the health and safety of consumers), specific activities to meet Core 25 vary by the type of organization. Examples include (but are not limited to): • A health network immediately suspending the participation status of a physician who is practicing in an unsafe manner; or • A utilization management organization notifies the patient and treating provider of a possibly harmful drug interaction.

CARF 2003 Behavioral Health Standards Manual; JCAHO 2001–2002 Comprehensive Accreditation Manual for Behavioral Health Care; NCQA 2003 Standards and Guidelines for the Accreditation of MBHOs; URAC 2002 Health Utilization Management Standards, Version 4.1.

and the Academy for Child and Adolescent Psychiatry. Available guidelines address these disorders: Attention Deficit Hyperactivity Disorder, Autism, Bipolar Disorder, Eating Disorders, Major Depressive Disorders, and Schizophrenia (see the Web Resources section at the end of this chapter).

In the absence of an appropriate guideline available through recognized sources, organizations may consider scientific evidence, professional standards, and expert opinion in drafting guidelines for use by practitioners in contracted networks (see chapter 4). Prior to internal or external adoption or dissemination, guidelines should be reviewed for consistency with policies and procedures, consumer education materials, and utilization management criteria used by an organization. Before guidelines are adopted or adapted, practitioners, consumers, and community agencies should be invited to provide feedback on any issues related to application in treatment. Finally, in addition to the workforce, guidelines should be made available to consumers, caregivers, and practitioners through contracts with service providers, by direct mail, or upon request, in links to association guidelines on the behavioral health organization's Web site, and through user-friendly summaries in consumer newsletters.

Monitoring for adherence may help an organization appreciate the extent to which practice guidelines are used in practice. Many managed care organizations monitor for adherence to guidelines. As an example, adherence to bipolar disorder guidelines can be monitored through routine reporting of performance on the following indicators.

Appropriate Medication

- Percentage of persons with bipolar disorder who have been prescribed a mood stabilizing medication prior to exception management
- Percentage of persons with bipolar disorder not on mood stabilizing medications who have received exception management
- Percentage of persons with bipolar disorder on appropriate medication or treatment is reviewed through an exception management process

Appropriate Treatment for Comorbid Chemical Dependency (CD)

- Percentage of persons with bipolar disorder and a comorbid substance abuse problem who have been referred for CD treatment prior to exception management

- Percentage of persons with bipolar disorder and a comorbid substance abuse problem not initially referred for CD treatment who have received exception management
- Percentage of persons with bipolar disorder and a comorbid substance abuse problem who were appropriately referred for CD treatment or treatment is reviewed through an exception management process

The biggest operational challenge is monitoring exception management. Exception management is an explicit process to assure that appropriate treatment is rendered when clinical practice guideline parameters are not used in the course of treatment. An example would be bipolar disorder and appropriate medications. It is developed as an explicit process for the management of exceptions to clinical practice guidelines that allows reasonable flexibility to be applied to clinical decision-making. Available resources required for data gathering, analysis, and reporting (e.g., people and information technology) could limit the acquisition of concurrent treatment information.

Continuity, Collaboration, and Coordination of Care

If medical fallibility is accepted, errors can occur within and between delivery systems, such as the accurate diagnosis of delirium and dementia in the emergency room that results in the appropriate transfer of the patient to the correct care setting. Poor information transfer and faulty communication can compromise patient safety (see chapter 1). Providers work to promote collaboration between behavioral health and medical care. This includes exchange of information, review of pharmacy benefits and formularies, collaboration when either the primary care practitioner (PCP) or another practitioner is prescribing psychotropic medication or when the patient has a coexisting medical diagnosis, and the implementation of preventive health guidelines.

Behavioral health care services are coordinated and integrated with general medical care throughout the continuum of care. Appropriate assessment and treatment and follow-up with consumers as they use multiple practitioners and providers, service sites, and levels of care are ensured. Additionally, when a consumer is affected by the termination of a practitioner or provider site for any reason other than quality of care issues, he or she should be notified prior to the effective termination date and assisted in selecting a new practitioner or site. A frequent complaint related to coordination of care between delivery systems is sharing information without breaching confidentiality, an error itself in behavioral health where trust between the consumer and treating provider is integral to successful engagement in treatment. To address this concern, an organization or delivery system can develop and implement a *Health Care Coordination Form (HCCF)* (see Appendix 14.1).

Discharge Planning and Transition of Care

According to the National Alliance for the Mentally Ill (NAMI), developing an individual treatment plan should include the consumer, the consumer's service manager, medical personnel, and family members, if appropriate. As the consumer progresses, the plan must be changed as needed to include appropriate psychosocial rehabilitation, education, and prevocational skills training compatible with the combined goals of the consumer and the community. The hospital discharge plan must ensure adequate housing, medical care, and continuation of the individual treatment plan with community support services (NAMI, 2001).

Continuity of care upon discharge from any level of care is an important area of treatment, which is sometimes neglected. Treatment frequently focuses on reduction or elimination of acute psychiatric symptoms. Is suicidal ideation reduced? Is harm to self or others no longer observed? Is the client responding to medications? While assuring that level of care is least restrictive and correlates with a person's clinical and psychosocial needs, near- and long-term safety needs might be missed. To provide seamless treatment, Silver and Burack (2002) suggest that service delivery in behavioral health must be a broad, fluid continuum of services to minimize adverse events after treatment is terminated. An example of this is medication adherence, a frequent hurdle to successful community treatment of persons with chronic disorders such as schizophrenia and bipolar disorder. Without clear plans for self-management, there is risk of deterioration and readmission. It is also important to ensure that level of care is least restrictive and correlates with a person's clinical and psychosocial needs.

Consumer and Provider Satisfaction

Patient safety, when considered from the point of view of the behavioral health provider, includes physical and mental well-being. Mental well-being encompasses satisfaction with services. If a consumer is dissatisfied, it means that he or she may not be receiving the quality of services that he or she should be receiving. If a provider is dissatisfied, this may translate into treatment for the service users not meeting acceptable standards and practices. Additionally, written policies and procedures should support thorough, appropriate, and timely resolution of complaints, including how a consumer can voice a complaint. Decision documentation, prompt resolution, and notification of complaint resolution as well as data analysis are critical to promote consumer satisfaction and proactively address potential quality problems (see chapter 9).

Quality of Care, Adverse Event, and Sentinel Event Monitoring

Quality of care delivered to consumers is in accordance with professionally recognized standards of practice. Any quality of care (QoC) issue is identified, reviewed, and addressed. A QoC concern can be defined as an issue that impacts a consumer's clinical treatment or involves actual or potential clinical risk to a consumer including, but not limited to, inappropriate clinical care. continuity of care, medication management, coordination of care, safety, and unethical behavior that places the consumer at risk of psychological or physical harm.

Organizations maintain programs to prevent and reduce risk and assure the safety of the consumer through ongoing processes of risk identification, risk analysis, action implementation and action evaluation. While monitoring quality of care concerns may be part of normal behavioral health care operations, sentinel or adverse events are critical because immediate investigation and response is required. While there are many kinds of sentinel events in behavioral health, the type of error most critical for RCA is death—due to suicide or secondary to restraint use. As demonstrated by JCAHO through sentinel event monitoring, the need for case identification, trending, and outcomes at the organizational and provider levels is necessary. See Figure 14.1 for JCAHO findings on suicide and restraint deaths in health care setting with primary root causes noted. Lack of orientation, communication, and patient assessment are consistent themes in the RCA for these deaths.

Determining optimal approaches to suicide prevention and reduction requires a multidisciplinary effort within institution and community-based care. One difference between suicide and an error performed in surgery

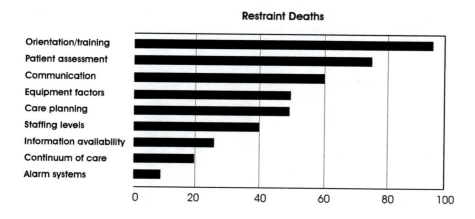

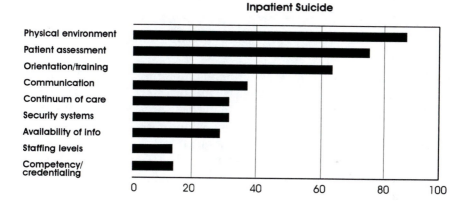

FIGURE 14.1   Root cause analysis for restraint deaths and inpatient suicide (1995–2002).

Copyright © Joint Commission on Accreditation of Healthcare Organizations, 2003. Reprinted with permission.See also, http://www.jcaho.org/accredited+organizations/ambulatory+care/sentinel+events/set+restraint+deaths.htm; and http://www.jcaho.org/accredited+organizations/ambulatory+care/sentinel+events/rc+inpatient+suicides.htm

is that it is the action of the individual harmed, not necessarily the health care professional, that results in death. Balancing the rights and freedom of the individual versus the potential errors of jurisprudence is no easy feat when the person is assessed to be a danger to self or others. Consumers are often critical that involuntary hospitalizations may be overused, robbing them of their freedom. Perhaps the person needs to be held involuntarily for his or her own protection and did not fully meet the intent of state-level voluntary hold requirements. Or the individual does not express suicidal ideation. Accountability for safety is clinically and professionally vexing.

It is important from treatment planning and risk management perspectives to have established policies and procedures, defined review criteria, and tools for data collection. Sample policy and procedure, data collection tool, and evaluation criteria for sentinel events are provided as Appendices 14.2 and 14.3, and Table 14.3 to assist the reader in this endeavor. Efforts to manage the risk of suicide attempts or completed suicide while clients are in treatment are critical. RCA can help the organization determine causal factors for active errors (human-system interface) or latent errors (system design).

Medical Staff Privileging, Credentialing and Peer Review

At the organizational level, monitoring and assuring quality of care and altering the conditions for provider participation can be grounded in mechanisms for credentialing and recredentialing behavioral health practitioners with scope of authority and action. This includes actions taken at initial credentialing and medical staff appointment and subsequent recredentialing. Behavioral health facilities and delivery systems have an obligation to assure that practitioners are qualified, competent, and in good standing to exercise recognized clinical privileges. Medical staff development planning and exclusive contracting or credentialing by hospitals can advance quality of care by assuring the professional has the appropriate qualifications, is not a substandard performer, and demonstrates trustworthy and nondisruptive behavior. It can also reduce the likelihood of court intervention on behalf of aggrieved practitioners (Hershey, 2002).

Behavioral health credentialing committees might benefit from conducting careful RCAs whenever a failure, near miss, or close call is identified in the credentialing process. According to HCPro, Inc. (2003), the following events may be worthy of an RCA: any fair hearing, termination, or denial of medical staff appointment or clinical privileges; a corporate negligence suit alleging improper or inadequate credentialing; or a privileging turf battle. These might prompt the formation of a multidisciplinary team to determine root causes of a breakdown or near miss.

TABLE 14.3   Evaluation Criteria for Sentinel Event Review

Indicator	

Diagnosis/Assessment

DSM-IV-TR™ Axis I	*DSM-IV-TR*™ Axis I is used for reporting all clinical disorders with the exception of Personality Disorders and Mental Retardation. At least one Axis I disorder should be noted in the record.
DSM-IV-TR™ Axis II	*DSM-IV-TR*™ Axis II is used for reporting any personality disorders and mental retardation. It may also be used for noting prominent maladaptive personality features and defense mechanisms. If applicable, the Axis II disorder should be noted in the record.
Diagnosis supported by available clinical information	A clear relationship exists between the information documented and the diagnosis given by the treating practitioner. This includes the consideration of alternate diagnoses based on the biopsychosocial data or differential diagnosis processes.
Mental status exam present and complete	Basic elements of a mental status exam are present, including but not limited to orientation to time, place, person, cognitive contents, dangerousness, mood, behaviors, judgment, insight, and intelligence.
Specific symptoms clearly identified	Clear statement of the specific symptoms the member presents to the practitioner.
Clinical information specific and individualized	The clinical information present in the record indicates that the practitioner focused on the salient clinical elements relevant to the person and this episode of care, and that the practitioner was attuned to the unique aspects of the member.
Changes in diagnosis supported by clinical data	If there are documented changes in the diagnosis sufficient data are reported in the record to support those changes
Severity of illness/ disorder addressed	Severity of symptoms and their potential ramifications regarding effects on member's functioning are reflected as considerations in the documentation:

(continued)

TABLE 14.3 *(continued)*

Indicator	
	• Severity of Illness (SI) criteria for a given level of care represent signs, symptoms, and functional impairments of such a nature and severity as to require treatment at a specified level at a given point in time. These criteria address the question: *"What specific dysfunction exists as a result of a present DSM-IV-TR™ diagnosis?"* • Intensity of Service (IS) criteria should match the patient's dysfunction. These criteria represent therapeutic modalities that, by virtue of their complexity and/or attendant risks, require a specified level of care for their safe, appropriate, and effective application. These criteria address the question: *"Does the patient's condition (behavior, symptoms, etc.) warrant this level of care (is it medically necessary)?"*
Psychosocial issues addressed (e.g., family, school, workplace)	The social context in which the member lives is both explored and contacted as needed.
Any safety concerns clearly addressed in the assessment	Safety is addressed as it relates to danger to self or others: • Suicide Attempt—evaluate the seriousness of the attempt and of the risk of repetition • Suicidal Ideation—evaluate presence of risk elements associated with suicidal ideation • History of mental illness and/or substance abuse • Hopelessness • Impulsivity • Childhood trauma • Homicidal Potential—threats to harm or kill someone considered
Evidence of substance use/abuse assessment	There is clear evidence that the member was questioned about past and/or present abuse/misuse of alcohol/drugs, and if there was suspicion of denial the practitioner explored other data sources

TABLE 14.3 *(continued)*

Indicator	

Presenting Problems

Presenting problems and complaints identified	There is a comprehensive and clear list of the problems and complaints which brought the member to treatment.
Reason for treatment clearly evident	In addition to any history present in the record, it is clear why the member has sought and/or been referred to treatment for this episode of care.
Functional impairment to be addressed that precipitated treatment episode evident	The deficit areas in the member's life which have created problems and which need to be remedied are clearly indicated.
There is an intervention identified for each problem/complaint or explanation of why problem(s) was not addressed	The treatment plan clearly lists each problem and complaint the member and treating practitioner agreed to and connects each one to a reasonable intervention.
Each intervention relates to the problem/complaint	Interventions are clearly connected to the problem/complaint.
The interventions are individualized rather than formulaic	Interventions are customized to the combination of problem/complaint and member characteristics.
Interventions chosen have a reasonable probability of effectiveness	Interventions chosen are targeted and represent recognized standards of care for the particular disorder being treated.

Therapeutic Goals and Actions

Progress notes reflect forward movement or at least the therapeutic attempt to move the member forward	Documentation indicates that there is an active interest in helping the member solve/move on the problems/complaints rather than settle for the status quo.
Progress notes reflect a sensitivity to new issues/concerns that arise during treatment	The practitioner was able to respond to new information that was revealed during treatment in a constructive manner.

(continued)

TABLE 14.3 *(continued)*

Indicator	
Progress notes reflect an active partnership between member and provider	Documentation indicates that the practitioner and member worked in tandem, identifying areas to be worked on and jointly exploring options/solutions.
Coordination of care issues is addressed	There is evidence that PCP has been contacted or other specialist(s) as needed if there are active medical problems that may interact with behavioral healthcare treatment.
Failed or cancelled appointments are addressed	There is evidence that missed appointments are followed up by phone and/or letter.
Timing of the interventions related to goals and actions	Interventions are timely and well-received by consumer as evidenced by progress note pathways.
Discharge plan/treatment termination plan is present	A plan is present from the start of treatment that indicates criteria for the cessation of treatment and lists details of follow-up care.
Discharge planning process identifies criteria for discharge/termination	Throughout treatment there was attention paid to the nature of the discharge criteria and how the therapeutic dyad will know they have been met.
Discharge plan considers possible early warning signs of relapse recurrence for member/family/caregivers	Member and family/caregivers where appropriate were given psycho-education as to how to detect relapse/recurrence and what steps to take should such early warning signs appear.
Illness education is addressed in the discharge plan	The practitioner considered the future of the member and made a prognostic statement in the record as well as sharing this impression with member/family/caregivers.
Completion of treatment is addressed	A closing/discharge summary is present and it details the course of treatment.
Outcome salutary given the person's characteristics and treatment issues	The treatment episode appears to have been salutary given who the member is and what he/she came to treatment with.

Informed Consent

Individuals have the right to determine the course of treatment, whether consent is given orally or in a written document. This ensures that consumers are informed and understand all of the important aspects of their care and treatment (see chapters 5 and 9). Established policies assure practitioners and providers obtain consent from individuals when treatment is initiated. In behavioral health, for example, a second opinion is required in certain states for verification of the patient's capacity to give informed consent for electroconvulsive therapy (ECT), while other states mandate a second opinion to validate that the treatment is medically necessary. In addition, state regulations differ with regard to the required specialty and board certification status of the physician providing the second opinion. There should be specific documentation of the physician's licensure, specialty, and board certification status, as required by law, prior to the administration of ECT.

Another area of concern is informed consent for behavioral health research (see chapter 15 and the Consumer Advocacy Exemplar later in this chapter). While research may be conducted as part of health care operations, there are special considerations for persons with behavioral health disorders, whether acute or chronic in nature. There are also needs of vulnerable populations to consider. Sharav, from The Alliance for Human Research Protection, recently completed a study (2003) examining an overview of regulatory issues, clinical research trials conducted on children, and the ethical conflicts. She focused on psychoactive drug trials performed on both adults and children and provides a comprehensive list of reference sources useful to research and analysis.

Privacy and Confidentiality of Health Information

Information about a consumer's medical care, including mental health treatment and chemical dependency diagnosis and treatment, and other personal information about consumers, is highly confidential and protected by state and federal law. There are severe penalties for not following prescribed rules with respect to the disclosure of confidential patient information. Behavioral health providers treat obligations to preserve the confidentiality of patient health information and other personal information seriously and expect all departments and employees to do so also. This is in keeping with recognized rights to privacy and in accordance with the applicable standards of the Health Insurance Portability and Accountability Act (HIPAA) and accreditation organizations.

Health Literacy and Information Dissemination

Health literacy and successful oral and written communication can reduce complications associated with developing a satisfactory plan for behavioral health treatment (see chapter 5). When information is unavailable or available in forms not understood by the consumer or support system, safety and well-being may be compromised. JCAHO recognized communication as an important strategy to reduce errors when it established improving effective communication among caregivers as one of its 2004 National Patient Safety Goals (JCAHO, 2003). With health communication strategies, "there is always the opportunity for unintended consequences to occur (e.g., confusion, unwarranted anxiety), even with the most well-intentioned and well-executed health communication interventions" (IOM, 2002b). Barriers to communication and literacy in behavioral health include consumer and behavioral health organization factors. Consumer barriers include: lack of ability to read; lack of fluency in English (dominant language for medical information in the United States); impaired cognitive/mental status; and vision and hearing impairment. Behavioral health care organization barriers may include lack of awareness of cultural issues/concerns; use of medical jargon; and development of communication materials with only one audience in mind.

Health care providers can aid and inform consumers about issues pertaining to behavioral health disorders, safety needs, and quality. Consider including the following areas for consumer materials: consumer rights and responsibilities; confidentiality; ethics; guidelines for practice; criteria for clinical decision making and treatment planning; appeals, grievances, and complaints; and prevention. This information can be made available to consumers in provider offices, through member materials distributed by health plans, and on the behavioral health care organization's Web site. Written information about diagnosis, signs, symptoms, treatment, and specific instructions about medications are all information worth sharing.

EVALUATING EFFECTIVENESS OF PATIENT SAFETY ACTIVITIES

Behavioral health quality improvement (QI) practices might include the monitoring and altering of processes and structures associated with the delivery of mental health, substance abuse, and employee assistance program services. Organizational focus and priorities should be targeting activities with a high probability of impact to reduce behavioral health adverse outcomes, procedural breakdowns, and sentinel events. Data gathering from these activities inform quality improvement and process improvement initiatives to reduce potential for harm. Results from the Utilization Review Assessment Commission's (URAC) 2001 medical management survey showed health care companies used the following approaches to address patient safety:

- Formal committee or program to assess patient safety issues separate from the quality management program (13%)
- Conducting patient safety studies (14%)
- Patient safety addressed in the quality management process (65%)
- Tracking/information system has the capability to flag possible problems with patient safety (e.g., unexpected return to operating room, complications, extended LOS, or other sentinel events) (45%)
- Patient safety indicators tracked by physician or by facility (37%)
- Program to contact providers or facilities appearing to have high rates of possible patient safety problems (41%) (URAC, 2003).

With this work by URAC, it is hopeful that safety initiatives in behavioral health will be advanced. URAC primarily accredits managed behavioral health care organizations for core, case management, and health utilization management standards. These organizations touch the lives and behavioral health care of millions of Americans.

Some determination of the effectiveness of its practices for behavioral health patient safety activities needs to occur. Through at least an annual evaluation, an organization can provide evidence of the effectiveness of practices, determine if opportunities for improvement exist, note the degree of improvements, and identify any policies and procedures that require development or modification. In conducting the evaluation, an organization strives to maintain and enhance a framework for assessing the main elements of patient safety activities, document any barriers and limitations in current practice, and convey the results in an organized and accessible way, making sure the "take home" message is easily understood by personnel, behavioral health providers, and consumers.

Focusing on the structure, processes and outcomes of care, a behavioral health patient safety program continually emphasizes changing the system to make treatment safer for consumers through evaluation of the evidence.

Evaluation of evidence-based practice relies on the availability of timely, meaningful, reliable, and valid data. The Agency for Healthcare Research and Quality (AHRQ) and the Substance Abuse and Mental Health Services Administration (SAMHSA) have sponsored research focusing on improving the quality and safety of care provided to persons with mental health and substance use disorders. AHRQ has provided tools to help clinicians identify people at risk for certain disorders and problems and has also developed tools to assess the quality of mental health programs (AHRQ, 2002). Specific areas where AHRQ research is available include the areas of suicide prevention, depression diagnosis, schizophrenia treatment, and quality improvement resources.

In the area of suicide prevention, emergency department triage nurses can identify 98% of children at risk for suicide. Four questions about past and present thoughts of suicide, prior self-destructive behavior, and current stressors can identify at risk children and take less than two minutes to complete. Children reported that they felt it was more acceptable to discuss suicidal thoughts if asked these questions. For diagnosis of depression, a computerized screening tool helps diagnose depression. Physicians who consulted the Primary Care Evaluation of Mental Disorders (PRIME-MD) were more likely than others to make a medical chart notation of depression, begin their patients on antidepressant medication, or refer their patients to mental health specialists (AHRQ, 2002).

AHRQ's schizophrenia Patient Outcomes Research Team (PORT) developed evidence-based treatment recommendations. The PORT on schizophrenia made a comprehensive assessment of practice variations in the treatment and management of schizophrenia. The Commonwealth of Massachusetts, the National Alliance for the Mentally Ill, and the New York State Office of Mental Health, have adopted recommendations from this PORT (AHRQ, 2002).

Quality improvement programs for depression treatment have long-term benefits. AHRQ's Patient Outcomes Research Team (PORT) II on depression developed and tested a quality improvement (QI) program. When compared with patients not enrolled in the QI program, QI patients were more likely to visit a mental health specialist, receive counseling, and take antidepressant medication. At 6 and 12 months, QI patients were also less likely to have depression and were more likely to be employed (AHRQ, 2002).

The National Inventory of Mental Health Quality Measures (Center for Quality Assessment and Improvement in Mental Health, n.d.) provides a searchable database of process measures for quality assessment and improvement in mental health and substance abuse care. There is an inventory of quality measures for mental health and substance-related for more than 300 process measures in the domains of quality: access, assessment, treatment, continuity, coordination, patient safety, and prevention. Data include: clinical context for the measure; summary and rating of supporting research evidence; measure specifications; data requirements; domain of quality; treatment modality; population; and developer information. The measures are useful to clinicians and facilities, health plans, oversight groups, researchers, and others seeking to assess and improve quality of care. A toolkit of quality management tools for mental health care and a consumer guide to information on the quality of mental health care are also available (Center for Quality Assessment and Improvement in Mental Health, 2002). Other sources for patient safety and quality improvement data include NCQA and JCAHO.

EXEMPLARS IN PRACTICE

Public Policy for Restraints and Seclusion

Enforceable national standards often result from a combination of consumer advocacy, state and federal agency support, and congressional interest. Consumer protections on the use of restraint and seclusion were specified into law by The Children's Health Act of 2000, Division A and Division B; Title XXXI—Provisions Relating to Services for Children and Adolescents. Sections 3207 and 3208 P.L. 106–310 provided for a national government standard governing the use of restraints and seclusion for all facilities receiving federally appropriated funds and there are specialized requirements for nonmedical community-based facilities for children and youth (Ross, 2001). The law targeted avoidable deaths and injuries and provided for the following: All federally funded facilities may only impose seclusion and restraints for emergency circumstances for physical safety purposes; seclusion and restraints can only be imposed upon the written order of a physician or state licensed independent practitioner; orders must specify the duration and circumstances; and deaths associated with seclusion and restraint must be reported to public entities within 24 hours.

To establish skill and competency in this arena, Pettit and colleagues (2001) suggest state certification and skill sets that would reduce the likelihood of nonvalidated therapies entering the treatment milieu. These skills and competencies include, but are not limited to, prevention and use of restraint and seclusion, alternatives to restraints, seclusion, and de-escalation methods, physiological and psychological impact of restraints and seclusion, monitoring physical signs of distress and obtaining medical assistance, management of position asphyxia, and documentation and investigation of injuries and complaints.

Technology for Risk Tracking

Developing and implementing analytic and decision making tools, particularly those that are easily adopted in a clinical setting, is critical as behavioral health and medical delivery systems seek innovative technology to improve the assessment, referral, and treatment of behavioral disorders (see chapter 8). Integral to successful treatment is early risk detection, such as suicide and substance use risks. Managed care organizations also strive to develop systems that make it hard for people to do the wrong thing and easy to take the right clinical course.

In 1999, PacifiCare Behavioral Health (PBH) developed and implemented a technology strategy to improve the quality of suicide risk assessments by panel providers. Algorithms for Effective Reporting and Treatment (ALERT™) is an innovative program found to be especially effective at detecting patients at risk for chemical dependency and those at risk for suicidal behavior (Brown, Burlingame, Lambert, Jones, & Vaccaro, 2001). At-risk cases are identified by the patient's self-reported high frequency of suicidal ideation on a standardized outcome measure. The system tracks a number of clinical variables and brings at-risk cases to the attention of the treating clinician and the PBH care manager. The primary reasons for flagging at-risk cases are worsening of symptoms, substance abuse problems, and suicide risk.

Potential clinician assessment errors are identified when the clinician assessment of suicidal ideation appears to significantly underestimate risk as compared with the patient self-report of suicidal ideation and symptom severity. The ALERT™ program encourages behavioral health clinicians to use scientifically validated patient self-rating measures as part of the treatment process, rather than relying only on discussion during therapy sessions to assess the clinical condition of their patients. For example, ALERT™ identifies persons at risk for suicide when they indicate on the self-rating scale that they frequently think about suicide. The program then compares the consumer's rating of suicidal thinking with the clinician's assessment of suicidal thinking. The clinician's assessment, based on discussions during therapy sessions, is identified as probably erroneous if the patient's rating indicates a high frequency of suicidal thinking and the clinician's assessment of suicidal thinking is "none." ALERT™ provides feedback to clinicians whenever potential errors in assessment are found and encourages clinicians to review the patient self-report ratings and in addition to discussions during therapy sessions to assess risk for chemical dependency or suicide. It appears that this feedback has been especially successful in encouraging clinicians to include patient self-rating measures in the assessment of suicidal thinking.

Consumer Advocacy

Through its *Public Policy Platform*, the National Alliance for the Mentally Ill (NAMI) has established standards for protecting the well-being of mentally ill individuals participating in research (see also chapter 15). NAMI acknowledges the necessity for research using human subjects, but that research is conducted with the highest medical, ethical, and scientific standards. Of note are the recommendations related to persons with cognitive impairment or brain disorders (NAMI, 2001):

- National standards to govern voluntary consent, comprehensive exchange of information, and related protections of persons with cognitive impairments who become research subjects must be developed and they must include the interests of persons who become human subjects, families, and other caregivers.
- Whenever someone other than the research participant gives consent, the participant and involved family members must receive information on the same basis as the person actually giving consent.
- Research participants should be carefully evaluated before and throughout the research for their capacity to comprehend information and their capacity to consent to continue participation in the research.
- Someone shall make the determination of competence other than the principal investigator or others involved in the research. Except for research protocols approved by the institutional review board (IRB) as minimal risk, whenever it is determined that the subject is not able to continue to provide consent, consent to continue participation in the research shall be sought from families or others legally entrusted to act in the participant's best interests.

- IRBs that regularly review research proposals for brain disorders must include consumers and family members who have direct and personal experience with brain disorders.
- Members of IRBs approving research on individuals with brain disorders must receive specialized training about brain disorders and other cognitive impairments and the needs of individuals who experience these disorders.
- Persons with brain disorders and members of their families must be integrally involved in the development, provision, and evaluation of this training.
- NAMI endorses the development of a uniform, standard definition of "brain disorders" to help all states obtain priority funding and services for the population that suffers the most severe disabilities.

FUTURE DIRECTIONS IN RESEARCH, POLICY AND PRACTICE

If the quality chasm is to be crossed to promote safe and efficient care, changes in the health system are requisite to creating pathways to close the gap. Through combined research and policy and practice initiatives, system change is possible. Summarized below are initiatives currently underway.

Public Policy Initiatives

Behavioral health services and programs were overlooked in the original Institute of Medicine (IOM) patient safety reports. It is not that the six aims, ten rules, and thirteen principles do not apply. It is simply the case where the IOM approach to assessment, treatment, and quality improvement separated the head from the body. Currently the Center for Mental Health Services is addressing this gap by developing a behavioral health specific resource guide or tool kit for *Crossing the Quality Chasm* (Committee on Quality of Care in America, 2001). The inaugural meeting was held in May 2003. In attendance were representatives from state and federal mental health agencies, professional associations, direct service organizations, and consumers. The recommendations will be shared with the IOM as it moves forward with its *Crossing the Quality Chasm* initiative for behavioral health. The resource guide will translate the *Crossing the Quality*

Chasm for applicability to the behavioral health setting, providing a road-map for creating a new behavioral health system for the 21st century. There will also be linkages with the behavioral health priority areas that the IOM (2003) suggests the U.S. Department of Health and Human Services and public/private stakeholders focus on to bring about improvements in health care quality and delivery. Two of the priority areas are directly related to behavioral health services—major depression, and severe and persistent mental illness. However, there are related priorities that will potentially be considered in association with mental health issues—care coordination, children with special care needs, frailty associated with aging, medication management, and obesity.

In 2002, President Bush established the President's New Freedom Commission on Mental Health as part of his commitment to eliminate inequality for Americans with disabilities. The Commission would provide direction for the future policy directions for implementation by the federal, state, and local governments. The hope is to "maximize the utility of existing resources, improve coordination of treatments and services, and promote successful community integration for adults with a serious mental illness and children with a serious emotional disturbance" (President's New Freedom Commission on Mental Health, 2003). The Commission received feedback, comments, and suggestions from nearly 2,500 people from all 50 states including mental health recipients and consumers, families, advocates, public and private providers, and administrators and mental health researchers. Fifteen subcommittees examined specific aspects of mental health services and offered recommendations for improvement. The subcommittees addressed areas directly or indirectly relevant to patient safety that included: concomitant disorders, criminal justice, cultural competence, employment and income support, evidence-based practices, home-lessness/housing, medication issues, mental health interface with general medicine, rights and engagement, and suicide prevention. The report can be accessed on the "Reports" page of the Commission's Web site at http://www.mentalhealthcommission.gov.

Environmental Initiatives

At the end of 2002, the National Association of State Mental Health Program Directors (NASMHPD) launched an initiative to establish a national training curriculum for seclusion and restraints to create a violence and coercion free mental health treatment environment (National Technical Assistance

Center for State Mental Health Planning [NTACSHMP], 2003). The course of this national initiative will result in:

- Identifying the essential systemic changes that must occur when reducing the use of seclusion and restraints
- Identifying common barriers and obstacles that occur in mental health environments when attempting to reduce seclusion and restraints and how to resolve them
- Understanding how to apply the public health prevention paradigm to reducing the use of seclusion and restraints
- Identifying the components of the seclusion and restraint toolbox, and how to use them
- Collaborating with state teams on developing an individualized facility plan with time frames to reduce the use of seclusion and restraints
- Understanding how the collection, analysis, distribution, and application of data support and helps to drive the reduction of seclusion and restraints

Under the auspices of the NASMHPD, the National Technical Assistance Center for State Mental Health Planning developed a national curriculum for the reduction of seclusion and restraints using primary and secondary prevention principles. The training curriculum includes 16 modules touching on topics such as the assumptions associated with the use of seclusion and restraints, consumer experiences with seclusion and restraints, staff culture, witnessing, and use of tools designed to minimize the risk of trauma and retraumatization in treatment environments. The final toolkit is available online at the NASMHPD Web site.

Workforce Training

Often health care organizations turn to workforce training as one alternative to improving individual knowledge and organizational intelligence for innovation and competency in clinical practice. This is critical for mental health and substance use issues since the tendency may be to either focus on the medical or the behavioral issues based on one's discipline, while either or both could be the underlying etiology for the reason treatment was initially sought. Underway is a national initiative supported by the AHRQ, the SAMHSA, the Center for Mental Health Services, the American College of Mental Health Administration, and the Academic Behavioral

Health Consortium. The work undertaken by key individuals of these organizations was featured in the *Administration and Policy in Mental Health* (2002) special double issue dedicated to these issues. Topics in this issue range from gap analysis of behavioral health education to leap-frogging beyond the status quo. Guest editors Michael Hoge and John Morris suggest that strengths and weaknesses for improving the quality of content are important in the areas of graduate education, continuing education, and education of consumers, families, and frontline staff. In keeping with the spirit of the IOM report, *Crossing the Quality Chasm* (Committee on Quality of Care in America, 2001) the idea of creating a national education agenda through consensus building and change related to workforce training is reinforced. Specific workforce training recommendations from the special issue include:

- Establishing core competencies for practitioners: initial and ongoing assessment, family and support system involvement, social and cultural factors, recovery and empowerment, provider/client relationship, community resource management, and coordination of care (Morris & Stuart, 2002).
- Fostering general standards for clinical and training systems: use of structure diagnostic tools, evidence-based care, outcomes concepts, shared decision making paradigms, and community based systems of care and wellness (Huey, 2002).   .
- Creating consistency in continuing education on a national level where professional development is reliant on state requirements to drive learning. Organizations themselves should determine the required competencies for the roles/functions needed within the organization. Continuing education content should be developed to support these competencies and the professional disciplines employed by the organization (Daniels & Walter, 2002).

CONCLUSION

Persons with acute and/or persistent behavioral health disorders deserve a full life and safe care. Because general/medical health and behavioral health services are interconnected, reducing risk of error is a complex endeavor. As organizations and providers look to the future, system change requires innovation and collaboration to promote treatment with a firm biopsychosocial foundation. Teamwork within and between systems and multidisciplinary problem solving are critical to the goals of recovery, providing the full continuum of care, and continuous quality improvement. Every person who enters treatment, regardless of setting, should enter it with trust and confidence that the clinician(s) and treatment team value human dignity and are committed to error-free treatment. This chapter provides information about how to make this a reality.

ACKNOWLEDGMENTS

The author wishes to thank the following individuals for their assistance with providing materials, guidance, and/or support in the preparation of this chapter: Jacquie Byers, PhD, University of Central Florida; Gigi Mathew, DrPh, CPHQ, and Victoria Vigil, MPH, CHES, CPHQ, PacifiCare Behavioral Health; Kevin Ann Huckshorn RN, MSN, CAP, National Association of State Mental Health Program Directors; Nikki Migas, CARF; Mary Cesare-Murphy, PhD, JCAHO Behavioral Health Professional and Technical Advisory Committee; Kristin Goudreau and Liza Greenberg, RN, MPH, URAC; E. Clarke Ross, EdD, Children and Adults with Attention Deficit/ Hyperactivity Disorder (CHADD); and Michael Hoge, PhD, Yale University.

WEB RESOURCES

Name of Resource/URL	Description
Agency for Healthcare Research and Quality http://www.ahrq.gov/research/mentalix.htm	Provides resource information about mental health and substance use/addiction services and quality improvement initiatives
American Managed Behavioral Healthcare Association http://www.ambha.org	Information about managed behavioral healthcare organizations that offer individualized care management, specialty networks, a continuum of care, quality management programs, consumer orientations, and innovations in behavioral health care delivery

American Psychiatric Association
http://www.psych.org
American Psychological
Association
http://www.apa.org
The Carter Center
http://www.cartercenter.org/
Center for Quality Assessment and
Improvement in Mental Health
http://www.cqaimh.org/
quality.html
Centre for Evidence-Based Mental
Health
http://www.cebmh.com

Center for Mental Health Services
http://www.samhsa.gov/centers/
cmhs/cmhs.html

Commission on Accreditation of
Rehabilitation Facilities
http://www.carf.org
Institute of Medicine/National
Academies Press
http://www.iom.edu

Association information and practice guidelines for mental health
Association information, publications, and a consumer health
center
Information about domestic and international mental health issues
Searchable database of more than
300 measures for quality assessment and improvement in mental
health and substance abuse care
Resources for promoting and supporting the teaching and practice
of evidence-based mental
healthcare
Resources on mental health services and trends in the U.S.: in addition, an electronic version of
Mental Health 2000 is available
Information about behavioral
health accreditation standards

Read these helpful publications
online:
- Reducing Suicide: A National
  Imperative
- Suicide Prevention and Inter-
  vention: Summary of a
  Workshop
- Priority Areas for National Ac-
  tion: Transforming Health
  Care Quality
- Speaking of Health: Assessing
  Health Communication Strate-
  gies for Diverse Populations
- Unequal Treatment: Confront-
  ing Racial and Ethnic Dispari-
  ties in Health Care

Joint Commission on Accreditation of Healthcare Organizations http://www.jcaho.org	Information on accreditation for behavioral health organizations
National Association for State Mental Health Program Directors http://www.nasmhpd.org	Identifies and makes information available about public mental health policy issues and best practices in the delivery of mental health services
National Alliance for the Mentally Ill http://www.nami.org	Advocacy and public policy resources from the nation's largest organization dedicated to improving the lives of persons affected by serious mental illness
National Association of Social Workers http://www.naswdc.org/	Information about social work profession, a key profession in mental health services
National Committee for Quality Assurance http://www.ncqa.org	Accreditation information for managed behavioral health care organization accreditation
National Institute of Mental Health http://www.mentalhealth.gov/	Provides scientific tools and information to achieve better understanding, treatment, and eventually prevention of mental illness
National Library of Medicine/Surgeon General Reports http://hstat.nlm.nih.gov	Find these and other reports on mental health treatment and policy: • Children's Mental Health (2001) • Mental Health Services and Primary Health Care (2001) • Mental Health: Culture, Race, and Ethnicity (Supplement) (2001) • National Strategy for Suicide Prevention (2001)
National Strategy for Suicide Prevention http://mentalhealth.samhsa.gov/suicideprevention/default.asp	Information about suicide prevention in English and Spanish

President's New Freedom Commission on Mental Health
http://www.mentalhealthcommission.gov

Summary reports and presentations from the Commission's past two years of work targeting mental health services and public policy

Substance Abuse and Mental Health Services Administration
http://www.samhsa.gov

Resource site with clearinghouse, information on mental health and addiction services, prevention, and national statistics.

Utilization Review Assessment Commission/URAC
http://www.urac.org

Information on accreditation standards for behavioral healthcare organizations

HCPro, Inc.
http://www.credentialinfo.com

Resource site for credentialing and peer review activities

Clinical Practice Guidelines

Attention Deficit Hyperactivity Disorder
http://www.aacap.org

American Academy of Child and Adolescent Psychiatry. Others available: NIH Consensus Development Panel, American Academy of Pediatrics, Scottish Intercollegiate Guideline Network and Institute for Clinical Systems Improvement (ICSI).

Autism
http://www.aacap.org

American Academy of Child and Adolescent Psychiatry

Bipolar Disorder
http://www.psych.org/psych_pract/treatg/pg/bipolar_revisebook_index.cfm

American Psychiatric Association

Eating Disorders
http://www.psych.org/psych_pract/treatg/pg/eating_revisebook_index.cfm

American Psychiatric Association

Major Depressive Disorder
http://www.psych.org/psych_pract/treatg/pg/Depression2e.book.cfm

American Psychiatric Association's

Obsessive Compulsive Disorder
http://www.psychguides.com/ocgl.html

Expert Consensus Guideline

Panic Disorder http://www.psych.org/psych_pract/ treatg/pg/pg_panic.cfm	American Psychiatric Association
Schizophrenia http://www.psych.org/psych_pract/ treatg/pg/pg_schizo.cfm	American Psychiatric Association

APPENDIX 14.1

Health Care Coordination Form

Send completed form to the physician, not to PBH. Please have attending physician review prior to filing in patient's clinical record.

Dear _____   _____

Name of Health Care Practitioner   Address

In order to coordinate care, I wish to inform you that your patient _____ was referred to me for treatment on ____/____/____.

DSM-IV-TR™ diagnosis code is _____.

Outpatient care is being delivered and the treatment plan consists of the following modalities:
(Check all that apply)

❑ Individual Psychotherapy   ❑ Couples Therapy
❑ Family Psychotherapy   ❑ Medication Management
❑ Group Psychotherapy   ❑ Other

Medication(s) are being managed by: _____

Medications and Dosages:

1. _____

2. _____

If you need additional information, contact me at: _____

Sincerely,

_____   _____

Clinician's Name (print)   Signature

My primary care physician contact information:

_____

Primary Care Physician Name

_____

Address

_____ Fax Number (   ) _____

Phone Number (   ) _____

(Please complete both sides of this form)

Consent for Release of Confidential Information to Primary Care Physicians and/or Other Health Care Practitioners

Patient Name: _____   Consumer ID Number: _____

By initialing all information items I approve, I authorize release of the following medical information to the Health Care Practitioner:
(Check and initial all that apply)

❐ Mental Health Diagnosis _____
❐ Medication Management Information _____
❐ HIV/AIDS Related Records (Except HIV Test Results) _____
❐ Other Mental Health Treatment Information _____
❐ Other Information Specified Here _____
❐ Substance Abuse (SA) Information _____
　　For SA Information, this authorization is:
　　　❐ Limited to the following treatment _____.
　　　❐ Limited to the following time period _____.

Confidentiality of alcohol and drug abuse patient records is protected under federal law. Federal regulations (42 CFR, part 2) prohibit anyone from making any further disclosure of the information without the specific written consent of the person to whom it pertains, or as otherwise permitted by such regulations. I understand that the release of this information is to permit my treating physician and other heath care practitioners to monitor my health status and to coordinate all the care, which I may receive. This authorization, unless otherwise indicated, becomes effective on the date signed and may be revoked by me at any time, except to the extent action has been taken in reliance hereon. If not earlier revoked or instructed, this authorization shall terminate automatically within one year of the date of execution. I understand that the information authorized by this release will be provided to the authorized recipient(s) only. Additional information may be provided to those recipients only with signed consent from me. I further understand that I have a right to receive a copy of this authorization upon my request.

_____   _____
Signature of Patient or Legal Guardian   Date

APPENDIX 14.2

Sample Sentinel Event Policy and Procedure

Title:	Sentinel Event Reporting and Review	Policy No:
Responsibility:	Director, Quality Improvement	No. of Pages:
Effective Date:		Revised:
Approved: (Committee)		Date:
Approved: (President and CEO)		Date:

POLICY

Mental Health (MH) Organization maintains programs that reduce and prevent risk and assure the safety of the consumer through ongoing processes of risk identification, risk analysis, action implementation and action evaluation. Sentinel events are defined as unexpected occurrences involving death or serious physical or psychological injury, or risk thereof. Serious injury includes loss of limb or function. "Risk thereof" includes process variation for which a recurrence would carry a significant chance of a serious adverse outcome (Source: Joint Commission on the Accreditation of Healthcare Organizations. SBHC 1999–2000 Standards for Behavioral Health Care, Chicago: JCAHO, 1999). There is a sentinel event review process to:

- Identify unusual or untoward occurrences that could result in risk/liability;
- Investigate whether standards of care were met.

Sentinel events are reviewed by MH Organization Clinical Staff and are investigated by MH Organization Quality Improvement (QI) staff. Appropriate action/interventions are taken in consultation with the Regional Medical Director or his/her physician designee. The quality improvement practices undertaken within this policy are protected from discovery as per state regulations.

PURPOSE

To delineate the mechanisms used to identify potential areas of clinical risk and implement actions to reduce or eliminate identified risk factors.

PROCEDURES

1. Sentinel events are identified by Regional Customer Service Associates, Care Managers, or other MH Organization staff in a variety of ways including, but not limited to telephone interaction with Providers and/or consumers, written correspondence from a Provider or consumer, or through the review of Provider Assessment Reports (PARs) or medical records.

    1.1 Upon the identification of a sentinel event, the MH Organization Clinical Operations/Clinical Services staff completes a *Sentinel Event Report* (Sections I. through IV.) in MS Outlook, and sends the form to the mailbox assigned to a designated staff person in the Regional QI Department.

2. The Regional QI Lead or designee ensures that the case is logged in the QI Database and is assigned to the QI Lead or a licensed designee. The licensed Regional QI Lead or designated licensed QI Specialist assigned to review and investigate the case, reviews the *Sentinel Event Report* and other *pertinent* information including, but not limited to the following, *as determined to be necessary through the case review process*:

    - Care Manager or Team Lead interviews;
    - Medical records;
    - Provider/facility response;
    - Member's treatment record.

3. These materials are forwarded to the assigned licensed Regional QI Lead/designated licensed QI Specialist within 24 hours of receipt of the *Sentinel Event Report* in the QI Department.

    3.1 Additional materials may be requested. All reviews are completed in a timely manner. MH Organization defines timely as within 30 days of receipt of all medically necessary information required to complete the review and make a determination of appropriate action/intervention.

4. The licensed QI Lead/designated licensed QI Specialist also determines whether the:

- Level of care/treatment authorized by MH Organization appears to have been inconsistent with MH Organization medical necessity and patient placement guidelines;
- Incident may have been caused by failure of the Provider to meet community/safety practice standards;
- Provider's response to the incident was inappropriate or inadequate in addressing the concerns raised.

5. If the licensed Regional QI Lead/designated licensed QI Specialist determines that one or more item is relevant, (e.g., the standard of care did not meet community/safety practice standards), he/she documents the rationale for the determination in the applicable portion of the *Sentinel Event Report*.

    5.1 The case is then reviewed with a senior clinical staff (e.g., Regional Director, Regional Director, Clinical Manager or Supervisor or QI Lead) and with a Regional Medical Director.

    5.2 Special Circumstances may require review by corporate-level personnel such as the Corporate Medical Director, Corporate Clinical Director, or the Director of QI.

6. The Regional QI Lead/designee presents all sentinel event cases involving death (even if by natural causes), services provided by an M.D., or serious suicide attempts to the MH Organization Regional Medical Director or his/her physician designee for review.

    6.1 The QI Lead/designated QI Specialist completes a review of the sentinel event summarizing relevant case findings for cases presented to an M.D. The M.D. completes a section of the *Sentinel Event Report*, designating his/her review.

    6.2 Summary information is documented in the QI Database, and the case is filed.

7. Cases reviewed by the Regional Medical Director or his/her physician designees that do not meet standards of care may be presented to the respective Regional Peer Review Committee. In addition to those cases not meeting standards of care, the Regional Medical Director, at his/her discretion may select other cases for presentation to the Regional Peer Review Committee.

8.   If necessary, the Regional Peer Review Committee makes recommendations regarding corrective action. (Refer to relevant MH Organization Clinical policies and procedures for credentialing).
9.   Practitioners providing treatment for MH Organization consumers are contractually required to report sentinel events that occur, which meet the criteria listed in the guidelines delineated herein.
10. Aggregate data are reported on a quarterly basis to the Regional Member Services, Regional
11. Quality Improvement, and Corporate Member Services Committees.

Sentinel Event Report Guidelines

Death/Completed Suicide

Any death that occurs during treatment provided under authorization from MH Organization, or within twelve (12) months of the individual receiving care authorized by MH Organization. For cases that appear to be medical in nature, review with a Regional Medical Director to ascertain potential relevancy of coexisting behavioral health issues (such as type of authorized care or lack of authorization/care).

Homicide

Any act of a consumer currently in treatment authorized by MH Organization or of a consumer for whom treatment was authorized by MH Organization within the twelve (12) months prior to the incident, who kills another individual.

Suicide Attempt Requiring Medical Intervention

An act of self-harm, which may result in a life-threatening situation. Consideration must be given to lethality of suicide attempt, intent of consumer, and potential pattern of behavior. If there is any doubt as to whether the attempt should be reported and/or investigated, review the incident with a licensed Team Leader and/or Senior Clinical staff; if so directed, the report should be completed and submitted to the Regional QI Department. Suicide attempts should only be reported, however, if the person is currently in treatment authorized by MH Organization or within twelve (12) months of the individual receiving care authorized by MH Organization. It is not necessary to complete a report if the person has neither been previously assessed by MH Organization nor authorized for treatment by MH Organization.

Other

An occurrence other than those defined by death, completed suicide, homicide or suicide attempt requiring medical attention, that is a process variation for which its occurrence or recurrence would carry a significant chance of a serious adverse outcome for the consumer.

APPENDIX 14.3

Sample Sentinel Event Report

Date of Report _____   Region _____
(mm/dd/yyyy)

I. CONSUMER INFORMATION

Reference ID Number _____   Consumer Name _____

Street Address _____   Date of Birth _____

City _____   State _____

Zip Code _____   SS # _____

Medical Insurance _____   Employer _____

II. PROVIDER INFORMATION

Practitioner Name _____   ID Number _____

Practitioner Name _____   ID Number _____

Facility Name _____   ID Number _____

III. OCCURRENCE TYPE (Check all that apply)

Death/Completed Suicide ☐   Homicide ☐

Suicide Attempt Requiring Medical   Other ☐
Intervention ☐

Mental Health ☐   Inpatient
Chemical Dependency ☐   Acute ☐
EAP ☐   Residential ☐
                                          PHP ☐
                                          Detoxification ☐
                                       Outpatient ☐

Other ❑

Date of Occurrence (mm/dd/yyyy, if known) _____

IV. REPORT OF OCCURRENCE

Please provide an objective summary of known facts including what happened, who witnessed the occurrence, measures taken by the provider in response to the occurrence, etc.

Submitted By: _____ Date: _____
(include licensure)

V. REVIEW BY LICENSED QI
SPECIALIST/QI STAFF MEMBER

Level of Care/Treatment Authorized by MH Organization *appears to have been* inconsistent with UM Criteria for Mental Health Disorders and/or Substance Use Disorders.   YES ❑ NO ❑ UNSURE ❑

Incident *may have been* caused by failure of the provider to meet accepted community standards for practice and/or safety.
YES ❑ NO ❑ UNSURE ❑

The provider's response to the concerns raised by the incident *was* inappropriate or inadequate.   YES ❑ NO ❑ UNSURE ❑

If the licensed QI Specialist/QI staff responds YES or UNSURE to any of the above, he/she must document facts to substantiate this determination:

Signature: _____ Date: _____
(include licensure)

VI. REVIEW BY SR. CLINICAL STAFF

Signature: _____ Date: _____

(include licensure)

VII. REVIEW BY MH ORGANIZATION MEDICAL DIRECTOR

If indicated following review by Regional QI Department

Refer to Regional Peer Review Committee: YES ☐   NO ☐

Signature: _____ Date: _____

(include licensure)

VIII. CORRECTIVE ACTION OR OTHER FOLLOW-UP

Refer to Provider Network Management due to Provider/Practitioner non-compliance with request for information: YES ☐   NO ☐

Signature: _____ Date: _____

(include licensure)

REFERENCES

Agency for Healthcare Research and Quality (AHRQ). (2002). *AHRQ focus on research: Mental health.* Retrieved April 18, 2003, from http://www.ahrq.gov/news/focus/focmental.htm.

Agency for Healthcare Research and Quality (AHRQ). (2003). *Information on medical errors.* Retrieved May 28, 2003, from http://www.ahrq.org/browse/mederrbr.htm

American Psychiatric Association. (2000). *Diagnostic and statistical manual of mental disorders,* Fourth Edition Text Revision *(DSM-IV-TR*™*).* Arlington, VA: Author.

Bazelon Center. (2003). *Disability rights and the Americans with Disabilities Act.* Retrieved May 21, 2003, from http://www.bazelon.org/issues/disabilityrights/index.htm

Brown, G. S., Burlingame, G. M., Lambert, M. J., Jones, E., & Vaccaro, J. (2001). Pushing the quality envelope: A new outcomes management system. *Psychiatric Services, 52*(7), 925–934.

Center for Quality Assessment and Improvement in Mental Health. (n.d.). *National inventory of mental health quality measures.* Retrieved May 28, 2003, from http://www.cqaimh.org/quality.html

Center for Quality Assessment and Improvement in Mental Health. (2002). *Selecting process measures for quality improvement in mental health care.* Retrieved May 28, 2003, from http://www.cqaimh.org/toolkit.website.pdf

Commission on Accreditation of Rehabilitation Facilities (CARF). (2003). *2003 behavioral health standards manual.* Tucson, AZ: Commission on Accreditation of Rehabilitation Facilities.

Committee on Quality of Care in America. (2001). *Crossing the quality chasm: A new health system for the 21st century.* Washington, DC: National Academy Press.

Daniels, A. S., & Walter, D. A. (2002). Current issues in continuing education for contemporary behavioral health practice. *Administration and Policy in Mental Health, 29*(4/5), 359–376.

Gerald, G. N. (2001). Mental Health Policy in 20th Century America. *Mental Health, United States 2000.* Rockville, MD: Center for Mental Health Services.

Grob, G. N. (1994). *The mad among us: A history of the care of America's mentally ill.* New York: Free Press.

HCPro, Inc. (2003). *Use root-cause analysis to improve credentialing.* Retrieved January 17, 2003, from http://www.credentialinfo.com/new/swedish_american.cfm

Hershey, N. (2202). A different perspective on quality. *American Journal of Medical Quality, 17*(6), 242–247.

Hritz, R. W., Everly, J. L., & Care, S. A. (2002). Medication error identification is key to prevention: A performance improvement approach. *Journal for Healthcare Quality, 24*(2), 10–17.

Huey, L. (2002). Problems in behavioral health care: Leap-frogging the status quo. *Administration and Policy in Mental Health, 29*(4/5), 403–419.

Institute of Medicine. (2003). *Priority areas for national action: Transforming health care quality.* Washington, DC: National Academies Press.

Institute of Medicine. (2002a). *Reducing suicide: A national imperative.* Washington, DC: National Academies Press.

Institute of Medicine. (2002b). *Speaking of health: Assessing health communication strategies for diverse populations.* Washington, DC: National Academies Press.

Joint Commission on Accreditation of Healthcare Organizations (JCAHO). (2001). *2001–2002 Comprehensive accreditation manual for behavioral health care.* Oakbrook Terrace, IL: Author.

Joint Commission for Accreditation of Healthcare Organizations (JCAHO). (2003). *2004 Patient safety goals.* Retrieved December 12, 2003, from http://www.jcaho.org/accredited+organizations/patient+safety/04+npsg/04_npsg.htm

Joint Commission on Accreditation of Healthcare Organizations (JCAHO). (2001, February). *Joint commission perspectives, 21* (2), 1, 3.

Joint Commission on Accreditation of Healthcare Organizations (JCAHO). (2003). *Voluntarily reportable sentinel events.* Retrieved April 27, 2003, from http://www.jcaho.org/accredited+organizations/home+care/sentinel+events/voluntarily+reportable+sentinel+events.htm

Mandescheid, R. W., Atay, J. E., Hernández-Cartagena, M. R., Edmond, P. Y., Male, A., Parker, et al. (2001). Highlights of organized mental health services in 1998 and major national and state trends. *Mental Health, United States 2000.* Rockville, MD: Center for Mental Health Services.

Morris, J. A., & Stuart, G. W. (2002). Training and education needs of consumers, families and frontline staff in behavioral health practice. *Administration and Policy in Mental Health, 29*(4/5), 377–402.

National Alliance for the Mentally Ill (NAMI). (2001). *NAMI public policy platform* (Revised Sixth Edition). Arlington, VA: Author.

National Committee for Quality Assurance (NCQA). (2002). *2003 standards and guidelines for the accreditation of MBHOs.* Washington, DC: Author.

National Technical Assistance Center for State Mental Health Planning. (2003). *Training curriculum for the reduction of seclusion and restraint.* Alexandria, VA: National Association of State Mental Health Directors.

Paget, M. A. (1988). *The unity of mistakes.* Philadelphia: Temple University Press.

Pettit, T. A., Mohr, W. K., Somers, J. W., & Sims, L. (2001). Perceptions of seclusion and restraint by patients and staff in an intermediate-term care facility. *Journal of Child and Adolescent Psychiatric Nursing, 14*(3), 115–127.

Pizzi, L. T., Goldfarb, N. I., & Nash, D. B. (2001). Promoting a culture of safety. In *Making health care safer: A critical analysis of patient safety practices.* Rockville, MD: Agency for Healthcare Research and Quality.

President's New Freedom Commission on Mental Health. (2003). *Web site.* Retrieved May 18, 2003, from http://www.mentalhealthcommission.gov

Ross, E. C. (2001). Seclusion and restraint. *Journal of Child and Adolescent Psychiatric Nursing, 14*(3), 103–104.

Sharav, V. H. (2003). Children in clinical research: A conflict of moral values. *The American Journal of Bioethics, 3*(1), In Focus. Retrieved May 9, 2003, from http://bioethics.net/in_focus/sharav.pdf

Silver, M. S., & Burack, O. R. (2002). Inpatient psychiatry incident management: Part I, special issues. *Journal for Healthcare Quality, 24*(2), 4–7.

Utilization Review Accreditation Commission (URAC). (2002). *Health utilization management standards, version 4.1.* Washington, DC: Author.

Utilization Review Accreditation Commission. (2003). *Patient safety practices in utilization management programs.* Retrieved April 22, 2003, from http://www.urac.org/urac.asp?id=46.

Chapter **15**

Promoting the Safety of Research Participants

Jacqueline Fowler Byers

INTRODUCTION

The ever-increasing volume of clinical research trials is critical to the advancement of health care, and to evidence-based practice. Research funding from the National Institutes of Health (NIH) is over $14 billion a year, and pharmaceutical and device companies fund an additional $17 billion annually (Rettig, 2000). Clinical research ultimately promotes patient safety by providing the foundation for evidence-based practice (see chapter 4). However, involvement in research frequently involves risks to the research participants. In the early phases of research these risks may be significant. Phase one (safety trials) pose the greatest risk, because safety profiles of the drug or device are not yet known. Nonetheless, there are steps that can be taken to minimize the risk for the research participants and to ensure that potential research subjects have a full understanding of potential risks prior to informed consent. Figure 15.1 illustrates how research supports patient safety, as well as the steps at which research subjects need safety protections.

In order to promote patient safety during the research process, scientific integrity must be an overarching concern of all persons involved with the research process. The Institute of Medicine's (2002) report, *Scientific*

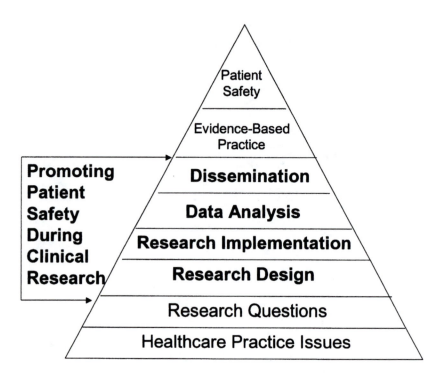

FIGURE 15.1   Phases of promoting patient safety during clinical research.

Integrity in Research, states, "For a scientist, integrity embodies above all the individual's commitment to intellectual honesty and personal responsibility. It is an aspect of moral character and experience. For an institution, it is a commitment to creating an environment that promotes responsible conduct by embracing standards of excellence, trustworthiness, and lawfulness, and then assessing whether researchers and administrators perceive that an environment with high levels of integrity has been created" (p. 4). This chapter discusses strategies to promote scientific integrity and patient safety during the clinical research process. Research safety strategies will be discussed sequentially from research study proposal development through study completion and dissemination.

FEDERAL REGULATIONS FOR RESEARCH PROTECTIONS

Federal regulations have been established in response to historical violations of the rights of human subjects. Current regulations include the

National Research Act, 45 CFR 46 (1974), 45 CFR 46 revised (1981), and 21 CFR 50 (1981) (*45 CFR 46 Protection of Human Subjects*, 1981; Food & Drug Administration, 1981). Federal statutes include special protections for vulnerable populations that are considered most at risk during human subject research. These populations include children, elders, prisoners, pregnant women, handicapped or mentally disabled, economically or educationally disadvantaged, and fetuses (*21 CFR 56 Institutional Review Boards*).

INSTITUTIONAL REVIEW BOARDS

Key to enforcing these statutes is the use of Institutional Review Boards (IRBs) to protect human subjects (21 CFR 56 Institutional Review Boards). IRBs are charged with reviewing all research protocols using human subjects. IRB membership regulations require at least five members of both genders with varied backgrounds including at least one nonscientist, one scientist, and one nonaffiliated member. Usual members include physicians, researchers, pharmacists, social workers, chaplains, risk managers, and community lay persons. Membership diversity is designed to ensure adequate ethical and scientific review of the study as well as to provide expertise regarding diverse and vulnerable populations. All members of IRBs are required to understand federal regulations including IRB purposes, functions, and membership responsibilities (*21 CFR 56 Institutional Review Boards*).

Federal criteria for IRB review are listed in Table 15.1. These requirements address both the scientific integrity of the proposed study and protection of human subjects during the process. Through the review of a proposal based on the criteria in the table, IRB members attempt to ensure that the proposed study meets scientific and ethical standards. There are several levels of IRB review, based on the level of risk to the subjects. These levels include exempt, expedited, and full review. All research involving human subjects must be reviewed by an IRB prior to study implementation (*21 CFR 56 Institutional Review Boards*).

HUMAN SUBJECTS RIGHTS VIOLATIONS

Despite these statutes, not all researchers in the United States follow research ethics and regulations. There has been significant media coverage of research violations at prominent universities. A 19-year-old Asian American

TABLE 15.1   Federal Requirements for IRB Protocol Review

During convened meeting with quorum present (full review only), protocol review including:

- Risk/benefit analysis
- Informed consent/assent
- Subject selection
- Privacy and confidentiality
- Research design/data analysis
- Protection of vulnerable populations
- Publicity/recruitment materials
- Qualifications of researchers
- Compliance with regulations
- Research-related financial interests or other potential conflicts of interest

(21 CFR 56 Institutional Review Boards)

consented to a bronchoscopy study to harvest alveolar macrophages in 1996 and died of lidocaine overdose. Research violations included facts that the subject was not observed following bronchoscopy, and that concentrations of lidocaine were increased without IRB approval. In 1999, a patient with a rare metabolic disorder died following a gene therapy trial (University of Miami, 2001). This subject was controlled with medication and diet prior to the trial. IRB violations included a conflict of interest of the investigators, lack of safety monitoring, and lack of informed consent (University of Miami, 2001). In 2001, a 24-year-old healthy female volunteer died during a research study. Violations included conflicts of interest of IRB members that were not documented, informed consent that did not state that the study drug was experimental and emphasized getting expensive tests for free, and Food and Drug Administration (FDA) approval of the study was not obtained (Keiger & De Pasquale, 2002). In 2003, a civil and class action suit was filed against researchers at the Veterans Affairs (VA) Medical Center in Albany, New York. Alleged violations included enrollment of subjects with known exclusion criteria, falsification of diagnostic test completion and test results, and administration of the wrong drug doses. This and other research irregularities resulted in a nationwide review of VA research practices (Otto, 2003a; *Steubing vs. Kornak, et al.,* 2003).

These events, and the concern raised regarding patient safety have put clinical investigators and their methods under increased governmental and media scrutiny. Researchers are no longer automatically trusted (Institute of Medicine Committee on Assessment of Integrity in Research Environments, 2002). The issues listed above and others must be addressed at each research phase to protect the safety of research subjects.

RESEARCH STUDY DESIGN

The first step in protecting research safety is to ensure that the researchers are knowledgeable regarding the research process and qualified to perform the research. They should be current in the science in their research area, as well as experienced researchers. The investigators should also have no conflict of interests. Most clinical research studies have an interdisciplinary research team to provide expertise in different aspects of the study, such as biochemists, physicians, and biostatisticians. However, the principal investigator is ultimately responsible for the work of the research team.

Another design consideration is to maximize benefit and minimize risks to the research subjects (*45 CFR 46 Protection of Human Subjects*, 1981). Study design is based on the research questions. Double-blind, randomized clinical trials with control groups are considered the "gold standard" in research. However, it is frequently not possible in clinical research. For instance, one cannot ethically randomize a pregnant woman to a no prenatal care group. However, you could randomize the woman to one of two different types of prenatal care programs. Similarly, using a placebo (inert substance) in a pain management study would also be unethical. As a result, clinical research is frequently designed to compare a new treatment with an existing FDA approved drug or device. An example of this is that a new antibiotic could be compared with a similar product currently on the market. Double blinding of investigators may not be possible due to the nature of the intervention. The key to research study design is to be as rigorous as possible without denying the research subject needed medical care or exposing the subject to unnecessary risks.

Study sample sizes should have adequate, but not excessive, statistical power. This allows the researchers to determine statistical significance, if it exists, but not to find differences artificially through overpowered studies (Burns & Grove, 2001). Study designs, procedures, and measurement should be the strongest possible to answer the research questions. For instance, minimizing confounding variables should be part of the study design. Research methods must include specific steps for maintaining data safety and integrity, as well as spell out all procedures to ensure confidentiality of the data. Scientific rigor minimizes the exposure to risk and protects the research subject from going through the trouble of participating in a research study that will not advance the science regarding the research question.

Vulnerable populations are also a design consideration. In addition to the vulnerable populations identified by federal statute, patients in general are vulnerable due to their illness, their placement in an institutional settings, language and communication limitations, or possible impaired cognitive status (Phipps, 2002). Study designs must not exclude certain populations such as women of childbearing age or various ethnic groups unless there is a scientific rationale for doing so. For instance, a phase-one (safety) trial could exclude women of childbearing age because the safety of the drug to fetuses would be unknown. On the other hand, an ethnic group, age range, or socioeconomic group shouldn't be specifically targeted unless there is a scientific rationale. If a disease only occurs in Native Americans, for instance, then that group could be specifically targeted. However, if it occurs across ethnicities, then all ethnic groups should be sampled (University of Miami, 2001).

MAINTAINING THE PRIVACY OF PROTECTED HEALTH INFORMATION

The Health Insurance Portability and Accountability Act (HIPAA) has requirements related to protecting the privacy of patient information, including that obtained during research studies. This involves deidentification of protected health information (PHI), for example, coding for any potential identifiers such as the subject's name, and the removal of all other PHI such as address, phone number, and birth date prior to research data being taken out of the practice setting. The procedure for maintaining confidentiality of the PHI of the subject must be explicitly stated in the informed consent. If PHI is needed for research purposes, a privacy board or IRB approval is required prior to initiation of the study. A PHI waiver may be obtained from an IRB or privacy board under the following circumstances:

- the use of the PHI involves no more than minimal risk to the privacy of individuals
- an adequate plan is in place to protect the PHI from improper use and disclosure

- a plan exists to destroy the PHI data at the first opportunity
- there is adequate written assurance that the PHI will not be reused in the future
- the research can not be reasonably conducted without the waiver
- the PHI is critical to the research study (USCFR 160, 164, 2002)

Informed consent of the patient may be required to obtain certain information if a waiver is not possible, as in the instance of sensitive information such as sexually transmitted disease status (USCFR 160 & 164, 2002).

HUMAN SUBJECTS APPROVAL

All research studies must submit their proposal and recruitment materials to an IRB and receive IRB approval prior to recruitment or study implementation (*21 CFR 56 Institutional Review Boards*). Some agencies also have additional layers of human subjects review. If an organization does not have an IRB, a local university or freestanding IRB are possible alternatives. The IRB may approve the study, determine it exempt from IRB review, or deny approval. If the study is not approved, the IRB will inform investigators about the human subjects and scientific issues to be addressed in order to protect the study subjects and to make the study potentially approvable.

RESEARCH TEAM TRAINING AND MONITORING

To ensure good science, research protocols must be strictly followed. The principal investigator (PI) is responsible for training and supervising the research team. The team must be educated regarding the study protocol and all statutory and IRB requirements. Inter-rater reliability must be established prior to data collection and periodically during the study (Burns & Grove, 2001). PI supervision and monitoring of the research team is an ongoing responsibility from study design to dissemination of the study findings.

RECRUITMENT AND INFORMED CONSENT

Recruitment

Although advertising for study subjects is permissible, all recruitment materials must be approved by the IRB approving the study. General principles of advertisements require that they not be misleading or coercive (Department of Health and Human Services Office of the Inspector General (DHHSOIG), 2000). In June 2000, the DHHSOIG issued a report in response to a rash of research violations. Industry-sponsored research recruitment pressures and resultant financial incentives to investigators were cited as a contributing factor to the violations. The DHHSOIG reported finding potential subjects being contacted repeatedly in attempts to recruit for research; a nursing home resident who was threatened with expulsion from the nursing home if study participation was declined; and a subject who died and was later found to have been ineligible for study enrollment. The report discussed the erosion of the informed consent process, concern about financial incentives, and the need for more federal oversight. It was also noted that IRBs were not exercising their responsibility to oversee recruitment practices (DHHSOIG, 2000).

Informed Consent

Once potential subjects are identified, the informed consent process begins. Informed consent is a critical element of protecting patient's rights during the research process. The importance of clear, positive communication in patient safety is critical and is discussed further in chapter 9. Informed consent requires full disclosure of research-related information by the researcher (Bosk, 2002). Key aspects of informed consent for potential research participants include competence (legal definition) or mental capacity (clinical definition) to understand the study, actual understanding of the study, and voluntary participation by the study participant (Food and Drug Administration, 1981; *45 CFR 46 Protection of human subjects*, 1981). In clinical practice, capacity is the primary criterion for informed consent. Capacity is determined subjectively based on patient assessment. If there is questionable mental capacity for any reason, consent must be obtained from the legal health care surrogate.

Required elements of informed consent of the potential research subject or legal surrogate are listed in Table 15.2. These elements are intended to ensure that the potential study participant has an accurate understanding of the research study, the risks and benefits, and possible alternatives. All known risks and potential benefits must be objectively described. Informed consent requires clear, simple, unbiased, and noncoercive communication in a language and reading level the patient and/or family can understand. To promote understanding of the research study and the informed consent

TABLE 15.2   Required Elements for Informed Consent

- Purpose of the research
- Experimental procedures
- Potential alternative treatments
- Duration of study participation
- Potential risks and benefits
- Steps to maintain confidentiality of study data
- Cost or compensation for participating
- Contact information for questions or for reporting a research-related injury
- Choice to participate or not will not impact their other treatment
- Freedom to withdraw at any time without penalty

Food and Drug Administration, 1981; *21 CFR 56 Institutional Review Boards.*

process, informed consent documents should be translated into the most common languages prevalent at the study sites. Font sizes should be enlarged for the elderly and vision impaired. Medical terminology should be avoided if possible and explanations provided in lay terms (see the Web Resources section at the end of this chapter). Recommended reading levels range from fourth to eighth grade (Centers for Disease Control, 1998; Johns Hopkins Medical Institutions, 2003). Reading levels can be determined using most word processing programs (see chapter 5). Adequate time for the patient or his family member to review the informed consent, consider the study, and ask questions is necessary to ensure that the consent be truly informed. To ensure true informed consent, the researcher enrolling the subject assesses for understanding of study details. If the patient is age 7–17, consent of the parent is required, as well as assent from the child if the child is capable. Following informed consent, research subjects should be given a copy of the consent form for future reference. For longitudinal studies, it is important to review the study protocol, reevaluate capacity, and reestablish consent of subjects verbally at every data collection point.

Despite good intentions, research provides evidence that the informed consent process is frequently not a true informed consent. There are known issues with capacity, understanding, and voluntariness. Since informed consent is key to ensuring ethical study participation and for the potential research subject to be aware of all potential safety risks, strategies must be implemented to improve this process.

Capacity

Capacity issues are common in clinical research. Capacity exists along a continuum from full capacity to no capacity. Capacity may vary based on the complexity of the decision to be made (Chen, Miller, & Rosenstein, 2002).

The very nature of clinical research is that frequently the potential subjects are very ill and possibly at the end of life. Young and elderly research subjects may have diminished capacity due to their developmental level or dementia. Trauma patients may be unconscious. Illness-related fatigue and anxiety might also diminish capacity (Bosk, 2002). Although legally and ethically problematic, the only alternative in these situations is to obtain informed consent from the legal surrogate if allowed by state law (Chen et al., 2002; Lawton, 2001; Nelson & Merz, 2002). The surrogate should base decisions on substituted judgment using the patient's previously stated wishes, or promoting the best interests of the incapacitated person (Chen et al., 2002). Individuals with diminished capacity may be able to agree to study participation and have their legal surrogate provide informed consent (Chen et al., 2002).

It is unethical to enroll an incapacitated individual into a research study if there is no scientific need to do so (Chen et al., 2002). For instance, antibiotic trials do not need to enroll incapacitated individuals. However, Alzheimer's clinical trials need to enroll subjects with diminished capacity, as this is the nature of the disease, and there is no other way to answer the research questions. If there is any way to predict future diminished capacity, initiating the conversation about study participation at the earliest opportunity is recommended (Bosk, 2002).

Understanding

Even when research subjects report understanding of a research study following consent, post-testing studies have not found this to be true. Joffe and colleagues post-tested oncology research trial participants a median of 16 days following informed consent. Although 90% of participants reported satisfaction with the informed consent process, 74% of respondents did not recognize the nonstandard treatment, 74% did not know the unproven nature of the treatment for their cancer, 63% did not recognize the incremental risk related to study participation, and only 29% realized that they might not receive direct benefit from participation. An average of one hour was spent to obtain informed consent for the study. In this study, increased understanding of research was related to English spoken at home, college education, use of a consent form template, presence of a nurse, careful reading of the consent, and not signing the consent at the time of initial discussion (Joffe, Cook, Cleary, Clark, & Weeks, 2001). Similarly, Agard and colleagues found that acute myocardial infarction patients who had consented to a clinical trial had little recall of the study, did not think that informed consent was necessary, and were willing to have a physician decide for them regarding study participation (Agard, Hermeren, & Herlitz, 2001). Use of a condensed consent form versus a standard IRB-approved, industry-written consent form in asthma patients yielded better understanding of every aspect of the consent form process (Dresden & Levitt, 2001). Enhanced understanding of the study occurs with reflective, patient-centered, supportive, and responsive communication (Albrecht, Blanchard, Ruckdeschel, Cooven, & Strongbow, 1999). Cultural competence is another factor to incorporate into the informed consent process in order to improve understanding (Terry & Terry, 2001).

Frequently, there is a "therapeutic misconception" on the part of participants or their legal proxies regarding research studies (Chen et al., 2002). Therapeutic misconception occurs when research subjects believe that they are going to receive individually focused treatment when, in reality, it is not the case (Lidz & Appelbaum, 2002). Subjects are randomized to treatment and the interventions are standardized, so individualization of treatment is not possible. The scientific rigor needed in a study to create valid, generalizable data conflicts with maximizing the benefit to an individual (Lidz & Appelbaum, 2002). Younger and better educated subjects are more likely to accurately understand a research study, and very ill subjects are more likely to believe there is a therapeutic benefit when there is none (Lidz & Appelbaum, 2002). Lidz and Appelbaum (2002) propose including the differences between research and treatment as the first part of the consent process to decrease therapeutic misconception. A key idea for potential research subjects to understand is the difference between an intervention and research on an intervention. Clinical interventions are routinely individualized, whereas research interventions are standardized in order to answer the research questions regarding intervention safety and efficacy. Therefore, in research trials, subjects may not receive the best treatment for their clinical situation (Lidz & Appelbaum, 2002). This is particularly important in phase-one trials (safety trials) where patients frequently have exhausted all other treatment options, and the chance of benefit is minimal (Susman, 2001). Interestingly, only 28% of health care providers in Joffe and colleagues' (2001) study realized that the primary goal of clinical research is to benefit future patients, thus they apparently share the therapeutic misconception bias.

Voluntariness

Research subjects report trust in the health care provider as a rationale for consenting to study participation (Bosk, 2002). The status of the researcher and recommendations by physicians also increase the probability of study participation (Nelson & Merz, 2002). This paternalistic approach to health care by the research subjects could be due to perceived coercion on the subject's part, i.e., "my physician wants me to participate". Whether real or perceived, persuasion, manipulation, and coercion have all been proposed as deterrents to voluntariness. This is more likely to occur with vulnerable or very ill populations (Bosk, 2002; Nelson & Merz, 2002). Deferment to the family's wishes by the desperately ill patient is also a threat to voluntariness (Bosk, 2002). Desire for treatment, improved health, understanding, and/or attention can provide further psychological pressure for subjects to consent to study participation, again limiting voluntary participation (Terry & Terry, 2001).

Awareness of all the issues related to the informed consent process allows researchers to monitor their behaviors to ensure that potential research subjects understand all possible alternatives and their right to refuse to participate without consequence. Not rushing the consent process and allowing a processing period following initial discussion supports voluntariness (Bosk, 2002; Pronovost, Wu, Dorman, & Marlock, 2002).

Informed Consent Oversight

The IRB has the right to monitor the informed consent process including interactions with patients and informed consent documentation, and to halt a research study if it is not being done correctly (*21 CFR 56 Institutional Review Boards*). This has not been done routinely in the past, but is a recommendation based on recent informed consent violations (DHHSOIG, 2000).

CONDUCT OF RESEARCH

Despite the best research design, research team training, and pilot research, conducting clinical research is fraught with challenges. Like every other phase of research, scientific integrity is key in order to promote valid, generalizable data. The principal investigator continues monitoring and provides oversight to assure 100% compliance with the research protocol. Data integrity, safety, and confidentiality must be maintained at all times.

If the research protocol needs to be modified in any way, the revised protocol and informed consent form must be approved by an IRB prior to implementation (*21 CFR 56 Institutional Review Boards*). If the consent form is changed due to new known risks or benefits, all prior subjects must reconsent to ensure they are aware of the new facts. Adverse events, protocol deviations and unanticipated problems must be reported to the IRB in a timely manner (*21 CFR 56 Institutional Review Boards*). Annually and at study termination, the principal investigator must provide a report to the IRB. The IRB has the right to review research records at any time and to withdraw IRB approval if significant violations exist. Principal investigators must allow unrestricted data access at any time (*21 CFR 56 Institutional Review Boards*).

Researchers are expected to terminate a study early if, based on interim data analysis, their results are much better or worse than expected. If the results are better than expected the researchers can show significant differences with fewer subjects than initially projected using prospective power analysis. If the results are worse than expected, or there are serious adverse reactions, the only ethical and safe course is to close the study. Recent examples of this were the Alzheimer's vaccine trial, where there was unexpected brain inflammation in 12 out of 360 study subjects worldwide. The sponsoring company stopped the clinical trial in early 2002 (British Broadcasting Corporation, 2002). In January 2003, gene therapy studies for the "Bubble Boy" immune defect were suspended due to the incidence of a leukemia type cancer in gene therapy recipients (Associated Press, 2003).

DATA ANALYSIS AND DISSEMINATION OF RESULTS

Thoughtful data analysis and dissemination of results are critical to ensure accurate, generalizable data and good science. If scientific integrity is not maintained at this stage, inaccurate conclusions may be drawn from the study, causing a risk to patient safety.

At this phase, the collected data are reviewed for accuracy and completeness, and are entered into a statistical software package for data analysis. Biostatistician support is needed to ensure that the most appropriate and robust statistical analyses are used to answer the research questions. Once the research results are known, dissemination of findings begins. The three most common venues for dissemination of research findings include health care journal articles, scientific presentations, and press releases. Scientific reports have more credibility if they are peer reviewed prior to dissemination (Burns & Grove, 2001).

Miller and Rosenstein (2002) advocate that, in addition to discussing human subjects review and approval in a manuscript, all ethical considerations during study design and implementation be discussed. This would potentially avoid undue criticism of a study design and promote more ethical accountability of researchers. Specific areas for inclusion in manuscripts include the ethical rationale for the use of placebos, the withdrawal of medications (drug washout), the use of cognitively impaired subjects or subjects from less developed countries, and the use of deception or provocation in the study design. In-depth discussion of the informed consent process is also recommended (Miller & Rosenstein, 2002).

The research team must be careful during this phase to use the results only as a trigger for discussion and conclusions of the study. Taking leaps beyond what the findings tell the researchers is a common research flaw (Burns & Grove, 2001). If leaps are taken, the goal of evidence-based practice will be hindered because the conclusions and recommendations are not based on empirical findings (see chapter 4).

FUTURE RESEARCH DIRECTIONS

Although clinical research is based on scientific and ethical principles, there are several areas for future research in order to promote patient safety and scientific integrity during the research process. Some areas for future research include:

- Development of scientific integrity measures (Institute of Medicine Committee on Assessment of Integrity in Research Environments, 2002)
- Determination of evidence-based approaches to scientific integrity (Institute of Medicine Committee on Assessment of Integrity in Research Environments, 2002)
- Development and evaluation of risk/benefit analysis models
- Determination of the best evidence-based approach to manage enrollment of persons with diminished capacity (Chen et al., 2002)

• Determination of the best evidence-based approach to having true informed consent in emergent situations (Bosk, 2002)

CONCLUSION

Scientific integrity, or good science, is everyone's responsibility. Table 15.3 summarizes the shared responsibilities of the patient/proxy, the research team, all health care providers, and the organizational administration to promote patient safety during clinical research. Scientific integrity is lost if each party does not do their part (Institute of Medicine Committee on Assessment of Integrity in Research Environments, 2002). Scientific integrity during the research process supports minimization of risks, maximization of benefits, and valid results to provide the foundation for evidence-based practice. Collectively, this promotes patient safety.

TABLE 15.3   Responsibilities for Patient Safety During Clinical Research

Responsibility	Patient/ Subject	Investigators	Health Care Providers	Administration
Clear communication	X	X	X	X
Ask questions if unsure	X	X	X	X
Use attentive listening	X	X	X	X
Advocate for patient rights	X	X	X	X
Support the informed consent process	X	X	X	X
Ensure protocol compliance		X		X
Follow all statutory and IRB requirements		X		X
Terminate study immediately if safety concerns arise		X	X	
Communicate concerns at any time in the research process	X	X	X	X
Ensure a culture of scientific integrity		X	X	X

WEB RESOURCES

Name of Resource/URL	*Description*
Applied Research Ethics National Association (ARENA) http://www.primr.org/arena.html	Organization for professionals interested in protecting the rights of human subjects
Code of Federal Regulations, Title 45, Public Welfare http://ohrp.osophs.dhhs.gov/ humansubjects/guidance/ 45cfr46.ht m	Federal regulations
Consent for CDC Research http://www.cdc.gov/od/ads/dscs/ consent.pdf	Guide to writing informed consents and oral scripts
Glossary of lay terms for use in preparing consents forms for human subjects http://ovcr.ucdavis.edu/ HumanSubjects/HSDefinitions/ HSGlossary.htm	From the University of California, Davis
Office for Civil Rights—Health Insurance Portability and Accountability Act (HIPAA) http://www.hhs.gov/ocr/hipaa/	Excellent HIPAA resources
Office for Human Research Protections. Department of Health and Human Services http://ohrp.osophs.dhhs.gov/	Web site
Office of Human Subjects Research, National Institutes of Health http://ohsr.od.nih.gov/	Online training and home page
The HIPAA Privacy Rule and Research http://privacyruleandresearch. nih.gov/	Booklet and PowerPoint presentation on the use of personal health information in clinical research are available.

REFERENCES

21 CFR 56 Institutional Review Boards. Retrieved December 12, 2003, from http://www.access.gpo.gov/nara/cfr/waisidx_00/21cfr56_00.html

45 CFR 46 Protection of Human Subjects. (1981). Retrieved December 12, 2003, from http://ohsr.od.nih.gov/mpa/45cfr46.php3

Agard, A., Hermeren, G., & Herlitz, J. (2001). Patients' experiences of intervention trials on the treatment of myocardial infarction: Is it time to adjust the informed consent procedure to the patient's capacity? *Heart, 86*(6), 632–637.

Albrecht, T. L., Blanchard, C., Ruckdeschel, J. C., Cooven, M., & Strongbow, R. (1999). Strategic physician communication and oncology clinical trials. *Journal of Clinical Oncology, 17*, 3324–3332.

Associated Press. (2003). "*Bubble boy" gene therapy halted*. Retrieved January 20, 2003, from http://www.wired.com/news/business/0,1367,57216,00.html

Bosk, C. L. (2002). Obtaining voluntary consent for research in desperately ill patients. *Medical Care, 40 (supplement)*, V64–V68.

British Broadcasting Corporation. (2002). *Safety fears halt Alzheimer's trial*. Retrieved January 20, 2003, from http://news.bbc.co.uk/hi/english/health/newsid_1836000/1836281.stm

Burns, N., & Grove, S. K. (2001). *The practice of nursing research: Conduct, critique & utilization* (4th ed.). Philadelphia: W. B. Saunders.

Centers for Disease Control. (1998). *Consent for CDC research: A reference for developing consents and oral scripts*. Retrieved March 7, 2003, from http://www.cdc.gov/od/ads/hsrconsent.pdf

Chen, D. T., Miller, F. G., & Rosenstein, D. L. (2002). Enrolling decisionally impaired adults in clinical research. *Medical Care, 40 (supplement)*, V20–V29.

Department of Health and Human Services Office of the Inspector General. (2000). *Recruiting human subjects pressures in industry sponsored clinical research*. Retrieved March 1, 2003, from http://oig.hhs.gov/oei/reports/oei-01-97-00195.pdf

Dresden, G. M., & Levitt, A. (2001). Modifying a standard industry clinical trial consent form improves patient information retention as part of the informed consent process. *Academic Emergency Medicine, 8*(3), 246–252.

Food and Drug Administration. (1981). *FDA 21 CFR 50 Protection of human subjects*. Retrieved February 26, 2003, from http://www.access.gpo.gov/nara/cfr/waisidx_00/21cfr50_00.html

Institute of Medicine Committee on Assessment of Integrity in Research Environments. (2002). *Integrity in scientific research: Creating an environment that promotes responsible conduct*. Washington, DC: National Academies Press.

Johns Hopkins Medical Institutions. (2003). *Consent form language too complex for many*. Retrieved March 7, 2003, from http://www.hopkinsmedicine.org/press/2003/February/030219.htm

Joffe, S., Cook, F., Cleary, P. D., Clark, J. W., & Weeks, J. C. (2001). Quality of informed consent in cancer clinical trials: A cross-sectional survey. *The Lancet, 358*, 1772–1777.

Keiger, D., & De Pasquale, S. (2002). *Trials & tribulations*. Retrieved March 04, 2002, from http://www.jhu.edu/~jhumag/0202/trials.html

Lawton, J. (2001). Pearls, pith, and provocation: Gaining and maintaining consent; Ethical concerns raised in a study of dying patients. *Qualitative Health Research, 11*(5), 693–702.

Lidz, C. W., & Appelbaum, P. S. (2002). The therapeutic misconception: Problems and solutions. *Medical Care, 40 (Supplement)*, V55–V63.

Miller, F. G., & Rosenstein, D. L. (2002). Reporting of ethical issues in publication of medical research. *The Lancet, 360,* 1326–1328.

Nelson, R. M., & Merz, J. F. (2002). Voluntariness of consent for research: An empirical and conceptual review. *Medical Care, 40 (Supplement),* V69–V80.

Otto, M. A. (2003a). *Health care researchers under criminal investigations for VA cancer study deaths in New York.* Retrieved March 28, 2003, from http://www.naim.org/wwwboard/messages/359.htm

Otto, M. A. (2003b). *Researcher hired despite revoked licens:; Feds launch probe of VA hiring practices.* Retrieved December 12, 2003, from http://www.sskrplaw.com/bioethics/researcherhired.pdf

Phipps, E. J. (2002). What's end of life got to do with it? Research ethics with populations at life's end. *The Gerontologist, 42* (Special issue III), 104–108.

Pronovost, P., Wu, A. W., Dorman, T., & Marlock, L. (2002). Building safety into ICU care. *Journal of Critical Care, 17*(2), 78–85.

Rettig, R. A. (2000). The industrialization of clinical research. *Health Affairs, 19*(2), 129–146.

Steubing vs. Kornak, et al. (2003). *Complaint for damages and class action.* Retrieved December 12, 2003, from http://www.sskrplaw.com/gene/steubing/complaint.pdf

Susman, E. (2001). Improving informed consent for phase I trials. *Oncology Times, 23*(3), 6, 8.

Terry, S. F., & Terry, P. F. (2001, Fall). A consumer perspective on informed consent and third-party issues. *Journal of Continuing Education in the Health Professions, 21*(4).

University of Miami. (2001). *IRB Training: Human Subjects Research Educational Module.* Retrieved February 26, 2003, from http://www.ci4.miami.edu/courses/IRB training/coursedocuments

U.S. CFR parts 160 and 164. (2002). *Standards for privacy of individually identifiable health information: Final rule.* Retrieved December 12, 2003, from http://www.hipaadvisory.com/regs/regs_in_PDF/finalprivmod.pdf

Glossary of Terms

Accident: An event that involves damage to a defined system that disrupts the ongoing or future output of the system (Kohn, Corrigan, & Donaldson, 2000).

Accreditation Watch: An attribute of an organization's Joint Commission accreditation status. A health care organization is placed on Accreditation Watch when a sentinel event has occurred and a thorough and credible root cause analysis of the sentinel event has not been completed within a specified time frame. Although Accreditation Watch is not an official accreditation category, it can be publicly disclosed by the Joint Commission (JCAHO, 2002).

Action plan: The product of a root cause analysis that identifies the strategies that an organization intends to implement to reduce the risk of similar events occurring in the future. The plan should address responsibility for implementation, oversight, pilot testing as appropriate, time lines, and strategies for measuring the effectiveness of the actions (Department of Veterans Affairs, 2002).

Active error: An error that occurs at the level of the frontline operator and whose effects are felt almost immediately (Kohn, Corrigan, & Donaldson, 2000; Reason, 1990).

Adverse drug event/drug error (ADE): Any incident in which the use of a medication (drug or biologic) may have resulted in an adverse outcome in a patient (Kohn, Corrigan, & Donaldson, 2000).

Adverse drug reaction (ADR): An undesirable response associated with use of a drug that either compromises therapeutic efficacy, enhances toxicity, or both (JCAHO, 2002).

Adverse event: An injury resulting from a medical intervention (Kohn, Corrigan, & Donaldson, 2000).

Advocate: A person who represents the rights and interests of another individual as though they were the person's own, in order to realize the rights to which the individual is entitled, obtain needed services, and remove barriers to meeting the individual's needs (JCAHO, 2002).

Bad outcome: Failure to achieve a desired outcome of care (Kohn, Corrigan, & Donaldson, 2000).

Blunt end: The multiple system issues and defense systems that contribute to error. The blunt end shapes the environment and influences behavior by the way resources, constraints, incentives, and demands are handled (Reason, 1990).

Causation/causality: The act by which an effect is produced. In epidemiology, the doctrine of causation is used to relate certain factors (predisposing, enabling, precipitating, or reinforcing) to disease occurrence. The doctrine of causation is also important in the fields of negligence and criminal law (JCAHO, 1998).

Criticality: The seriousness of the failure, related to FMEA (VA National Center for Patient Safety, 2001).

Disclosure: Communication of information regarding the results of a diagnostic test, medical treatment, or surgical intervention.

Effective control measure: A barrier that eliminates or substantially reduces the likelihood of a hazardous event occurring (Department of Veterans Affairs, 2002).

Error: Failure of a planned action to be completed as intended or use of a wrong plan to achieve an aim; the accumulation of errors results in accidents (Kohn, Corrigan, & Donaldson, 2000).

Error of commission: An error that occurs as a result of an action taken (JCAHO, 1998).

Error of omission: An error that occurs as a result of an action not taken (JCAHO, 1998).

Evidence based practice: Conscientious, explicit and judicious use of current best evidence in making decisions about the care of individual patients (Sackett, Rosenberg, Gray, Hayanes & Richardson, 1996).

Exception management: An explicit process to ensure that appropriate treatment is rendered when clinical practice guideline parameters are not used in the course of treatment. An example would be bipolar disorder and appropriate medications. It is developed as an explicit process for the management of exceptions to clinical practice guidelines that allows reasonable flexibility to be applied to clinical decision making.

Failure mode: Different ways that a process or subprocess can fail to provide the anticipated result (Department of Veterans Affairs, 2002).

Failure mode and effects analysis (FMEA): A systematic way of examining a design prospectively for possible ways in which failure can occur. It assumes that no matter how knowledgeable or careful people are, errors will occur in some situations and may even be likely to occur (JCAHO, 2000).

Flow chart/diagram: A pictorial summary that shows with symbols and words the steps, sequence, and relationship of the various operations involved in the performance of a function or a process (JCAHO, 1998).

Hazard analysis: The process of collecting and evaluating information on hazards associated with the selected process. The purpose of the hazard analysis is to develop a list of hazards that are of such significance that they are reasonably likely to cause injury or illness if not effectively controlled (Department of Veterans Affairs, 2002).

Health care failue mode and effects analysis (HFMEA): A prospective assessment that identifies and improves steps in a process thereby reasonably ensuring a safe and clinically desirable outcome. A systematic approach to identify and prevent product and process problems before they occur (Department of Veterans Affairs, 2002).

Human factors: Study of the interrelationships between humans, the tools they use, and the environment in which they live and work (Kohn, Corrigan, & Donaldson, 2000).

Incident report: The documentation of any unusual problem, incident, or other situation that is likely to lead to undesirable effects, or that varies from established policies and procedures or practices (JCAHO, 1998).

Injury: Physical or psychological harm occurring to a patient (Kohn, Corrigan, & Donaldson, 2000).

Latent error: Errors in design, organization, training, or maintenance that lead to operator errors and whose effects typically lie dormant in the system for lengthy periods of time (Kohn, Corrigan, & Donaldson, 2000).

Malpractice: Improper or unethical conduct, or unreasonable lack of skill by a holder of a professional or official position; often applied to physicians, dentists, lawyers, and public officers to denote negligent or unskillful performance of duties when professional skills are obligatory. Malpractice is a legal cause of action for which damages are allowed (JCAHO, 1998).

Medication error: Any preventable event that may cause or lead to inappropriate medication use or patient harm while the medication is in the control of the health care professional, patient, or consumer. Such events may be related to professional practice, health care products, procedures, and systems including prescribing, order communication, product labeling, packaging, and nomenclature, compounding, dispensing, distribution, administration, education, monitoring, and use (NCCMERP, 2001).

Near miss/close call: Used to describe any process variation which did not affect the outcome, but for which a recurrence carries a significant chance of a serious adverse outcome (Department of Veterans Affairs, 2002).

Negligence: Failure to use such care as a reasonably prudent and careful person would use under similar circumstances (JCAHO, 1998).

Patient safety: Freedom from accidental injury; ensuring patient safety involves the establishment of operational systems and processes that minimize the likelihood of errors and maximize the likelihood of intercepting them when they occur (Kohn, Corrigan, & Donaldson, 2000).

Patient safety practice: A type of process or structure whose application reduces the probability of adverse events resulting from exposure to the health care system across a range of diseases and procedures (University of California at San Francisco, Stanford University Evidence-Based Practice Center, 2001).

Plan-do-study-act (PDSA)/Deming/Shewhart cycle: A four-part method for discovering and correcting assignable causes to improve the quality of processes (JCAHO, 1998).

Probability: Likelihood of an event occurring (or, in FMEA, the likelihood of a failure) (JCAHO, 1998).

Process: A goal-directed, interrelated series of actions, events, mechanisms, or steps that transform inputs into outputs (JCAHO, 2002).

Proximate cause/factors: An act or omission that naturally and directly produces a consequence. It is the superficial or obvious cause for an occurrence. Treating only the "symptoms," or the proximate special cause, may lead to some short-term improvements, but will not prevent the variation from recurring (JCAHO, 1998).

Quality of care: The degree to which health services for individuals and populations increase the likelihood of desired health outcomes and are consistent with current professional knowledge (Kohn, Corrigan, & Donaldson, 2000).

Risk containment: Immediate actions taken to safeguard patients from a repetition of an unwanted occurrence. Actions may involve removing and sequestering drug stocks from pharmacy shelves, and checking or replacing oxygen supplies or specific medical devices (JCAHO, 2000).

Risk management: Clinical and administrative activities undertaken to identify, evaluate, and reduce the risk of injury to patients, staff, and visitors, and the risk of loss to the organization itself (JCAHO, 1998).

Root cause: The most fundamental reason for the failure or inefficiency of a process that if eliminated or corrected would prevent an undesirable event from occurring (Spath, 1999a).

Root cause analysis (RCA): A systematic process for identifying the basic or causal factor(s) that underlie variation in performance, including the occurrence of death, serious physical or psychological injury, or the risk thereof. Serious injury specifically includes loss of limb or function. The phrase "or the risk thereof" includes any process variation for which a recurrence would carry a significant chance of a serious adverse outcome. Such events are called "sentinel" because they signal the need for immediate investigation and response (JCAHO, 2002).

Safety: The degree to which the risk of an intervention and risk in the care environment are reduced for a patient and other persons, including health care practitioners (JCAHO, 2002).

Sentinel event: An unexpected occurrence of death, serious physical or psychological injury, or the risk thereof. Serious injury specifically includes loss of limb or function. The phrase "or risk thereof" includes any process variation for which a recurrence would carry a significant chance of a serious adverse outcome. Such events are called "sentinel" because they signal the need for immediate investigation and response (JCAHO, 2002).

Severity: The seriousness of the failure, related to FMEA (VA National Center for Patient Safety, 2001).

Sharp end: Patient and caregiver interface, where an error usually is visible (Reason, 1990).

System: Set of interdependent elements interacting to achieve a common aim. These elements may be both human and nonhuman (equipment, technologies, etc.) (Kohn, Corrigan, & Donaldson, 2000).

Unanticipated outcome: The result of a treatment or procedure that differs significantly from what was anticipated (JCAHO, 2002).

Variation: The differences in results obtained in measuring the same phenomenon more than once. The sources of variation in a process over time can be grouped into two major classes: common causes and special causes. Common-cause variation, also called endogenous-cause variation or systemic cause variation, in a process is due to the process itself, is produced by interactions of variables of that process, and is inherent in all processes, not a disturbance in the process. It can be removed only by making basic changes in the process. Special-cause variation, also called exogenous-cause variation or extrasystemic cause variation, in performance results from assignable causes. Special-cause variation is intermittent, unpredictable, and unstable. It is not inherently present in a system; rather, it arises from causes that are not part of the system as designed and results in an occurrence or possible occurrence of a sentinel event (JCAHO, 2002).

REFERENCES

Department of Veterans Affairs. (2002). *VHA National Patient Safety Improvement Handbook*. Retrieved January 12, 2003, from http://www.patientsafety.gov/NCPShb.pdf

Joint Commission on Accreditation of Healthcare Organizations (JCAHO). (1998). *Lexikon* (2nd ed.). Oakbrook Terrace, IL: Author.

Joint Commission on Accreditation of Healthcare Organizations (JCAHO). (2000). *Glossary of terms*. Retrieved January 10, 2003, from www.jcaho.org

Joint Commission on Accreditation of Healthcare Organizations (JCAHO). (2001). *Revisions to Joint Commission standards in support of patient safety and medical/health care efforts*. Retrieved January 13, 2003, from www.jcaho.org/standard/fr_safety.html

Joint Commission on Accreditation of Healthcare Organizations (JCAHO). (2002a). *Sentinel event policy and procedures*, Revised July 2002. Retrieved January 12, 2003, from www.jcaho.org/accredited+organizations/hospitals/sentinel+events/se_pp.htm.

Kohn, L. T., Corrigan, J. M., & Donaldson, M. S. (Eds.). (2000). *To err is human: Building a safer health system*. Washington, DC: National Academy Press.

National Coordinating Council for Medication Error Reporting and Prevention (NCCMERP). (2001). *Types of medication errors*. Retrieved December 4, 2003, from http://www.nccmerp.org/medErrorCatIndex.html

Reason, J. T. (1990). *Human error*. Cambridge: Cambridge University Press.

Spath, P. (1999a). *Investigating sentinel events: How to find and resolve root causes.* Forest Grove, OR: Brown-Spath and Associates.

University of California at San Francisco Stanford University Evidence-Based Practice Center. (2001). *Making health care safer: A critical analysis of patient safety practices.* Rockville, MD: Agency for Healthcare Research and Quality.

VA National Center for Patient Safety. (2001). *Healthcare Failure Mode and Effect Analysis Course Materials (HFMEA™).* Retrieved December 4, 2003, from http:// www.patientsafety.gov/HFMEAIntro.pdf

Index